DIAGNOSTIC AND THERAPEUTIC ALGORITHMS

in internal medicine
for dogs and cats

Federico Fracassi

DIAGNOSTIC AND THERAPEUTIC ALGORITHMS

in internal medicine for dogs and cats

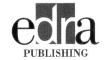

edra PUBLISHING

Federico Fracassi, DIAGNOSTIC AND THERAPEUTIC ALGORITHMS in internal medicine for dogs and cats
©2022 Edra Publishing US LLC – All rights reserved

ISBN: 978-1-957260-21-1
eISBN: 978-1-957260-40-2

Book Publishing Manager: Costanza Smeraldi, Edra S.p.A.
Paper, Printing and Binding Manager: Paolo Ficicchia, Edra S.p.A.
Cover: Gaetano Altamura, Edra S.p.A.
Layout: Fulvio Martello, Como, Italy
Copyediting: Mercedes González Fernández de Castro – Science & Health Publications

Knowledge and best practice in this field are constantly changing: As new research and experience broaden our knowledge, changes in practice, treatment, and drug therapy may become necessary or appropriate. Readers are advised to check the most current information provided (i) or procedures featured or (ii) by the manufacturer of each product to be administered, to verify the recommended dose or formula, the method and duration of administration, and contraindications.

It is the responsibility of the practitioners, relying on their own experience and knowledge of the patient, to make diagnoses, to determine dosages and the best treatment for each individual patient, and to take all appropriate safety precautions. To the fullest extent of the law, neither the Publisher nor the Editors assume any liability for any injury and/ or damage to persons or property arising out of or related to any use of the material contained in this book.

This publication contains the author's opinions and is intended to provide precise and accurate information.

The processing of the texts, even if taken care of with scrupulous attention, cannot entail specific responsibilities for the author and / or the publisher for any errors or inaccuracies. Readers should be aware that websites listed in this work may have changed or disappeared between when this work was written and when it is read.

The Publisher has made every effort to obtain and cite the exact sources of the illustrations. If in some cases he has not been able to find the right holders, he is available to remedy any inadvertent omissions or errors in the references cited. Product or corporate names may be trademarks or registered trademarks, and are used only for identification and explanation without intent to infringe. All registered trademarks mentioned belong to their legitimate owners.

Edra Publishing US LLC
3309 Northlake Boulevard, Suite 203
Palm Beach Gardens, FL, 33403
EIN: 844113980
info@edrapublishing.com
www.edrapublishing.com

Printed in Italy by "LegoDigit" Srl., Lavis (TN) - August 2022

EDITOR

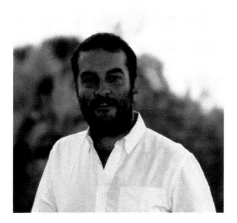

Federico Fracassi graduated in Veterinary Medicine (DVM) "cum laude" at the University of Bologna, Italy. He did an internship and started a Ph.D. at the same veterinary school, and defended his Ph.D. thesis in 2005. After the Ph.D., he became a permanent staff member at the Department of Veterinary Medical Sciences – University of Bologna (Italy) where at present he is Associate Professor of Internal Medicine and Head of the Unit of Internal Medicine. He completed a Residency in Internal Medicine at the Clinic for Small Animal Internal Medicine, University of Zurich, Switzerland, and gained his status of European Specialist in Internal Medicine in 2012 (Diplomate ECVIM-CA-internal medicine). Dr. Fracassi's duties include patient care, education (to students, postgraduate training, and training of interns and residents), and research in internal medicine of companion animals, with special emphasis on endocrinology. He is the past-president of the European Society of Veterinary Endocrinology (ESVE), past-president of the Italian Society of Veterinary Internal Medicine (SIMIV), and board member of the executive committee of the ECVIM-CA congress. He is editor of "Veterinaria", a peer-review journal, and associate editor of the Journal of Small Animal Practice. His publication list consists of journal articles, research abstracts, case reports, and book chapters. His main research focus is the field of small animal endocrinology.

CONTRIBUTORS

Chiara Agnoli, DVM, PhD
Department of Veterinary Medical Sciences
Alma Mater Studiorum - University of Bologna
Ozzano Emilia (BO), Italy

Francesco Albanese, Med Vet
Centro Dermatologico Veterinario Toscano,
Arezzo, Italy
MYLAV Veterinary private laboratory
Passirana di Rho (Milan), Italy

Federica Alessandrini, DVM
Department of Veterinary Medical Sciences
Alma Mater Studiorum - University of Bologna
Ozzano Emilia (BO), Italy

Carolina Arenas, DVM, PhD, DECVIM-CA
(Internal Medicine)
AniCura Valencia Sur Veterinary Hospital
Valencia, Spain

Federica Balducci, DVM, DECVN
Veterinary Hospital AniCura I Portoni Rossi
Bologna, Italy

Emma Bellei, DVM, PhD
Veterinary Hospital AniCura I Portoni Rossi
Bologna, Italy

Elsa Beltrán, DVM, DECVN, PGDipVetEd,
FHEA, MRCVS
Department of Clinical Science and Services
Royal Veterinary College
Hawkshead, United Kingdom

Andrea Boari, DVM, PhD
Faculty of Veterinary Clinical Sciences
University of Teramo, Italy

Domenico Caivano, DVM, PhD
Department of Veterinary Medicine
University of Perugia, Italy

Veronica Cola, DVM
Department of Veterinary Medical Sciences
Alma Mater Studiorum - University of Bologna
Ozzano Emilia (BO), Italy

Silvia Colombo, DVM, DECVD
Servizi Dermatologici Veterinari
Legnano, Italy

Andrea Corsini, DVM, PhD, DECVIM-CA
(Internal Medicine)
Department of Veterinary Medical Sciences
University of Parma, Italy

Paolo Emidio Crisi, DVM, PhD
Faculty of Veterinary Clinical Sciences
University of Teramo, Italy

Serena Crosara, DVM, PhD, DECVIM-CA
(Cardiology)
Department of Veterinary Sciences
University of Parma, Italy

Marco Cunto, DVM, PhD
Department of Veterinary Medical Sciences
Alma Mater Studiorum - University of Bologna
Ozzano Emilia (BO), Italy

Francesca Del Baldo, DVM, MRCVS, PhD,
DECVIM-CA (Internal medicine)
Department of Veterinary Medical Sciences
Alma Mater Studiorum - University of Bologna
Ozzano Emilia (BO), Italy

Sara Del Magno, DVM, PhD, Resident ECVS
Department of Veterinary Medical Sciences
Alma Mater Studiorum - University of Bologna
Ozzano Emilia (BO), Italy

Lucy Davison, MA, VetMB, PhD, DSAM, DECVIM-CA, MRVCS
Department of Clinical Science and Services
Royal Veterinary College
Hawkshead, United Kingdom

Francesco Dondi, DVM, PhD
Department of Veterinary Medical Sciences
Alma Mater Studiorum - University of Bologna
Ozzano Emilia (BO), Italy

Eugenio Faroni, DVM, resident ECVIM (Oncology)
Department of Veterinary Medical Sciences
Alma Mater Studiorum - University of Bologna
Ozzano Emilia (BO), Italy

Luca Ferasin, DVM, PhD, CertVC, PGCert(HE), DipECVIM-CA (Cardiology), GPCert(B&PS), FRCVS
Specialist Veterinary Cardiology Consultancy, Hampshire, United Kingdom

Armando Foglia, DVM, PhD
Department of Veterinary Medical Sciences
Alma Mater Studiorum - University of Bologna
Ozzano Emilia (BO), Italy

Teresa Gagliardo, DVM, PhD, DECVN
Centro Diagnostico Veterinario PalermoVet, Palermo, Italy

Sara Galac, DVM, PhD
Department of Clinical Sciences
Utrecht University
Utrecht, The Netherlands

Antonella Gallucci, DVI, PhD, DECVN
Centro Veterinario Neurologico - La Fenice
Cagliari, Italy

Gualtiero Gandini, DVM, PhD, DECVN
Department of Veterinary Medical Sciences
Alma Mater Studiorum - University of Bologna
Ozzano Emilia (BO), Italy

Alexander German, BVSc(Hons), PhD, CertSAM, DECVIM-CA, SFHEA, FRCVS
Institute of Life Course and Medical Sciences
University of Liverpool
Neston, United Kingdom

Massimo Giunti, DVM, PhD, Dipl DECVECC
Department of Veterinary Medical Sciences
Alma Mater Studiorum - University of Bologna
Ozzano Emilia (BO), Italy

Stefania Golinelli, DVM
Department of Veterinary Medical Sciences
Alma Mater Studiorum - University of Bologna
Ozzano Emilia (BO), Italy

Rosanne E. Jepson, BVSc, MVetMed, PhD, DACVIM-SAIM, DECVIM-CA
Department of Clinical Science and Services
Royal Veterinary College
Hawkshead, United Kingdom

Andrea N. Johnston, DVM, PhD, DACVIM
School of Veterinary Medicine
Louisiana State University, USA

María C. López, DVM, MRCVS
Hospital Clínic Veterinari
Universitat Autònoma de Barcelona, Spain

Francesco Lunetta, DVM
Department of Veterinary Medical Sciences
Alma Mater Studiorum - University of Bologna
Ozzano Emilia (BO), Italy

Federica Marchesotti, DVM, DECVIM-CA (Cardiology)
Department of Cardiology AniCura,
Istituto Veterinario Novara, Italy

Laura Marconato, DVM, DECVIM-CA (Oncology)
Department of Veterinary Medical Sciences
Alma Mater Studiorum - University of Bologna
Ozzano Emilia (BO), Italy

Marika Menchetti, DVM, PhD, DECVN
Clinica Veterinaria San Marco
Veggiano (Padova), Italy

Erika Monari, DVM
Department of Veterinary Medical Sciences
Alma Mater Studiorum - University of Bologna
Ozzano Emilia (BO), Italy

Rodolfo Oliveira Leal, DVM, PhD, DECVIM-CA
(Internal Medicine)
Centre for Interdisciplinary Research in Animal
Health, University of Lisbon, Portugal
Associate Laboratory for Animal and Veterinary
Sciences (AL4AnimalS), Portugal

Manuela Perego, DVM, DECVIM-CA (Cardiology)
Clinica Veterinaria Malpensa
Samarate (Varese), Italy

Dolores Pérez Alenza, DVM, PhD
Small Animal Internal Medicine Service
Veterinary Teaching Hospital
Complutense University of Madrid, Spain

Marco Pesaresi, DVM
Ospedale Veterinario Portoni Rossi
Zola Predosa (Bologna), Italy
Ospedale veterinario San Francesco
Milan, Italy

Matteo Petini, DVM, DECVIM-CA
(Internal Medicine)
Clinica Veterinaria San Marco
Veggiano (Padova), Italy

Andrea Petrelli, DVM, MRCVS
Small Animal Teaching Hospital
University of Liverpool, United Kingdom

Marco Pietra, DVM
Department of Veterinary Medical Sciences
Alma Mater Studiorum - University of Bologna
Ozzano Emilia (BO), Italy

Francesco Porciello, DVM
Department of Veterinary Medicine
University of Perugia, Italy

Fabio Procoli, DMV, MVetMed, DACVIM,
DECVIM-CA, MRCVS
Veterinary Hospital AniCura I Portoni Rossi
Bologna, Italy

Giovanni Romito, DVM, SMIPPV, MSc, PhD,
DECVIM-CA (Cardiology)
Department of Veterinary Medical Sciences
Alma Mater Studiorum - University of Bologna
Ozzano Emilia (BO), Italy

Xavier Roura, DVM, DECVIM-CA
Hospital Clínic Veterinari
Universitat Autònoma de Barcelona, Spain

Roberto Santilli, DVM, PhD, DECVIM-CA
(Cardiology)
Clinica Veterinaria Malpensa
Samarate (Varese), Italy

Fabia Scarampella, Med Vet, MSc, DECVD
Studio Dermatologico Veterinario
Milan, Italy

Johan P. Schoeman, BVSc, MMedVet, PhD,
DSAM, DECVIM, FRCVS
Department of Companion Animal Clinical
Studies
University of Pretoria, South Africa

Sofia Segatore, DVM
Department of Veterinary Medical Sciences
Alma Mater Studiorum - University of Bologna
Ozzano Emilia (BO), Italy

Paolo Silvestrini, DVM, PhD, DECVIM-CA
School of Veterinary Medicine
University of Pennsylvania, USA

Harry Swales, BVSc, CertAVP(SAM), PgCert,
VPS, DECVIM-CA (Internal Medicine), MRCVS
Moorview Referrals, Northumberland,
United Kingdom
Veterinary Postgraduate Unit
University of Liverpool, United Kingdom

Antonio Maria Tardo, DVM
Department of Veterinary Medical Sciences
Alma Mater Studiorum - University of Bologna
Ozzano Emilia (BO), Italy

Alessandro Tirolo, DVM
Department of Veterinary Medical Sciences
Alma Mater Studiorum - University of Bologna
Ozzano Emilia (BO), Italy

Roberta Troìa, DVM, PhD, DECVECC
Department of Veterinary Medical Sciences
Alma Mater Studiorum - University of Bologna
Ozzano Emilia (BO), Italy

Michele Tumbarello, DVM, Ph.D. student
Department of Veterinary Medical Sciences
Alma Mater Studiorum - University of Bologna
Ozzano Emilia (BO), Italy

Kateryna Vasylyeva, DVM
Department of Veterinary Medical Sciences
Alma Mater Studiorum - University of Bologna
Ozzano Emilia (BO), Italy

Panagiotis G. Xenoulis, DVM, Dr.med.vet.,
PhD, ECVCN Candidate
Faculty of Veterinary Sciences
University of Thessaly, Greece
College of Veterinary Medicine and Biomedical
Sciences
Texas A&M University, USA

Daniele Zambelli, DVM, PhD, DECAR
Department of Veterinary Medical Sciences
Alma Mater Studiorum - University of Bologna
Ozzano Emilia (BO), Italy

Andrea Zoia, DVM, PhD, CertSAM,
DECVIM-CA
Clinica Veterinaria San Marco
Veggiano (Padova), Italy

FOREWORD

Veterinary clinicians who provide care for dogs and cats are asked numerous minor-to-serious questions every day: "What should I feed my kitten?", "What vaccinations should my dog be given?", "Why is my old cat limping?", "Why does my four-year-old dog have diarrhea?", "Why is my dog suddenly thirsty and hungry?" While veterinarians often have ready answers to these and other questions, it is understood that veterinarians, themselves, often seek answers for simple to difficult questions.

The most common question we veterinarians ask ourselves: "What diagnosis, test, or treatment am I forgetting?"

This book of easily used algorithms provides answers for most of our most common questions and reminds us of what we may have forgotten. Each algorithm guides the reader step by step with logical, practical, cost-effective options to proceed from a general concern, laboratory abnormality, or imaging finding to a specific diagnosis or treatment. A concise summary is provided on the first page of each topic, the algorithm follows, and then succinct explanations are provided for many of the recommended steps within each algorithm.

Advice is only as good as the advisor. Federico Fracassi has become one of the world's most outstanding veterinary endocrinologists and internists, first by learning well the lessons taught by his Veterinary School Professors in Bologna, then by Dr. Claudia Reusch and her colleagues in Zurich, and since by the many colleagues from around the world with whom he collaborates. Federico Fracassi has committed himself to teaching, by first being committed to learning. The foundation of his expertise is being objectively analytical when assessing his experiences and those of his colleagues. He is dedicated to reminding his audiences to rely on solid evidence-based diagnostics and therapeutics. But he also reminds us that the owner must be fully educated and in agreement with any plan regarding their pet. Federico understands the single most important diagnostic tool in internal medicine is the owner history. Physical examination, extremely important, is far behind in second place. Laboratory testing, imaging recommendations, and treatment options must be based on the history, physical examination, and the owner's goals. Federico would remind us to maintain open minds and rely on the evidence provided before giving advice or making decisions.

Federico Fracassi and the outstanding group of experts he assembled to author each topic in this book have provided clear insights rarely available in the veterinary literature. Using this book will improve our ability to answer questions and enhance our confidence in making decisions. The information in the algorithms assure that we will not forget.

Edward C. Feldman
DVM, DACVIM (Small Animal Internal Medicine)
Emeritus Professor of Small Animal Internal Medicine
University of California, Davis
Davis, California, USA

PREFACE

The problem-oriented approach (POA) is the method recommended by the College of Internal Medicine to address and resolve medical questions and problems. Proponents of POA are attracted to algorithms. I have always thought that algorithms allow proceeding in a logical, orderly, and above all, efficient manner. However, some limitations of many algorithms are that they omit information that is considered obvious, they do not detail diagnostic investigations, and often neglect the therapeutic aspects.

Hence, the idea of creating a book based on algorithms dealing with the main clinical and laboratory canine and feline clinical abnormalities, using an innovative perspective.
Each of the 85 chapters begins with a short introduction which includes the basic pathophysiological and classification information. By means of each algorithm, the clinician is guided, step by step, in carrying out diagnostic investigations in a sequential manner, reaching a diagnosis, and setting up treatment.

In this book, two useful and innovative aspects were included: color codes and links for additional information within the algorithm. Yellow indicates the diagnostic path, red the diagnosis, and blue the therapy; this allows the veterinarian to be guided through the diagnostic labyrinth in order to reach the most appropriate therapy. Inside the red boxes, the list of differential diagnoses for each problem can quickly be identified. By following the yellow boxes, one can understand how to reach these diagnoses and optimize the diagnostic protocol. Frequently, one can read algorithms lacking in information; they may suggest carrying out a certain diagnostic test without explaining how it should be done. This limitation was overcome by inserting numbers inside the main boxes of each algorithm. The numbers refer to a short text that gives more details regarding a specific diagnostic investigation, a particular disease, or the therapy recommended.

This book is for veterinarians who have to deal with various canine and feline internal medicine problems as well as for students of veterinary medicine who have to learn rigorous methods which are, at the same time, simple and efficient.

I want to thank Professor Edward Feldman for supporting and helping me in setting up this text; the initial idea was to work together on this project; however, reasons beyond our control did not allow it. Thanks, Ed, for being a great example to me every day.

I thank the 62 authors of the chapters for their outstanding contributions. Your competence and experience have made it possible to obtain a rich, in-depth, and, above all, practical book. Finally, thanks to EDRA, a high-level publishing company that knows how to best support the ideas of those who want to create a scientific text. In particular, I want to thank Costanza Smeraldi, who gave me the initial idea and let me read the book on human medicine by Professor Violi. Thanks also to Gerald Goldsmith and Mercedes González for their kindness and professionalism.

Federico Fracassi

ABBREVIATIONS

ACE	Angiotensin-converting enzyme
AChR	Acetylcholine receptor
ACIP	Acute idiopathic polyradiculoneuritis
ACTH	Adrenocorticotropic hormone
ADH	Antidiuretic hormone
Afib	Atrial fibrillation
Afl	Atrial flutter
AHDS	Acute hemorrhagic diarrhea syndrome
AKI	Acute kidney injury
ALP	Alkaline phosphatase
ALT	Alanine aminotransferase
ANA	Antinuclear antibodies
ARB	Angiotensin receptor blocker
ARE	Antibiotic responsive enteropathy
AST	Aspartate aminotransferase
BCS	Body condition score
BMBT	Buccal mucosal bleeding time
BOAS	Brachycephalic obstructive airway syndrome
BPH	Benign prostatic hyperplasia
bpm	Beats per minute
BUN	Blood urea nitrogen
CBC	Complete blood count
CHF	Congestive heart failure
CK	Creatine kinase
CKD	Chronic kidney disease
CNS	Central nervous system
cPLI	Canine pancreatic lipase immunoreactivity
CPSE	Canine prostate-specific esterase
CRP	C-reactive protein
CRTZ	Chemoreceptor trigger zone
CSF	Cerebrospinal fluid
CT	Computed tomography
DDAVP	Desmopressin
DGGR	1,2-O-dilauryl-rac-glycero-glutaric acid (6'-methylresorufin) ester
DIC	Disseminated intravascular coagulation
DJD	Degenerative joint disease
DKA	Diabetic ketoacidosis
ECF	Extracellular fluid
ECG	Electrocardiogram
EDTA	Ethylenediaminetetraacetic acid
ERG	Electroretinography
FCoV	Feline coronavirus
FCV	Feline calicivirus

FDPs	Fibrin degradation products
FeHV-1	Feline herpes virus 1
FeLV	Feline leukemia virus
FeNa	Fractional excretion of sodium
FFP	Fresh frozen plasma
FIC	Feline idiopathic cystitis
FIP	Feline infectious peritonitis
FIV	Feline immunodeficiency virus
FNA	Fine-needle aspiration
FRE	Food-responsive enteropathy
fT4	Free thyroxine
FUO	Fever of unknown origin
GDV	Gastric dilatation and volvulus
GFR	Glomerular filtration rate
GI	Gastrointestinal
GORD	Gastro-oesophageal reflux disease
H	Human medicine
Hb	Hemoglobin
HCT	Hematocrit
HDDSt	High dose dexamethasone suppression test
HHS	Hyperglycemic hyperosmolar syndrome
IBD	Inflammatory bowel disease
IGF-I	Insulin growth factor-I
IMHA	Immune-mediated hemolytic anemia
IMT	Immune-mediated thrombocytopenia
IRE	Immunosuppressant-responsive enteropathy
IRIS	International Renal Interest Society
JT	Junctional tachycardia
LDDSt	Low dose dexamethasone suppression test
LES	Lower esophageal sphincter
LGN	Lateral geniculate nucleus
MCHC	Mean corpuscular hemoglobin concentration
MCS	Muscle condition score
MCV	Mean corpuscular volume
MGUS	Monoclonal gammopathy of unknown significance
MRI	Magnetic resonance imaging
MUO	Meningomyeloencephalitis of unknown origin
NDI	Nephrogenic diabetes insipidus
NRE	Non responsive enteropathy
NSAID	Nonsteroidal anti-inflammatory drugs
NT-proBNP	NT-proB-type natriuretic peptide
OA	Osteoarthritis
OAVRT	Orthodromic atrioventricular reciprocating tachycardia
PARR	PCR for antigen receptor rearrangement
PAWP	Pulmonary artery wedge pressure
PB	Phenobarbital
PCR	Polymerase chain reaction
PCV	Packed cell volume
PDA	Patent ductus arteriosus
PHF	Primary hyperfibrinolysis
PIMA	Precursor-targeted immune-mediated anemia
PJRT	Permanent junctional reciprocating tachycardia

PLE	Protein-losing enteropathy
PLN	Protein-losing nephropathy
PLR	Pupillary light reflex
PLT	Platelets
PNDS	Post-nasal drip syndrome
PRA	Progressive retinal atrophy
PTRV	Peak tricuspid regurgitation velocity
PU/PD	Polyuria/polydipsia
RAAS	Renin-angiotensin-aldosterone system
ROTEM	Rotational thromboelastometry
RRT	Renal replacement therapy
SARDS	Sudden acquired retinal degeneration syndrome
SBP	Systolic blood pressure
SDMA	Symmetric dimethylarginine
SIADH	Syndrome of inappropriate antidiuretic hormone secretion
SIRS	Systemic inflammatory response syndrome
SLE	Systemic lupus erythematosus
TEG	Thromboelastography
TGL	Triglyceride
TLI	Trypsin-like immunoreactivity
TnI	Troponin I
TP	Total proteins
TS	Total solids
TSH	Thyroid-stimulating hormone
TT4	Total thyroxine
TXA	Tranexamic acid
UA	Urinalysis
UCCR	Urinary corticoid to creatinine ratio
UP/C	Urine protein/creatinine
US	Ultrasonography
USG	Urinary specific gravity
UTI	Urinary tract infection
VFSS	Videofluoroscopic swallowing study
VSH	Ventricular septal defect
VT	Ventricular tachycardia
vWD	von Willebrand disease
vWF	von Willebrand factor
vWf:Ag	von Willebrand factor antigen test
WBC	White blood cells

TABLE OF CONTENTS

ABDOMINAL EFFUSION

Andrea Zoia

The mesothelium is a membrane composed of a monolayer of flattened squamous-like epithelial cells that form the lining of the abdominal cavity (peritoneum). The luminal surface of the mesothelium is covered with microvilli. The main purpose of these cells is to produce a lubricating fluid providing a slippery, non-adhesive, and protective surface for internal organs to slide past one another. Lymphatic stomata are the main structures responsible for peritoneal fluid drainage and are mainly located in the diaphragmatic peritoneum. Stomata drain into the lymphatic vessels, and these pass through the parasternal lymph nodes until they end up in the terminal thoracic duct. Diaphragmatic movement produces a change in hydrostatic pressure, which moves the peritoneal fluid forward. These stomata are the only way for cells and larger particles to exit the cavitary spaces, whereas proteins may also exit via active cell transport (i.e., electrolyte-coupled liquid absorption and transcytosis) through the parietal and visceral mesothelial cells.

Peritoneal fluid is a low-protein ultrafiltrate of plasma, and its production and its removal from the peritoneal space is a continuous process. The Starling forces at the visceral mesothelium (i.e., gradients of hydrostatic and oncotic pressures between the vessels and the body cavities), the degree of mesothelial and endothelial permeability, and the integrity of the lymphatic drainage regulate the volume and composition of the peritoneal fluid. In the case of ascites associated with liver cirrhosis, which represents 80% of the causes of ascites in humans (but is rare in small animals), the pathophysiology of fluid formation is more complicated. Several factors are involved, including portal hypertension, splanchnic arterial vasodilatation, activation of vasoconstrictor, and antidiuretic factors, such as norepinephrine, angiotensin II, aldosterone, and ADH. Renin-angiotensin-aldosterone system (RAAS) activation leads to sodium retention, which causes additional fluid accumulation and expansion of the extracellular fluid contributing to the formation of ascites.

Finally, hypoalbuminemia, due to decreased liver synthesis, which reduces the oncotic plasma pressure, also contributes to the loss of fluid from the vascular compartment into the peritoneal cavity.

ABDOMINAL EFFUSION

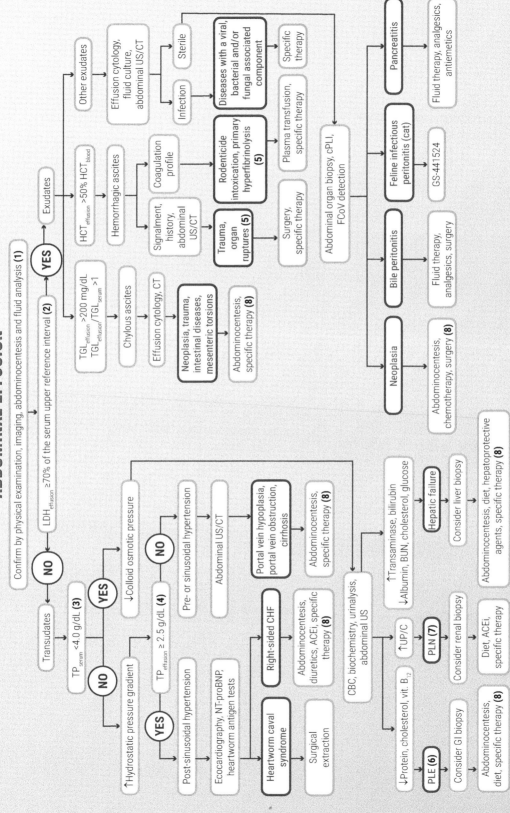

DIAGNOSTIC PROTOCOL

1. The diagnosis of ascites can be reached using clinical findings, imaging, and abdominal fluid centesis. If the volume is significant enough, the presence of a fluid wave can be appreciated by palpating the abdomen. A careful general examination may also reveal signs that direct the diagnostic approach. For example, cardiac murmur, tachycardia or arrhythmia, and jugular distension are suggestive of right-sided congestive heart failure (CHF), while muffled heart sounds are consistent with pericardial effusion; jaundice is consistent with liver failure or a ruptured biliary system. Decreased appetite, chronic weight loss, and diarrhea may be present in chronic enteropathies. Abdominal ultrasound and/or CT are indicated in ascites of non-cardiac origin and also allow identification of low-volume ascites. Abdominal centesis and fluid analysis allow fluid classification.

2. Traditionally, ascites are classified according to their pathophysiology of formation into a transudate (due to decreased colloid osmotic pressure or increased venous hydrostatic pressure with portal hypertension), an exudate (due to the increased permeability of the peritoneal surface), and hemorrhagic. In veterinary medicine, specific gravity, total protein (TP) in fluid, and total nucleated cell count in fluid have historically been used to identify the nature of the effusion; however, there are no studies validating this type of classification, which is no longer used in human medicine. A study has recently found that, in dogs, a simplified version of the Boyer's criteria allowed a correct classification (94% accuracy) of the ascitic fluid in the transudate and the exudate. In this study, hemorrhagic effusion and uroperitoneum were considered exudates. According to these criteria, ascitic lactic dehydrogenase (LDH) ≥70% of the serum upper reference limit identifies exudative ascites.

3. In the case of a transudate, serum total protein concentration ≥4.0 g/dL will differentiate a transudate due to increased hydrostatic pressure (i.e., portal hypertension) from a transudate due to decreased colloid osmotic pressure, which generally has a serum total protein concentration <4.0 g/dL. Notably, if a transudate is found, additional fluid analysis other than ascitic total protein in the case of portal hypertension is not necessary, and other tests, such as bloodwork, abdominal ultrasound, and echocardiography, are indicated according to the suspected underlying disease.

4. In the case of transudative ascites due to increased hydrostatic pressure measurement, total proteins in fluid differentiate a transudate due to post-sinusoidal hypertension (ascitic total proteins ≥2.5 g/dL) from a transudate due to pre-or sinusoidal hypertension, which generally has an ascitic total protein concentration <2.5 g/dL.

DIAGNOSIS

5. Hemorrhagic ascites occurs secondary to trauma, spontaneous ruptures of pathologicalorgans containing haematoma or being infiltrated by tumours or amyloidosis. Coagulopathies causing hemothorax include primary hyperfibrinolysis (PHF) due to angystrongylosis androdenticide poisoning.

6. Protein-losing enteropathy (PLE) causing ascites due to decreased colloid osmotic pressure is common in dogs but rare in cats. In the vast majority of cases, it is associated with

inflammatory bowel disease, intestinal lymphoma, or intestinal lymphangiectasia.

7. Protein-losing nephropathies (PLNs) include glomerulonephritis, glomerulopathy, and amyloidosis; they are fairly common in dogs but not in cats. Diseases associated with glomerulonephritis include infectious, neoplastic, and inflammatory diseases. In many cases, the cause of glomerulonephritis remains idiopathic. Amyloidosis can be a familial disorder in Shar Pei dogs and Abyssinian cats, and it can also occur in conjunction with chronic antigenic stimulation. Familial glomerulopathy has been reported in soft-coated Wheaton Terriers and English Cocker Spaniels but less commonly in other breeds.

TREATMENT

8. Removal of the ascitic fluid by abdominocentesis should be performed for therapeutic reasons only for large abdominal volumes that impair breathing function, and it is rarely curative. Treatment of the underlying disease is therefore required to prevent fluid re-accumulation. This can require medication or even surgery. See the algorithm for specific treatment of the multiple underlying disorders.

SUGGESTED READINGS

-   Balfe A, Cannon D. Ascitic/peritoneal fluid. In McGing P, O'Kelly R, O'Meara Y (editors). The Biochemistry of Body Fluids. Association of Clinical Biochemists in Ireland, 2009, pp 17-19.
-   Busato F, Gianesini G, Drigo M, Zoia A. Discriminating transudates and exudates in dogs with ascites: comparison of diagnostic utility of serum ascites albumin gradient (SAAG), Boyer's criteria, simplified Boyer's criteria and two traditional veterinary classifications based on ascites total protein (TPascites) and total nucleated cell count (TNCCascites). Proceedings of the 30th ECVIM-CA Congress, 2020.
-   Dempsey SM, Ewing PJ. A review of the pathophysiology, classification, and analysis of canine and feline cavitary effusions. *J Am Anim Hosp Assoc* 47:1-11, 2011.
-   Isaza-Restrepo A, Martin-Saavedra JS, Velez-Leal JL, et al. The peritoneum: beyond the tissue – A review. *Front Physiol* 9:1-12, 2018.
-   Stokol T. Fluid analysis: thoracic, abdominal, joint. In Ettinger SJ, Feldman EC, Côté E (editors). Textbook of Veterinary Internal Medicine 8th edition. St. Louis, Elsevier, pp 872-882.

ABDOMINAL ENLARGEMENT

Stefania Golinelli

Abdominal enlargement is a common clinical sign of many diseases in dogs and cats and requires a thorough and systematic medical approach. An animal's owner may describe abdominal distension or may describe some other clinical signs, such as exercise intolerance, weight gain, increased respiratory rate and effort, lethargy, weakness, decreased appetite, or clinical signs specific to the underlying disease process (e.g., collapse with cardiac tamponade, or retching with gastric dilation/volvulus).

Some patients with abdominal enlargement require emergency intervention. A thorough history is essential to assess the need for such urgent intervention and develop a complete list of differential diagnoses. Physical examination findings are related to the etiology, and they can include a fluid wave on ballottement of the abdomen, gas distension of the abdomen or gastrointestinal tract, abdominal pain, organomegaly, or palpation of a soft tissue mass.

The causes of abdominal enlargement can be classified into the following categories: organomegaly or abdominal mass (tissue), abdominal effusion (liquid), gas, and other diseases such as hypercortisolism (reduced abdominal musculature and fat accumulation), obesity, pregnancy, and constipation.

Due to the number of etiologies causing abdominal enlargement, the diagnostic approach should be thorough and stepwise. After using a thorough history and physical examination to formulate an initial differential diagnosis list, a minimum database (including complete blood count [CBC], a serum biochemistry profile, and urinalysis) should be set up. Diagnostic imaging of the abdomen is mandatory and can involve using multiple modalities and identifying several abnormalities, such as an abdominal mass, cavitary effusions, or gas.

The treatment of abdominal enlargement should be targeted to the underlying cause. This may involve interventions specific to a disease process, such as medical management of hypercortisolism, a surgical correction of gastric dilatation/volvulus, or palliative care.

ABDOMINAL ENLARGEMENT

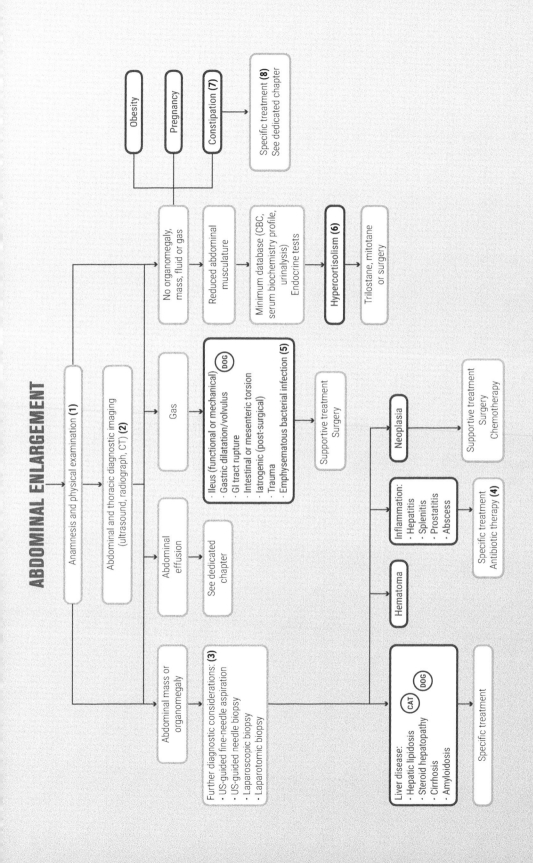

Anamnesis and physical examination (1)

Abdominal and thoracic diagnostic imaging (ultrasound, radiograph, CT) (2)

Abdominal mass or organomegaly

Abdominal effusion

See dedicated chapter

Gas

- Ileus (functional or mechanical)
- Gastric dilatation/volvulus
- GI tract rupture
- Intestinal or mesenteric torsion
- Iatrogenic (post-surgical)
- Trauma
- Emphysematous bacterial infection (5) **DOG**

Supportive treatment
Surgery

No organomegaly, mass, fluid or gas

Reduced abdominal musculature

Minimum database (CBC, serum biochemistry profile, urinalysis)
Endocrine tests

Hypercortisolism (6)

Trilostane, mitotane or surgery

Obesity

Pregnancy

Constipation (7)

Specific treatment (8)
See dedicated chapter

Further diagnostic considerations: (3)
- US-guided fine-needle aspiration
- US-guided needle biopsy
- Laparoscopic biopsy
- Laparotomic biopsy

Hematoma

Inflammation:
- Hepatitis
- Splenitis
- Prostatitis
- Abscess

Specific treatment
Antibiotic therapy (4)

Neoplasia

Supportive treatment
Surgery
Chemotherapy

Liver disease:
- Hepatic lipidosis **CAT**
- Steroid hepatopathy **DOG**
- Cirrhosis
- Amyloidosis

Specific treatment

1. Abdominal enlargement often develops insidiously. However, in some cases such as gas accumulation in the stomach during gastric distension and volvulus or bleeding from a ruptured splenic neoplasia, it may be an acute event. A thorough history is vital for assessing the need for such urgent intervention and developing a complete differential diagnosis list. The history should include the pet's previous medical history, the description and duration of the clinical signs, environment, travel history, and drug administration. If the patient is relaxed and not obese, abdominal palpation can directly detect intra-abdominal masses, organomegaly, gas, or fluid accumulation.

2. The abdomen can be imaged using a variety of methods (plain and contrast radiographs, ultrasound, CT, or MRI scans). Abdominal ultrasound is probably the highest-yielding test if fluid or organomegaly is present, if hypercortisolism is suspected or if no abnormalities are detected on physical examination. Abdominal radiographs can identify the presence of abdominal gas and gastric volvulus.

3. Dogs and cats with abdominal masses or diffuse organomegaly should undergo fine-needle aspiration or biopsy of the tissue(s) involved to identify the underlying abnormality (e.g., neoplasia, inflammation). Cytology is less invasive than a biopsy; it does not require general anesthesia and usually does not require a clotting study. However, although it may allow assessment of the cell types present, it does not identify structural changes in an organ such as fibrosis, cirrhosis, dysplasia, and hyperplasia, and it does not permit diagnosing neoplasia if the tissue involved does not exfoliate.

DIAGNOSIS

5. Gas accumulation can cause abdominal distension and may occur within the abdominal organs or freely in the peritoneal or retroperitoneal spaces. Distension of the gastrointestinal (GI) tract with gas can be seen with gastric dilation/volvulus or mesenteric torsion. Gas accumulation in the GI tract can also be secondary to mechanical and/or functional ileus. Emphysematous bacterial infections can result in gas production within the liver, gallbladder, or urinary bladder. Finally, free gas in the peritoneal and retroperitoneal spaces could result from GI perforation, secondary to gas-producing bacteria in bacterial peritonitis, perforating trauma, or it can be iatrogenic in origin after surgical intervention.

6. Progressive wasting and weakening of the abdominal musculature commonly occur due to inappropriate and chronic high glucocorticoid concentrations (hypercortisolism). Hypercortisolism, also called Cushing's syndrome, can cause hepatic enlargement due to glycogen accumulation in the liver and abdominal fat accumulation. Muscle wasting and hepatic enlargement combine to produce the classical "pot-bellied" appearance in the patient. This is a major complaint in hypercortisolism, along with polyuria, polydipsia, polyphagia, bilaterally symmetrical hair loss, thin skin, comedones, prominent abdominal vessels, and excessive panting.

7. Abdominal enlargement can also be due to feces accumulation. Constipation is defined as the infrequent or difficult evacuation of feces but does not necessarily imply a permanent loss of the ability to defecate. Several predisposing factors can contribute to constipation,

such as megacolon, pelvic fracture, foreign bodies, prostatomegaly in an intact male dog, perineal hernia, and tumors.

TREATMENT

4. Use antibiotics only if an infection is present and the tissue culture tests positive. The choice of antibiotics should be based on susceptibility tests.

8. The specific therapeutic plan for constipation depends upon the severity of constipation and its underlying cause. Hydration, dietary modification, warm water enemas, oral or suppository laxatives, colonic prokinetic agents, or a combination of these treatments are usually used. Severe cases of constipation usually require brief periods of hospitalization to correct dehydration and metabolic abnormalities and to evacuate impacted feces using water enemas, manual extraction of retained feces, or both. Subtotal colectomy is necessary in some severe cases with recurrences.

SUGGESTED READINGS

-   Nelson RW, Couto CG. Clinical manifestations of gastrointestinal disorders. In Nelson RW, Couto CG (editors). Small Animal Internal Medicine. St. Louis, Elsevier, 2013, pp 388-389.
-   Walter J. Abdominal enlargement. In Ettinger SJ, Feldman EC, Côté E (editors). Textbook of Veterinary Internal Medicine 8th edition. St. Louis, Elsevier, 2017, pp 450-4550.

ACID-BASE ANOMALIES: ACIDOSIS

Marco Pesaresi

Maintaining a blood pH within the normal range is essential for normal organic function. Acidemia is defined as a reduction in the blood pH due to the increase in H^+ ions in the extracellular fluid (ECF). This may be due to the accumulation of volatile acid CO_2 (respiratory acidosis) or fixed acids (metabolic acidosis).

Metabolic acidosis is a very common syndrome, characterized by a reduction in standard bicarbonate ($stHCO_3^-$) and base excess (BE) values, and can result from an increase in acid or the loss of bicarbonate. Many situations can lead to metabolic acidosis, such as hypoperfusion, diarrhea, kidney disease, toxicosis, and other conditions; it is very important to differentiate between acid load and bicarbonate loss. This can be done by calculating the anion gap (AG) with the formula $(Na^+ + K^+) - (Cl^- + HCO_3^-)$. The AG corresponds to the sum of unmeasured anions and increases during acid gain conditions, such as lactic acidosis, ketoacidosis, or intoxication. When the AG is in the normal range, the acidosis is defined as hyperchloremic acidosis; it is due to the loss of bicarbonate, such as in diarrhea and renal tubular acidosis.

Respiratory acidosis is due to an accumulation of CO_2 in blood; it may be caused by an increase in its production, such as fever, sepsis, and malignant hyperthermia or, most frequently, by a reduction in the CO_2 elimination rate due to hypoventilation. Different situations can lead to a reduction in alveolar ventilation, such as central nervous system conditions, cervical disk disease, neuromuscular dysfunctions, chest wall and pleural diseases, and obstructive airway conditions.

Under normal conditions, the body tries to compensate for the alteration in pH with an opposite disturbance which mitigates the acidemia (e.g., metabolic alkalosis to compensate for respiratory acidosis). When the compensation is adequate, the acid-base disturbance is defined as simple; instead, when there is not adequate compensation, the disturbance is defined as a mixed acid-base disorder.

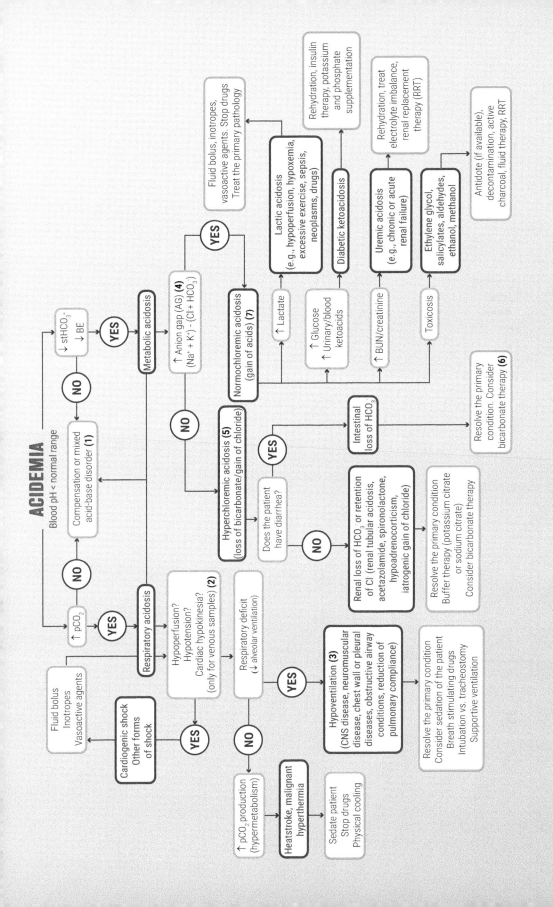

ACIDEMIA

Blood pH < normal range

↑ pCO₂ — **YES** → Respiratory acidosis

↑ pCO₂ — **NO** → Compensation or mixed acid-base disorder **(1)**

↓ stHCO₃⁻ / ↓ BE — **NO** → Compensation or mixed acid-base disorder **(1)**

↓ stHCO₃⁻ / ↓ BE — **YES** → Metabolic acidosis

Respiratory acidosis

Hypoperfusion? Hypotension? Cardiac hypokinesia? (only for venous samples) **(2)**

— **YES** → Cardiogenic shock / Other forms of shock → Fluid bolus / Inotropes / Vasoactive agents

Respiratory deficit (↓ alveolar ventilation)

— **YES** → Hypoventilation **(3)** (CNS disease, neuromuscular disease, chest wall or pleural diseases, obstructive airway conditions, reduction of pulmonary compliance) → Resolve the primary condition / Consider sedation of the patient / Breath stimulating drugs / Intubation vs. tracheostomy / Supportive ventilation

— **NO** → ↑ pCO₂ production (hypermetabolism) → Heatstroke, malignant hyperthermia → Sedate patient / Stop drugs / Physical cooling

Metabolic acidosis

↑ Anion gap (AG) **(4)**
$(Na^+ + K^+) - (Cl^- + HCO_3^-)$

— **NO** → Hyperchloremic acidosis **(5)** (loss of bicarbonate/gain of chloride)

Does the patient have diarrhea?

— **YES** → Intestinal loss of HCO₃⁻ → Resolve the primary condition. Consider bicarbonate therapy **(6)**

— **NO** → Renal loss of HCO₃⁻ or retention of Cl⁻ (renal tubular acidosis, acetazolamide, spironolactone, hypoadrenocorticism, iatrogenic gain of chloride) → Resolve the primary condition / Buffer therapy (potassium citrate or sodium citrate) / Consider bicarbonate therapy

— **YES** → Normochloremic acidosis **(7)** (gain of acids)

↑ Lactate → Lactic acidosis (e.g., hypoperfusion, hypoxemia, excessive exercise, sepsis, neoplasms, drugs) → Fluid bolus, inotropes, vasoactive agents. Stop drugs. Treat the primary pathology

↑ Glucose / ↑ Urinary/blood ketoacids → Diabetic ketoacidosis → Rehydration, insulin therapy, potassium and phosphate supplementation

↑ BUN/creatinine → Uremic acidosis (e.g., chronic or acute renal failure) → Rehydration, treat electrolyte imbalance, renal replacement therapy (RRT)

Toxicosis → Ethylene glycol, salicylates, aldehydes, ethanol, methanol → Antidote (if available), decontamination, active charcoal, fluid therapy, RRT

DIAGNOSTIC PROTOCOL

1. To evaluate the body compensatory response, the expected change in bicarbonates or pCO_2 should be calculated and then compared with that measured in the patient. If the difference between these numbers is less than 2 mmHg for pCO_2 or 2 mmol/L for HCO_3^-, the compensation is adequate, and the condition is defined as a simple acid-base disorder. If the measured value is not within two points of the expected value, the condition is defined as a mixed acid-base disorder. It is important to remember that compensation never normalizes the pH. Not enough data exist regarding compensation in cats; however, it seems that there is no respiratory compensation in metabolic disturbances in this species.

Primary disorder	Primary change	Timing	Expected compensation for dogs	Expected compensation for cats
Metabolic acidosis	↓ HCO_3^- ↓ Base excess		↓ 1 mmHg of pCO_2 every ↓ 1 mmol/L of HCO_3^-	pCO_2 does not change (few data)
Respiratory acidosis	↑ pCO_2	Acute (<3 days)	↑ 0.15 mmol/L of HCO_3^- every ↑ 1 mmHg of pCO_2	
		Chronic (>5 days)	↑ 0.35 mmol/L of HCO_3^- every ↑ 1 mmHg of pCO_2	No data
		Long-standing (>30 days)	↑ 0.55 mmol/L of HCO_3^- every ↑ 1 mmHg of pCO_2	No data

1. While the arterial value of pCO_2 depends only on alveolar ventilation and the cellular metabolic rate, the venous pCO_2 also depends on the cardiac output and peripheral perfusion. Therefore, a venous blood gas sample can have an increase in pCO_2 due to the reduction in peripheral perfusion.

4. The anion gap (AG) value reflects the unmeasured anions and increases under all conditions with fixed acid accumulation. Albumin concentration influences the AG, and the presence of hypoalbuminemia can result in a normal AG, even in the presence of an acid gain. To bypass this problem, this correction formula can be applied:
    a. For dogs: $AG_{alb} = AG + 0.42 \times (3.77 - [Alb])$
    b. For cats: $AG_{alb} = AG + 0.41 \times (3.3 - [Alb])$

DIAGNOSIS

3. Hypoventilation is the most common condition causing respiratory acidosis. Identification of the reason for the hypoventilation requires the evaluation of the physical examination (e.g., respiratory rate and pattern, neurological evaluation), CBC and biochemistry, and diagnostic imaging (e.g., thoracic X-ray or ultrasonography).

5. Hyperchloremic acidosis can be due to a loss of bicarbonate by the gastrointestinal system (such as in patients with diarrhea) or by the renal system (such as in proximal tubular acidosis,

diuretic therapy with acetazolamide, or with spironolactone, or in hypoadrenocorticism). This type of acidosis can also be secondary to a chloride gain, such as with the administration of an excess of chloride-rich fluids (e.g., normal saline, NaCl 0.9%).

7. In patients with normochloremic acidosis, the reduction in HCO_3^- is due to consumption to buffer the acids. When the acids are eliminated or metabolized by the body, the metabolic balance normalizes without any integration with HCO_3^-. There are some situations in which HCO_3^- therapy or the administration of buffer-rich solutions are required to mitigate the acidemia.

TREATMENT

6. Bicarbonate therapy is indicated every time the patient has a loss of bicarbonate or when the pH remains below 7.1 despite fluid administration. The dose of sodium bicarbonate that should be administrated is calculated using the formula:

$$NaHCO_3 \text{ (mmol)} = 0.3 \times BW(kg) \times (16 - HCO_{3\ patient}^-)$$

It is a common practice to give half of this dose as a bolus in 10-20 minutes and give the other half during the next 2-6 hours to prevent paradoxical cerebral acidosis or rebound alkalosis. Bicarbonate therapy is contraindicated in patients with hypercapnia since they cannot compensate for the net gain of CO_2 with hyperventilation.

SUGGESTED READINGS

- De Caro Carella C, de Morais HA. Compensation for acid-base disorders. *Vet Clin North Am Small Anim Pract* 47:313-323, 2017.
- DiBartola SP (editor). Fluid, Electrolyte, and Acid-Base Disorders in Small Animal Practice 4th edition. St. Louis, Elsevier, 2012.
- Funes S, de Morais HA. A quick reference on high anion gap metabolic acidosis. *Vet Clin North Am Small Anim Pract* 47:205-207, 2017.
- Kaae J, de Morais HA. Anion gap and strong ion gap: a quick reference. *Vet Clin North Am Small Anim Pract* 38:443-447, 2008.
- Torrente Artero C. A quick reference on anion gap and strong ion gap. *Vet Clin North Am Small Anim Pract* 47:191-196, 2017.

ACID-BASE ABNORMALITIES: ALKALEMIA

Marco Pesaresi

Alkalemia is an acid-base disorder and can be due to respiratory or metabolic disorders. Alkalemia is characterized by an increase in blood pH value above the normal range with a reduction in pCO_2 (respiratory alkalosis) or an increase in HCO_3^- values (metabolic alkalosis). Alkalemia is not as common as acidemia in dogs and cats. Still, it can have a deleterious effect on the patient's cerebral and coronary perfusion, reducing the release of oxygen into the tissues and decreasing the blood potassium concentration.

Respiratory alkalosis is not common as a primary disorder in small animals; it is usually secondary to metabolic acidosis as a compensatory pathway. The reduction in the pCO_2 value may be due to an increase in alveolar ventilation or a reduction in the metabolic rate (a very rare condition). The cause of the hyperventilation should be identified and, when possible, treated. In the case of respiratory alkalosis, the metabolic compensation can be very efficient, but it takes some days to be complete. Therefore, the pH can increase significantly in an acute situation, causing a dangerous condition for the patient.

Metabolic alkalosis is also not very common in veterinary medicine; it is characterized by an increase in blood pH associated with an increase in HCO_3^- or base excess (BE) values. This condition can be due to a loss of chloride-rich fluids (such as vomiting or removal of the gastric juice by a feeding tube, a net gain of alkali (such as bicarbonate therapy or the administration of citrate salt), or due to excessive mineralocorticoid activity (such as hyperadrenocorticism and hyperaldosteronism). When approaching a patient with primary metabolic alkalosis, it is important to evaluate the hydration status and blood volume since this information may help the clinician to understand the underlying mechanism causing the alkalosis and institute the correct treatment.

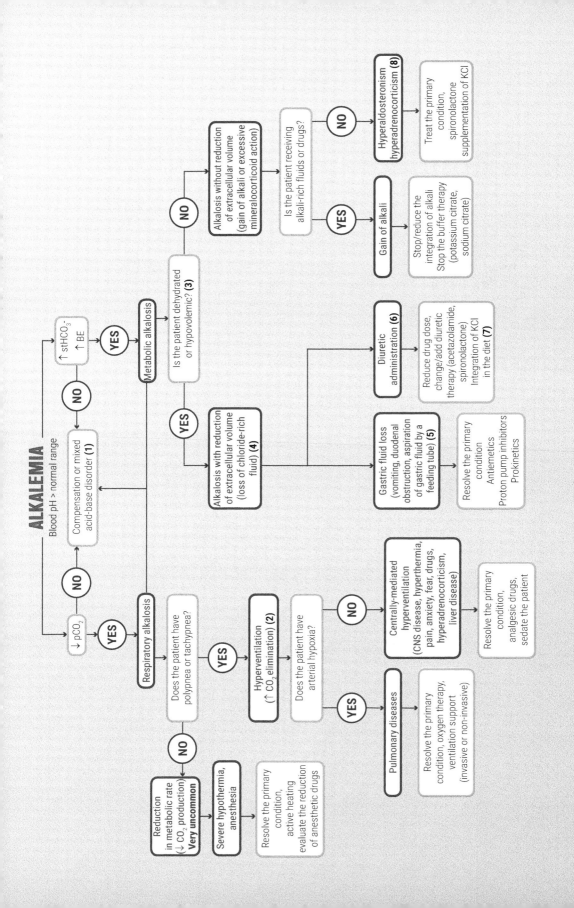

ALKALEMIA

Blood pH > normal range

Compensation or mixed acid-base disorder (1)

↓ pCO₂ — **(YES)** → **Respiratory alkalosis**

(NO) — ↑ stHCO₃⁻ ↑ BE — **(YES)** → **Metabolic alkalosis**

(NO)

Respiratory alkalosis

Does the patient have polypnea or tachypnea?

(YES) → **Hyperventilation (↑ CO₂ elimination) (2)**

Does the patient have arterial hypoxia?

(YES) → **Pulmonary diseases** → Resolve the primary condition, oxygen therapy, ventilation support (invasive or non-invasive)

(NO) → **Centrally-mediated hyperventilation** (CNS disease, hyperthermia, pain, anxiety, fear, drugs, hyperadrenocorticism, liver disease) → Resolve the primary condition, analgesic drugs, sedate the patient

(NO) → **Reduction in metabolic rate (↓ CO₂ production) Very uncommon** → **Severe hypothermia, anesthesia** → Resolve the primary condition, active heating, evaluate the reduction of anesthetic drugs

Metabolic alkalosis

Is the patient dehydrated or hypovolemic? **(3)**

(YES) → **Alkalosis with reduction of extracellular volume (loss of chloride-rich fluid) (4)**

- **Gastric fluid loss (vomiting, duodenal obstruction, aspiration of gastric fluid by a feeding tube) (5)** → Resolve the primary condition, Antiemetics, Proton pump inhibitors, Prokinetics

- **Diuretic administration (6)** → Reduce drug dose, change/add diuretic therapy (acetazolamide, spironolactone) Integration of KCl in the diet **(7)**

(NO) → **Alkalosis without reduction of extracellular volume (gain of alkali or excessive mineralocorticoid action)**

Is the patient receiving alkali-rich fluids or drugs?

(YES) → **Gain of alkali** → Stop/reduce the integration of alkali Stop the buffer therapy (potassium citrate, sodium citrate)

(NO) → **Hyperaldosteronism hyperadrenocorticism (8)** → Treat the primary condition, spironolactone supplementation of KCl

1. It is important to evaluate the body's compensatory response to alkalemia. The expected compensatory effect for metabolic and respiratory alkalosis is reported in the table below. If the difference between the expected number and the measured number is less than 2 mmHg for pCO_2 or 2 mmol/L for HCO_3^-, the compensation is adequate, and the disturbance is defined as a simple acid-base disorder; otherwise, it is a mixed acid-base disorder. Compensation never completely normalizes the pH.

Primary disorder	Primary change	Timing	Expected compensation for dogs	Expected compensation for cats
Metabolic alkalosis	↑ HCO_3^- ↑ Base excess		↑ 0.7 mmHg of pCO_2 every ↑ 1 mmol/L of HCO_3^-	
Respiratory alkalosis	↓ pCO_2	Acute (<3 days)	↓ 0.25 mmol/L of HCO_3^- every ↓ 1 mmHg of pCO_2	
		Chronic (>5 days)	↓ 0.55 mmol/L of HCO_3^- every ↓ 1 mmHg of pCO_2	

3. Evaluation of hydration and blood volume in patients with metabolic alkalosis is critical in differentiating between conditions. Hydration status can be estimated by clinical evaluation of skin turgor and elasticity, mucous membrane moisture, and weight changes, and by some laboratory values, such as hematocrit, total solids, blood urea nitrogen (BUN) value, and urine specific gravity. Evaluation of the blood volume can be extrapolated using clinical hemodynamic parameters, such as pulse quality, mucous color, capillary refill time, and blood pressure. However, the ultrasonography evaluation of the left ventricular end-diastolic diameter (LVEED) and the ratio between the caudal vena cava and the aorta (Cvc/Ao) are more accurate and specific investigations than the others.

DIAGNOSIS

2. Hyperventilation is undoubtedly the most common cause of respiratory alkalosis. It can be due to emotional activation of the respiratory center secondary to pain, anxiety, and fear. Other common conditions that can lead to an increase in the respiratory rate are stimulation of peripheral chemoreceptors by hypoxemia, activation of pulmonary stretch receptors or nociceptors, and direct activation of central respiratory centers. Activation of pulmonary stretch/nociceptors occurs in different pulmonary diseases, such as pneumonia, pulmonary thromboembolism, interstitial lung disease, and pulmonary edema, and can stimulate hyperventilation even in the absence of hypoxia. Direct activation of the central respiratory centers can be due to CNS diseases (e.g., trauma, tumors, inflammation), drugs (e.g., corticosteroids, salicylates, and xanthines), metabolic diseases (e.g., liver disease, hyperadrenocorticism), hyperthermia, fever, and sepsis.

4. Alkalosis due to the loss of chloride-rich fluids is the most common type of alkalosis in dogs and cats. It is also called chloride-responsive alkalosis since it can improve with an infusion of a solution having a high chloride concentration. This type of alkalosis is always associated with dehydration

and hypovolemia, and it is due to loss of gastric juice or the administration of loop diuretics.

5. The loss of gastric juice is one of the most common causes of alkalosis in dogs and cats. It is usually due to vomiting and gastrointestinal obstruction. Still, it can be secondary to gastric juice aspiration by feeding tubes, and it should be considered during the daily water balance for the patient. Generally, this type of loss is also associated with hypokalemia since gastric juice is rich in potassium.

6. Loop diuretics act on the Na^+-K^+-$2Cl^-$ pump in the nephron and inhibit the reabsorption of sodium, potassium, and chloride. Since the chloride loss is greater than the sodium loss, these drugs increase the strong ion difference (SID) that causes alkalosis.

8. Hyperadrenocorticism and hyperaldosteronism can cause chloride-resistant alkalosis in dogs and cats. Stimulation of the distal nephron Na^+-H^+ and Na^+-K^+ exchange is probably the most important pathophysiologic mechanism. This type of alkalosis does not respond to chloride-rich fluid administration, and it could be challenging to manage.

TREATMENT

7. To reduce the alkalosis associated with loop diuretic therapy, it is helpful to add other types of diuretics, such as acetazolamide or spironolactone, which can improve the H^+ restoration in the body and the excretion of HCO_3^-. Since many patients receiving loop diuretics also have hypokalemia, it can be helpful to integrate this electrolyte with a chloride salt (KCl) instead of a buffering salt, such as potassium citrate.

SUGGESTED READINGS

- De Caro Carella C, de Morais HA. Compensation for acid-base disorders. *Vet Clin North Am Small Anim Pract* 47:313-323, 2017.
- DiBartola SP (editor). Fluid, Electrolyte, and Acid-Base Disorders in Small Animal Practice 4th edition. St. Louis, Elsevier, 2012.
- Foy DS, de Morais HA. A quick reference on metabolic alkalosis. *Vet Clin North Am Small Anim Pract* 47:197-200, 2017.
- Ha YS, Hopper K, Epstein SE. Incidence, nature, and etiology of metabolic alkalosis in dogs and cats. *J Vet Intern Med* 27:847-853, 2013.
- Silverstein DC. Hopper K (editors). Small Animal Critical Care Medicine 2nd edition. St. Louis, Elsevier, 2015.

ACUTE DYSPNEA

Roberta Troìa

Dyspnea is defined as difficult or labored breathing.

Acute dyspnea may result from alterations in any portion of the respiratory system or be due to abnormal mechanics of the lung and chest wall. In this regard, acute dyspnea can be a sign of life-threatening hypoxemia (reduced SpO_2 or PaO_2 due to impaired gas exchange) or hypoventilation (increased $PaCO_2$ due to ineffective minute ventilation).

The five causes of hypoxemia include a low fraction of inspired oxygen (FiO_2), global hypoventilation, right-to-left shunt, diffusion impairment, and ventilation-perfusion mismatch. Hypoventilation is usually the consequence of neurological or muscular disease (e.g., peripheral neuropathy), thoracic wall or pleural space diseases, or upper airway obstruction. However, patients with problems not directly related to the cardiopulmonary system (e.g., pain, anemia, hypovolemia, metabolic acidosis, Cushing's syndrome, anxiety, or stress) may show a non-respiratory "look-alike", presenting with tachypnea or even apparent respiratory distress, but with normal SpO_2 or PaO_2.

Truly dyspneic patients have minimal tolerance for handling and restraint; they are critical and on the verge of respiratory decompensation and potentially respiratory arrest. Prompt recognition of respiratory distress and the ability to localize upper versus lower respiratory tract dysfunction are important for promptly initiating appropriate management. Most of the time, a rapid physical examination focused on the patient respiratory pattern, and breathing sounds allows for localizing the source of the respiratory disease and guiding supportive care and initial diagnostics. During triage, oxygen therapy should be provided to increase the FiO_2.

Diagnostic procedures and definitive treatment for patients with acute dyspnea depend on the underlying cause. Unfortunately, investigations may be hampered by the unstable condition of the animal.

For these reasons, it is important to combine clinical findings with minimally invasive diagnostics to confirm the source of the respiratory compromise and complete patient stabilization, while stressful or invasive procedures should be postponed until the patient is deemed stable.

ACUTE DYSPNEA

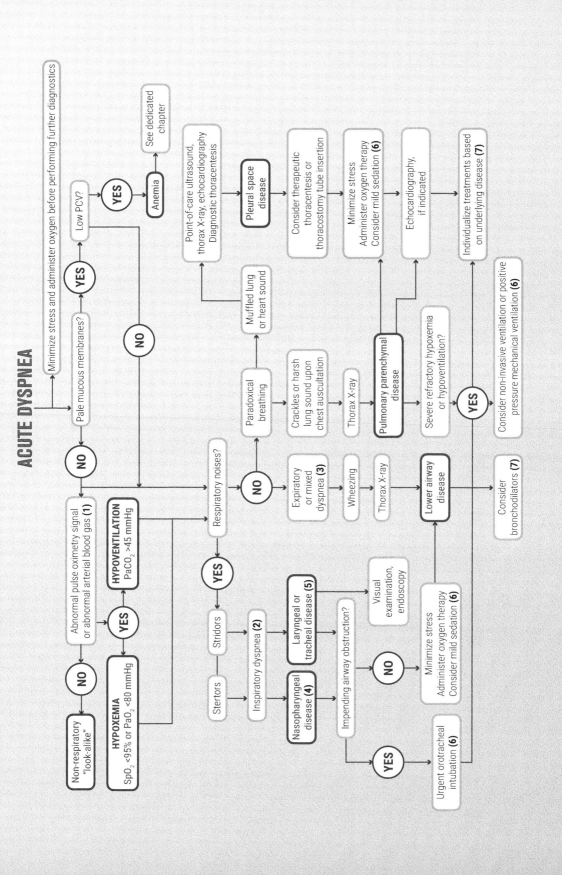

Minimize stress and administer oxygen before performing further diagnostics

Abnormal pulse oximetry signal or abnormal arterial blood gas (1)

NO → Non-respiratory "look-alike"

YES →

HYPOXEMIA SpO₂ <95% or PaO₂ <80 mmHg

HYPOVENTILATION PaCO₂ >45 mmHg

Pale mucous membranes?

YES → Low PCV?

YES → Anemia → See dedicated chapter

NO →

Respiratory noises?

YES → Stridors / Stertors

Stridors → Inspiratory dyspnea (2) → **Laryngeal or tracheal disease (5)** → Visual examination, endoscopy

Stertors → Inspiratory dyspnea (2) → **Nasopharyngeal disease (4)**

Impending airway obstruction?

NO → Minimize stress Administer oxygen therapy Consider mild sedation (6)

YES → Urgent orotracheal intubation (6)

NO →

Paradoxical breathing → Muffled lung or heart sound

Point-of-care ultrasound, thorax X-ray, echocardiography Diagnostic thoracentesis

Pleural space disease

Consider therapeutic thoracentesis or thoracostomy tube insertion

Minimize stress Administer oxygen therapy Consider mild sedation (6)

Echocardiography, if indicated

Individualize treatments based on underlying disease (7)

Crackles or harsh lung sound upon chest auscultation → Thorax X-ray → **Pulmonary parenchymal disease**

Severe refractory hypoxemia or hypoventilation?

YES → Consider non-invasive ventilation or positive pressure mechanical ventilation (6)

Expiratory or mixed dyspnea (3) → Wheezing → Thorax X-ray → **Lower airway disease** → Consider bronchodilators (7)

1. A pulse oximeter is a non-invasive device that measures the blood's oxygen saturation using spectrophotometric methods. A SpO_2 signal <95% in room air is usually indicative of hypoxemia. A normal SpO_2 level can indicate compensated respiratory disease (non-oxygen-dependent) or a non-respiratory look-alike disease. The gold standard for characterizing dyspnea is arterial blood gas analysis calculating the alveolar-arterial gradient (A-a). Hypoxemia (PaO_2 <80 mmHg), increased A-a (>14 mmHg), and normal PCO_2 should be documented in the case of venous admixture and problems in oxygen transfer. Hypoxemia with normal A-a and increased $PaCO_2$ are the features of dyspnea due to hypoventilation.

2. Clinically, pure inspiratory dyspnea implies a lesion in the respiratory tract outside the thorax. More specifically, noisy inspiratory dyspnea usually signals upper airway disease, with stertors mostly related to nasopharyngeal disease and stridor associated with laryngeal or tracheal compromise (e.g., laryngeal paralysis). Visual examination and endoscopy are useful tools for reaching a final diagnosis.

3. Expiratory and mixed dyspnea usually occur in patients with thoracic disease. The increased expiratory effort, or mixed efforts due to both inspiratory and expiratory components, are generally associated with lower airway disease or pulmonary parenchymal disease. In the case of lower airway diseases (e.g., asthma, severe intrathoracic tracheal collapse, bronchomalacia), patients usually cough, and wheezing is often audible at chest auscultation. Rapid/shallow breathing or paradoxical breathing associated with muffled heart and lung sounds are most often due to pleural space disease (pleural effusion, pneumothorax, mass effect within the pleural space). Rapid breathing or mixed dyspnea with inspiratory and expiratory effort usually signals pulmonary parenchymal disease (e.g., pneumonia, pulmonary edema, contusions). Auscultation reveals harsh lung sounds or crackles (noisy restrictive expiratory dyspnea). Point-of-care ultrasound is a non-invasive technique for rapidly assessing the thorax and the pleural space (e.g., to identify pneumothorax, effusion, "wet-lung", an intrathoracic mass). Thoracic radiographs can be used to observe the severity and distribution of lung disease.

DIAGNOSIS

4. Nasopharyngeal diseases usually present with stertorous breathing. They rarely cause severe inspiratory dyspnea unless associated with additional airway compromise (e.g., brachycephalic syndrome).

5. Laryngeal disease (laryngeal mass, laryngeal collapse) or severe tracheal collapse usually presents with inspiratory dyspnea, stridor, and signs of severe hypoxemia and hypoventilation. Animals may display cyanosis and hyperthermia.

6. Oxygen therapy should be immediately provided upon triage and during the initial clinical assessment. Flow-by oxygen therapy should be the initial choice. An oxygen mask, a

nasal cannula, an oxygen cage, or high-flow oxygen therapy are additional possibilities. The final choice for oxygen administration would ultimately depend on individual patient characteristics regarding tolerance and severity of hypoxemia. Intravenous access should be promptly obtained to administer rapidly acting drugs or anesthesia induction if emergency intubation is needed. Dyspneic patients have minimal tolerance for handling and restraint, and they can benefit from mild sedation (e.g., low dose butorphanol 0.2-0.3 mg/kg). Non-invasive ventilation (e.g., continuous positive airway pressure using a mask or helmet) may be an ideal choice for oxygen and partial ventilatory support in selected patients (e.g., brachycephalic syndrome, cardiogenic pulmonary edema) provided that control of the airways is maintained. For severe hypoxemia refractory to oxygen therapy, hypoventilation, or impending respiratory fatigue, positive pressure mechanical ventilation is required to provide respiratory support.

7. Definitive treatments for treating acute dyspnea vary according to the underlying respiratory disease. Injectable or inhalant bronchodilators (e.g., aminophylline 8 mg/kg IV) and steroids (dexamethasone 0.1 mg/kg IV) are useful drugs in the case of asthma or chronic bronchitis. Broad-spectrum antimicrobials (e.g., ampicillin-sulbactam 20 mg/kg IV) should be considered for treating bacterial pneumonia. Diuretics (e.g., furosemide 1-4 mg/kg IV) are emergency drugs for treating cardiogenic pulmonary edema.

SUGGESTED READINGS

-   Domínguez-Ruiz M, Reinero CR, Vientos-Plotts A, et al. Association between respiratory clinical signs and respiratory localization in dogs and cats with abnormal breathing patterns. *Vet J* 277, 2021.
-   Silverstein D, Hopper K (editors). Small animal critical care medicine, 2nd edition. St. Louis, Elsevier, 2014.
-   Tong CW, Gonzalez AL. Respiratory emergencies. *Vet Clin North Am Small Anim Pract* 50:1237-1259, 2020.

ADRENAL MASS

Sara Galac

An adrenal mass is defined as a focal enlargement of the adrenal gland leading to the loss of the typical adrenal gland shape. It can be unilateral or bilateral, benign or malignant, functional (hormonally active), or non-functional (hormonally silent).

A functional adrenal mass can originate from the adrenal cortex or medulla and oversecrete mineralocorticoids, glucocorticoids, sex steroids, or catecholamines. After identifying an adrenal mass, the contralateral adrenal gland should be evaluated carefully. Unilateral enlargement accompanied by an atrophic contralateral adrenal gland suggests a glucocorticoid-secreting adrenal mass. In other types, the contralateral adrenal should be of normal size. Bilateral adrenal masses are rare; however, they do occur. When an adrenal mass is found serendipitously during diagnostic imaging in the absence of clinical features suggestive of adrenal disease, endocrine testing is still warranted because the significance of the clinical signs may have been misinterpreted.

The aspects of malignancy of an adrenal mass assessed with diagnostic imaging include evaluating the size and appearance of the mass, invasive growth, and the presence of metastasis. There is no consensus on a size cut-off for malignancy of an adrenal mass; however, large adrenal masses that compress adjacent structures and invade blood vessels are potentially malignant. The only straightforward signs of malignancy of an adrenal mass are metastases. While the final diagnosis of the origin of the adrenal mass is reached using histopathology and immunohistochemistry, differentiation between benign or malignant adrenal masses remains challenging. An important differential diagnosis of an adrenal mass is metastatic disease, with pulmonary, prostatic, gastric, pancreatic, and mammary carcinomas being the most common. Other abnormalities which can present as an adrenal mass are (myelo)lipoma, hemorrhage, hematoma, cyst, and nodular hyperplasia.

When dealing with an adrenal mass, the essential question is whether it requires intervention (malignant and/or hormonally active) or whether it can be left untreated (benign and hormonally silent).

ADRENAL MASS DETECTED ON DIAGNOSTIC IMAGING

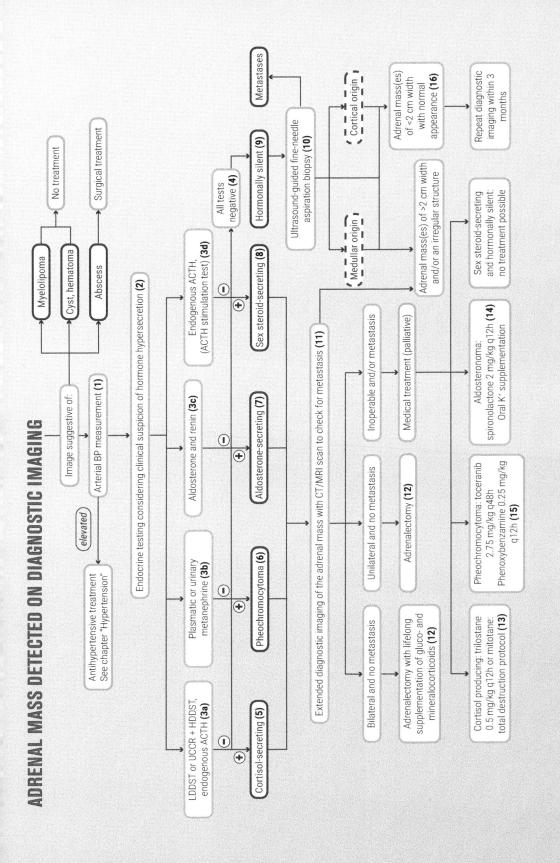

DIAGNOSTIC PROTOCOL

1. Blood pressure (BP) measurement: all hormonally active adrenal masses may cause arterial hypertension. Prompt treatment with antihypertensive drugs is advised to prevent target organ damage.

2. In a patient with an adrenal mass a thorough clinical evaluation to detect signs of underlying hormonal activity is of paramount importance. Medical history, physical examination, and clinical-pathological findings may give rise to a suspicion of endocrine activity that should be confirmed by endocrine testing.

3. Endocrine testing:
   3a. Adrenal-dependent hypercortisolism:
   positive low-dose dexamethasone suppression test (LDDST) or urinary corticoid creatinine ratios (UCCRs) combined with a high dose dexamethasone suppression test; endogenous plasma adrenocorticotropic hormone (ACTH) concentration is not detectable.
   3b. Pheochromocytoma:
   elevated plasma normetanephrine, or urinary normetanephrine: creatinine ratio.
   3c. Hyperaldosteronism:
   elevated plasma aldosterone concentration and low renin (activity).
   3d. Sex hormone excess:
   to date, no reliable endocrine testing is available; however, an ACTH stimulation test with measurement of sex steroids can be used. Endogenous ACTH may be suppressed.

4. Hormonally silent adrenal mass: when all the endocrine tests mentioned above are negative.

10. Ultrasound-guided fine-needle aspiration biopsy (FNAB) when metastasis to the adrenal gland is suspected. The FNAB is accurate in determining the cortical or medullary origin; however, it is not reliable for differentiating benign from malignant lesions. The FNAB is associated with certain risks.

11. Extended diagnostic imaging (preferentially CT scan) when surgery is intended and to check for the presence of metastases.

16. Hormonally silent adrenal masses represent a therapeutic challenge. Currently, adrenalectomy is recommended when the size of the adrenal mass is >2 cm due to potential malignancy. This advice is based on small case series. When the adrenal mass is less than 2 cm in width, regular monitoring of the size is recommended.

DIAGNOSIS

5. The most diagnosed is adrenal-dependent hypercortisolism (Cushing's syndrome) caused by a cortisol-secreting adrenocortical tumor.

6. Pheochromocytoma presents with a plethora of clinical signs and is commonly diagnosed after an adrenal mass has been detected incidentally.

7. Aldosteronoma is rare in dogs but rather common in cats. The typical presentation is arterial hypertension and hypokalemia.

8. Sex steroid-secreting tumors in cats are associated with sexual behavior. In dogs, the clinical signs are comparable to those of hypercortisolism.

9. The diagnosis of a hormonally silent adrenal mass can only be established by excluding the above-mentioned differential diagnoses.

TREATMENT

12. The preferred treatment for a hormonally active adrenal mass is adrenalectomy. Removal of the adrenal mass will reverse the clinical signs associated with excessive hormone release and avoid the complications of uncontrolled growth. In unilateral cortisol-secreting adrenocortical masses, temporary supplementation with glucocorticoids is needed postoperatively, while pheochromocytomas and aldosterone-secreting tumors usually require no supplementation. In bilateral adrenalectomy, life-long treatment with gluco- and mineralocorticoids is required.

13. Trilostane or mitotane are used to treat cortisol-secreting adrenal masses. Trilostane does not affect the growth of the adrenal mass; however, suppression of the cortisol concentration will improve the clinical signs of hypercortisolism. Trilostane is administered in a starting dose of 0.5 mg/kg PO q12h. When mitotane is used, a total-destruction protocol should be applied.

14. Spironolactone (2 mg/kg PO q12h) is used to treat a mineralocorticoid-secreting mass. Regular check-ups of electrolytes are needed during the therapy, and the dosage is titrated until a satisfactory effect is achieved, usually in combination with antihypertensive medication. This approach does not affect the growth of the adrenal mass.

15. Pheochromocytomas may be managed by the tyrosine kinase inhibitor toceranib (2.75 mg/kg PO q48h). This treatment requires close monitoring due to its side effects and the possibility of progression of the adrenal mass. It may be combined with phenoxybenzamine with an initial dose of 0.25 mg/kg PO q12h and antihypertensive medication, if indicated.

SUGGESTED READINGS

- Behrend EN. Non-cortisol-secreting adrenocortical tumors and incidentalomas In Ettinger SJ, Feldman EC, Côté E (editors). Textbook of Veterinary Internal Medicine 8th edition. St. Louis, Elsevier, 2017, pp 1819-1825.
- Cook AK, Spaulding KA, Edwards JF. Clinical findings in dogs with incidental adrenal gland lesions determined by ultrasonography: 151 cases (2007-2010). *J Am Vet Med Assoc* 244:1181-1185, 2014.
- Melián C. Investigation of adrenal masses. In Mooney CT, Peterson ME (editors). BSAVA Manual of Canine and Feline Endocrinology 4th edition. Gloucester, British Small Animal Veterinary Association, 2012, pp 272-277.
- Musser M, Taikowski KL, Johannes C, Bergman PJ. Retrospective evaluation of toceranib phosphate (Palladia) use in the treatment of inoperable, metastatic, or recurrent canine pheochromocytomas: 5 dogs (2014-2017) *BMC Vet Res* 14:272-279, 2018.
- Pey P, Rossi F, Mortier J, et al. Safety of percutaneous ultrasound-guided fine-needle aspiration of adrenal lesions in dogs: perception of the procedure by radiologists and presentation of 50 cases. *J Vet Intern Med* 34:626-635, 2020.

ALOPECIA IN CATS

Francesco Albanese

The term alopecia refers to the absence of hair in areas of the body where it is usually present. Other terms, such as hypotrichosis, are also used to define the lack of hair; however, some dermatologists prefer to reserve it for congenital alopecia. To confuse the nomenclature, the term alopecia is also incorrectly used to define a common hair disorder in cats known as self-induced symmetrical alopecia. The hair is numerically normal but shorter due to excessive grooming, giving a "false" aspect of alopecia.

The causes of alopecia include pruritic diseases (e.g., allergies), infectious and parasitic diseases of the hair follicle (e.g., dermatophytosis, demodicosis), physiological or functional abnormalities of the hair follicle (e.g., endocrinopathies, metabolic diseases), anatomical abnormalities (e.g., congenital alopecia), and paraneoplastic or neoplastic diseases (e.g., feline paraneoplastic alopecia, feline exfoliative dermatitis associated with thymoma, or epitheliotropic lymphoma).

Diseases in which alopecia is secondary to pruritus, such as allergic or ectoparasitic diseases, are not included in this chapter (see the chapter about "pruritus in cats").

In the following algorithm, alopecic problems are divided into two main groups: inflammatory and non-inflammatory, based on clinical presentation. Inflammatory alopecia includes all cases in which lesions on the skin, such as erythema, papules, scales, pustules, etc., are associated with hair loss; on the other hand, non-inflammatory alopecic diseases include cases in which alopecia is not associated with other skin lesions. In cats, diseases characterized by non-inflammatory alopecia are much less common than those of inflammatory alopecia.

Although these clinical features help dermatologists to reach a diagnosis, it should be emphasized that this subclassification is not definitive and can be modified with chronicity. In fact, a case of alopecia, starting as non-inflammatory, can appear inflamed when a secondary demodicosis or large ulcers due to skin atrophy occur; hypercortisolism is a typical example in cats.

Therefore, the following algorithm is based on the clinical aspect of alopecia since, from a histopathological point of view, alopecic diseases, which clinically do not show any inflammatory lesions on the skin but can be histologically characterized by inflammation, are recognized; pseudopelade is a clear example in which a lymphocytic attack on follicular components occurs.

ALOPECIA IN CATS

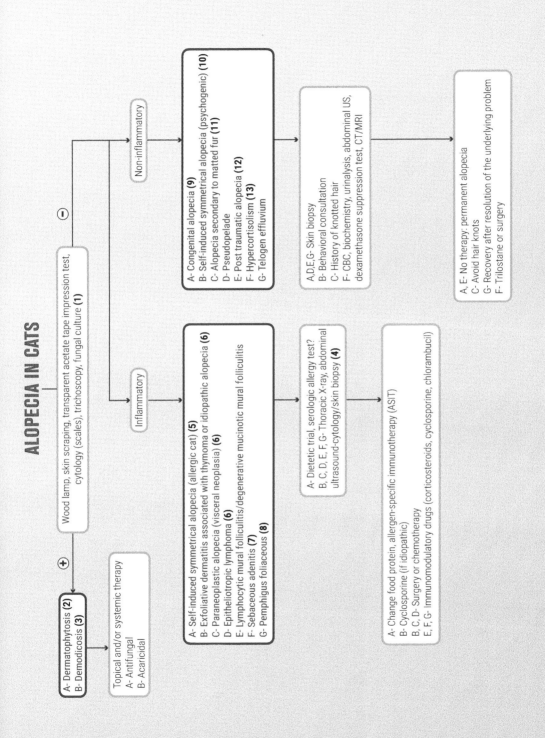

Wood lamp, skin scraping, transparent acetate tape impression test, cytology (scales), trichoscopy, fungal culture **(1)**

(–)

(+)

A- Dermatophytosis **(2)**
B- Demodicosis **(3)**

Topical and/or systemic therapy
A- Antifungal
B- Acaricidal

Inflammatory

A- Self-induced symmetrical alopecia (allergic cat) **(5)**
B- Exfoliative dermatitis associated with thymoma or idiopathic alopecia **(6)**
C- Paraneoplastic alopecia (visceral neoplasia) **(6)**
D- Epitheliotropic lymphoma **(6)**
E- Lymphocytic mural folliculitis/degenerative mucinotic mural folliculitis
F- Sebaceous adenitis **(7)**
G- Pemphigus foliaceous **(8)**

A- Dietetic trial, serologic allergy test?
B, C, D, E, F, G- Thoracic X-ray, abdominal ultrasound-cytology/skin biopsy **(4)**

A- Change food protein, allergen-specific immunotherapy (ASIT)
B- Cyclosporine (if idiopathic)
B, C, D- Surgery or chemotherapy
E, F, G- Immunomodulatory drugs (corticosteroids, cyclosporine, chlorambucil)

Non-inflammatory

A- Congenital alopecia **(9)**
B- Self-induced symmetrical alopecia (psychogenic) **(10)**
C- Alopecia secondary to matted fur **(11)**
D- Pseudopelade
E- Post traumatic alopecia **(12)**
F- Hypercortisolism **(13)**
G- Telogen effluvium

A,D,E,G- Skin biopsy
B- Behavioral consultation
C- History of knotted hair
F- CBC, biochemistry, urinalysis, abdominal US, dexamethasone suppression test, CT/MRI

A, E- No therapy: permanent alopecia
C- Avoid hair knots
G- Recovery after resolution of the underlying problem
F- Trilostane or surgery

DIAGNOSTIC PROTOCOL

1. The Wood's lamp test, trichoscopic examination, adhesive acetate tape test, cytology, skin scrapings, and fungal culture on DTM (dermatophyte test medium) should always be carried out in any cases of alopecia.

4. At the moment, a restrictive dietetic trial is the only way to rule out a food reaction. Since the role of IgE in cats with feline atopic syndrome is not yet clear, evidence of the reliability of an allergological serologic test is still low; nevertheless, many cats show good results with allergen-specific immunotherapy based on the results of these tests. When cats show clinical aspects of a paraneoplastic syndrome, diagnostic imaging is mandatory in order to discover a thymoma or visceral neoplasia. Cytology can be useful in the case of epitheliotropic lymphoma and pemphigus foliaceus. In most of these diseases, as in the case of immune-mediated adnexal diseases, such as mural folliculitis and sebaceous adenitis, a biopsy is the test of choice.

DIAGNOSIS

2. Dermatophytosis is the most common cause of focal and multifocal inflammatory alopecia in cats; alopecic lesions are mainly present on the extremities and head, with or without truncular lesions.

3. Demodicosis is rarely reported in feline patients; an underlying systemic disease or a history of chronic treatment with steroids is usually reported. Lesions, usually focal and less frequently multifocal, are mainly located on the face.

5. Self-induced symmetrical alopecia is very common in cats in the course of allergic or ectoparasitic diseases; in these cases, inflammatory signs, such as miliary dermatitis, eosinophilic dermatitis, and self-induced inflammatory lesions are frequently associated. Skin biopsy is not necessary for diagnosis; however, a correct diagnostic workup for hypersensitive diseases is mandatory. In rare cases, self-induced alopecia localized on the abdominal skin is linked to a painful sensation secondary to cystitis.

6. Two paraneoplastic skin disorders are well recognized in cats as the cause of inflammatory alopecia. Diffuse exfoliative dermatitis has been associated with thymoma; in the early stage of the disease, large white scales and erythema are observed on the head and trunk, which rapidly spread all over the body. Some cats can manifest the same clinical symptoms in the absence of thymic neoplasia. Symmetrical alopecia, shiny in appearance and ventral in location (axilla, groin, abdomen, and inner surface of legs), is associated with different malignancies. Pyoderma and *Malassezia* overgrowth contribute to severe inflammation of the alopecic skin. Epitheliotropic lymphoma is a very rare skin neoplasia in cats. Exfoliative dermatitis is the most observed skin presentation; however, since only a few cases have been reported, the clinical features of this neoplasia have not yet been well characterized.

7. A group of immune-mediated diseases that affect the adnexa, the follicles, and the sebaceous glands are clinically characterized by inflammatory and scaling alopecia. The name of these skin disorders arises from the nomenclature regarding histopathology (lymphocytic mural folliculitis, degenerative mucinotic mural folliculitis, sebaceous adenitis). These histopathological aspects

can be simultaneously present, creating great confusion in their classification; furthermore, their clinical presentation can also be very similar and impossible to differentiate. The head, face, and neck are the most involved body areas, and a skin biopsy is necessary for diagnosis. Alopecic areas are constantly covered by exfoliative dermatitis with fine scales, while swelling of the skin of the head, eyelids, and face with a shiny appearance of the skin are clinical aspects suggestive of degenerative mucinotic mural folliculitis.

8. Pemphigus foliaceous is an uncommon autoimmune pustular disease. Pustules are transient and are rapidly replaced by yellowish crusts that cause alopecia as the disease progresses. The face, the pinna, and the abdominal skin are the most commonly affected body sites. The presence of a multi-digital caseous paronychia is another common finding in feline pemphigus foliaceous. Furthermore, many cats manifest malaise and hyperthermia.

9. A focal or multifocal noninflammatory hair loss present from birth is diagnostic of congenital alopecia.

10. Self-induced alopecia due to behavioral disorders is usually not accompanied by inflammatory lesions on the skin. However, in the absence of signs of inflammation, ruling out allergic causes is also always recommended. When self-induced alopecia also involves the tail, a behavioral problem must first be suspected, followed by an allergic cause.

11. Long-haired cats can manifest an area of alopecia secondary to removing a large amount of knotted fur; usually, no inflammation is present on the alopecic skin.

12. In cats with a history of trauma to the lumbar region and hips, non-inflammatory alopecia may develop after some weeks. The hair falls out and leaves smooth and injury-free skin. A history of a previous traumatic event is fundamental for diagnosis.

13. Spontaneous hypercortisolism (Cushing's syndrome) is a rare endocrinopathy in cats. Cats with hypercortisolism commonly have secondary diabetes mellitus, showing polyuria and polydipsia. In the early stage, non-inflammatory truncal alopecia is observed since the skin is atrophic, and large skin tears secondary to skin fragility are frequently observed; demodicosis is another cause of the onset of inflammation of the skin in cats with hypercortisolism which can modify the initial non-inflammatory alopecic pattern.

SUGGESTED READINGS

- Miller WH, Griffin CE, Campbell KL. Muller and Kirk's Small Animal Dermatology 7th edition. St. Louis, Elsevier, 2021.
- Moriello K, Mason K. Handbook of Small Animal Dermatology 1st edition. Pergamon, 1995.
- Noli C, Colombo S. Feline Dermatology 1st edition. Springer, 2020.

ALOPECIA IN DOGS

Francesco Albanese

The term alopecia refers to the absence of hair in areas of the body where it is usually present; other terms, such as hypotrichosis, are also used to define the lack of hair: however, some dermatologists prefer to reserve it for congenital alopecia. To additionally confuse the nomenclature, the term alopecia is also incorrectly used to define a hair disorder known as post-clipping alopecia in which the hair, numerically normal but shorter, gives a "false" aspect of alopecia.

The causes of alopecia include pruritic diseases (e.g., allergies), infectious and parasitic diseases of the hair follicle (e.g., demodicosis, dermatophytosis, bacterial folliculitis), physiological or functional abnormalities of the hair follicle (e.g., endocrinopathies, alopecia X, metabolic internal diseases), anatomical abnormalities (e.g., congenital alopecia, follicular dysplasia), and immune-mediated vascular diseases (ischemic dermatopathy linked to low-grade vasculitis).

Diseases in which alopecia is secondary to pruritus such as allergic or ectoparasitic diseases are not included in this chapter (see the chapter about "pruritus in dogs").

In the following algorithm, alopecia is divided into two main groups: inflammatory and non-inflammatory, based on clinical presentation; inflammatory alopecia includes all cases in which lesions on the skin, such as erythema, papules, scales, pustules, etc., are associated with hair loss; on the other hand, non-inflammatory alopecic diseases include cases in which alopecia is not associated with other skin lesions.

Although these clinical features help dermatologists in formulating a diagnosis, it should be emphasized that this sub-classification is not definitive. It can be modified with chronicity; in fact, a case of alopecia that starts as non-inflammatory can appear inflamed when a secondary pyoderma occurs. Endocrinopathies, such as hypothyroidism or hypercortisolism, are two classic examples.

Therefore, the following algorithm is based on the clinical aspect of alopecia since, from a histopathological point of view, alopecic diseases that do not clinically show any inflammatory lesions on the skin but can be histologically characterized by inflammation, are recognized; alopecia areata is a clear example in which a lymphocytic attack of the follicular components occurs.

To streamline such a complex algorithm, alopecic diseases will be additionally divided into focal/multifocal and diffuse, based on the number and the spread of alopecic areas.

ALOPECIA IN DOGS

Wood's lamp, skin scraping, transparent acetate tape impression test, cytology (collarettes and pustules), trichoscopy, fungal culture **(1)**

①

(+)

Inflammatory

- Focal/multifocal
- Diffuse

Non-inflammatory

- Focal/multifocal
- Diffuse

A - Superficial pyoderma
B - Demodicosis
C - Dermatophytosis **(2)**

Topical and/or systemic therapy
A - Antibacterial
B - Acaricidal
C - Antifungal

Skin biopsy

(6)
A - Alopecia areata
B - Follicular lipidosis: Rottweiler
C - Recurrent "flank alopecia"
D - Familial trichomalacia: German Shepherds
E - Traction alopecia (hair ties)
F - Post-injection or spot-on

Skin biopsy

A - Corticosteroids, oclacitinib, spontaneous regression
B,C,D - Spontaneous regression
E - Irreversible (scar)
F - Spontaneous regression if not irreversible damage of follicle (scar)

(3)
Ischemic dermatopathies (low-grade vasculitis):
A - Leishmaniasis
B - Dermatomyositis
C - Post-vaccination
D - Idiopathic

CBC, biochemistry, UA, lymph nodes and/or bone marrow cytology, serology, PCR positive for leishmaniasis

YES

A - Antiprotozoal therapy: antimonial salts, miltefosine, allopurinol

NO

B, C, D - Oclacitinib, corticosteroids, cyclosporine, pentoxifylline **(5)**

(4)
A - Sebaceous adenitis
B - Epitheliotropic lymphoma

A - Vitamin A, cyclosporine, topical lipidic therapy
B - Chemotherapy, e.g. lomustine

With extracutaneous signs (7)

CBC, byochemistry, UA
A - ACTH stimulation test/LDDST, abdominal US, CT/MRI
B - T₄ and TSH, fT₄, TSH stimulation test
C - Genital ultrasound, preputial cytology

A - Hypercortisolism
B - Hypothyroidism
C - Hyperestrogenism

YES

A - Trilostane, mitotane, surgery adrenal or pituitary neoplasia
B - L-thyroxine supplementation
C - Surgery

Without extracutaneous signs

CBC, byochemistry, UA

Normal

NO

Skin biopsy

(8)
A - Congenital alopecia
B - X-linked ectodermal dysplasia
C - Follicular dysplasia (CDA, BHD, non-color linked, specific breed)
D - Alopecia X (hair cycle arrest)
E - Recurrent "flank" alopecia
F - Telogen effluvium
G - Post-clipping alopecia
H - Pattern baldness
I - Anagen effluvium

A, B, C - No therapy (irreversible)
D - Suprelorin, surgical castration, melatonin, trilostane, micro-needling
E, F, G - Spontaneous regression
H - Melatonin (anecdotally)
I - Regression after stopping therapy

1. The Wood' lamp test, trichoscopic examination, adhesive acetate tape test, cytology, skin scrapings, and fungal culture on DTM (dermatophyte test medium) should always be carried out in any cases of alopecia.

7. When non-inflammatory alopecia is associated with systemic signs, endocrinopathies must be considered. Polyuria, polydipsia, panting, and weight gain are frequent systemic symptoms associated with hypercortisolism along with thinning and loss of elasticity of the skin, comedones, and calcinosis cutis. Lethargy, exercise intolerance, and weight gain are suggestive of hypothyroidism. Vulvar enlargement with discharge and a prolonged estrus in females, and gynecomastia, preputial erythema/hyperpigmentation and bitch-like attitudes in male dogs are typical in animals with hyperestrogenism.

DIAGNOSIS

2. Pyoderma, dermatophytosis, and demodicosis are the most common causes of inflammatory focal and multifocal alopecia. When lesions are mainly or only present on the trunk, pyoderma must first be suspected; instead, if lesions are present on the extremities and head, along with or without truncal lesions, demodicosis, dermatophytosis, or low-grade vasculitis should be considered rather than pyoderma.

3. Ischemic dermatophytes refer to lesions due to low-grade vasculitis characterized by similar histopathological and clinical findings but linked to different causes. Early lesions are usually inflamed, showing erythema, erosions, small ulcers, scales, or crusts. In the chronic stage, multiple and variably large alopecic and cicatricial areas can have a residue, frequently appearing as shiny and hyperpigmented lesions. In endemic areas, in the case of multifocal cicatricial lesions, a complete blood test along with serology or PCR for *Leishmania* and lymph nodes and/or bone marrow cytology searching for amastigotes should always be carried out.

4. Both sebaceous adenitis (SA) and cutaneous epitheliotropic lymphoma (CEL) can start with multifocal alopecia and spread rapidly to more diffuse alopecia. In dogs with CEL erythema, scales, plaques, nodules, and both mucocutaneous junctions and nose depigmentation are the main lesions associated with alopecia. Sebaceous adenitis is an immune-mediated disease characterized by exfoliation and follicular casts. Akita Inus, Samoyeds, and Standard Poodles are among the more affected breeds. In the Vizla breed, multifocal alopecia without follicular casts or scales is well known as being the only clinical sign.

6. Some uncommon or rare diseases can be characterized by focal and multifocal non-inflammatory alopecia. Patient data, clinical presentations, and history orient to diagnosis or suggest which diagnostic test should be carried out. In focal lesions located in selected body areas, the anamnesis of infection or hair tie application is diagnostic. In the German Shepherd trichomalacia, the alteration of the hair shafts is pathognomonic. Multifocal areas of alopecia on the face and legs involving only the brown hair and sparing the black hair are suggestive of follicular lipidosis in young Rottweilers. For all diseases in which routinary diagnostic tools are not-diagnostic, a skin biopsy is necessary.

8. A broad group of diseases characterized by diffuse non-inflammatory alopecia not associated with systemic signs have been well recognized; although blood tests are unremarkable and only skin biopsy allows reaching a diagnosis, fundamental indications are obtained from the patient data, history, and clinical presentation. Loss of hair from birth is typical, apart from alopecic breeds, of congenital alopecia or X-linked ectodermal dysplasia; in the latter, defects of dentition are constantly associated with alopecia. Some breeds such as Chesapeake Bay Retrievers, Irish Water Spaniels, and Portuguese Water Dogs are predisposed to genetic follicular dysplasia. In dogs with a dilute haircoat, large clumps of melanin (named "macro-melanosome") are organized into the hair's cortex, causing fracture of the hair shaft. In many cases, these features are not so clearly evident at trichoscopy, and a biopsy is necessary to reach a diagnosis. In some breeds, such as Lagotto Romagnolo affected by "flank" recurrent alopecia, hair loss is not only localized to the flanks as in the majority of other breeds, but involves the back and the trunk, and can mimic endocrinopathy. Alopecia X is a common skin disorder of unknown origin, which is mainly observed in Pomeranians. Since clinical presentation is identical to endocrine alopecia, the diagnosis needs to rule out hormonal disorders via blood tests and it can be confirmed with a skin biopsy. A history of clipping is diagnostic of "post clipping alopecia", while the history of a stressful event (pregnancy, lactation, general anesthesia) or history of chemotherapy treatment are indicative of telogen and anagen effluvium, respectively. Finally, pattern baldness is typical of short-haired breeds such as Pinschers, Whippets, Dachshunds, etc.; miniaturized hair on the ventral neck, temporal and retroauricolar areas, and posterior thighs are the hallmarks.

TREATMENT

5. In vasculopathies not linked to canine leishmaniasis, skin lesions can only be treated with symptomatic drugs, especially when the underlying causes cannot be removed (e.g., post-vaccination). Immunomodulatory drugs, such as oclacitinib, corticosteroids, and cyclosporine, have been used with variable efficacy. Drugs with rheological activity (pentoxifylline) are also used in order to improve the vascularization of the skin.

SUGGESTED READINGS

- Mecklenburg L, Linek M, Tobin DJ. Hair loss disorders in domestic animals. Wiley Blackwell, 2009.
- Miller WH, Griffin CE, Campbell KL. Muller and Kirk's Small Animal Dermatology 7th edition. St. Louis, Elsevier, 2021.
- Moriello K, Mason I. Handbook of Small animal Dermatology 1st edition. Pergamon, 1995.

ANEMIA: NON-REGENERATIVE

Chiara Agnoli

Anemia is defined as a reduction in the oxygen-carrying capacity of the blood, resulting from a decrease in the hemoglobin (Hb) concentration, the red blood cell (RBC) number, and the hematocrit (HCT) value. In the evaluation of an anemic dog or cat, hydration status must be considered. Hematocrit reflects the severity of anemia only when the animal has normal hydration and blood volume. A drop in Hb concentration, in the number of RBCs, or in the HCT value can sometimes be observed without a real decrease in the erythrocyte mass (relative anemia). This can occasionally result from the splenic sequestration of erythrocytes, as it happens during anesthesia, and from overhydration, resulting in erythrocyte dilution.

Anemias with minimal or no increase in blood reticulocyte count are classified as poorly regenerative and non-regenerative, respectively, and are related to insufficient erythrocyte production in the bone marrow. Mild to moderate non-regenerative anemias are more likely due to secondary bone marrow suppression (e.g., anemia due to inflammatory/neoplastic diseases, also called anemia of chronic disease) while primary bone marrow problems (e.g., neoplastic myelophthisis, myelonecrosis or myelofibrosis) are associated with moderate to severe anemia.

Severe non-regenerative anemia or pancytopenia (concomitant non-regenerative anemia, neutropenia, and thrombocytopenia), always suggest a primary bone marrow problem, and bone marrow aspiration becomes a necessary step in the diagnostic workup. The clinical signs of anemia vary greatly depending on the rapidity of onset, type, and underlying cause. In nonregenerative anemia, blood RBCs usually decrease slowly, and the animals may have mild clinical signs as compared to those with the acute onset of anemia.

Non-specific clinical signs in these animals are anorexia, lethargy, and sometimes pica. Depending on the cause of non-regenerative anemia, the treatment needs to be addressed appropriately; however, the underlying cause sometimes remains unknown, and in disorders such as bone marrow aplasia, mortality rates are high, with most animals dying or being euthanized within a few weeks of diagnosis.

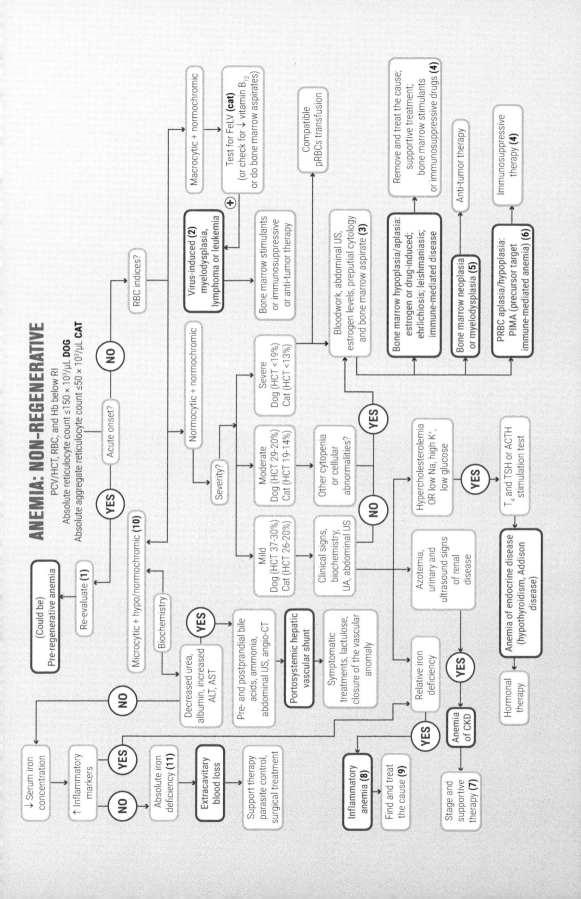

ANEMIA: NON-REGENERATIVE

PCV/HCT, RBC, and Hb below RI
Absolute reticulocyte count ≤150 × 10³/µL **DOG**
Absolute aggregate reticulocyte count ≤50 × 10³/µL **CAT**

(Could be)
Pre-regenerative anemia

Re-evaluate **(1)**

Acute onset?

YES

NO

RBC indices?

Macrocytic + normochromic

Test for FeLV **(cat)**
(or check for ↓ vitamin B₁₂
or do bone marrow aspirates)

Virus-induced **(2)** myelodysplasia,
lymphoma or leukemia

(+)

Bone marrow stimulants
or immunosuppressive
or anti-tumor therapy

Compatible
pRBCs transfusion

Normocytic + normochromic

Severity?

Severe
Dog (HCT <19%)
Cat (HCT <13%)

Bloodwork, abdominal US,
estrogen levels, preputial cytology
and bone marrow aspirate **(3)**

Remove and treat the cause;
supportive treatment;
bone marrow stimulants
or immunosuppressive drugs **(4)**

Bone marrow hypoplasia/aplasia:
estrogen or drug-induced;
ehrlichiosis; leishmaniasis;
immune-mediated disease

Anti-tumor therapy

Bone marrow neoplasia
or myelodysplasia **(5)**

Immunosuppressive
therapy **(4)**

PRBC aplasia/hypoplasia:
PIMA (precursor target
immune-mediated anemia) **(6)**

Moderate
Dog (HCT 29-20%)
Cat (HCT 19-14%)

Other cytopenia
or cellular
abnormalities?

YES

NO

Hypercholesterolemia
OR low Na, high K⁺,
low glucose

YES

T₄ and TSH or ACTH
stimulation test

Anemia of endocrine disease
(hypothyroidism, Addison
disease)

Hormonal
therapy

Mild
Dog (HCT 37-30%)
Cat (HCT 26-20%)

Clinical signs,
biochemistry,
UA, abdominal US

Azotemia,
urinary and
ultrasound signs
of renal
disease

YES

Anemia
of CKD

Stage and
supportive
therapy **(7)**

Microcytic + hypo/normochromic **(10)**

Biochemistry

Decreased urea,
albumin, increased
ALT, AST

YES

Pre- and postprandial bile
acids, ammonia,
abdominal US, angio-CT

Portosystemic hepatic
vascular shunt

Symptomatic
treatments, lactulose,
closure of the vascular
anomaly

Relative iron
deficiency

YES

NO

↓ Serum iron
concentration

↑ Inflammatory
markers

YES

Absolute iron
deficiency **(11)**

Extracavitary
blood loss

Support therapy
parasite control,
surgical treatment

NO

Inflammatory
anemia **(8)**

Find and treat
the cause **(9)**

1. Reticulocytes need time to reach the expected peak; this usually occurs approximately 3-5 days after the onset of the anemia (pre-regenerative anemia). If the course of the non-regenerative anemia seems to be acute, causes such as hemolysis and blood loss must be ruled out with a careful anamnestic, clinical and clinicopathological investigation. The hematologic course needs to be carefully monitored to confirm the absence of reticulocytes and other signs of regeneration (presence of polychromasia, nucleated red cells, or Howell-Jolly bodies).

3. Bone marrow evaluation is indicated in non-regenerative anemias that have had adequate time to respond, are moderate or severe, and are not attributable to other causes. This procedure is also necessary if other cytopenias are present, or other cell lines are abnormal in the peripheral blood. Typically, both aspirates for cytology and core biopsy for histopathology are recommended since they give complementary information. The morphology of the individual cells is more easily assessed with an aspiration sample while core samples allow for the architecture of the cells to be better detected. A complete blood count contextual to the bone marrow sampling is always recommended.

10. Blood loss anemia becomes progressively less regenerative over time due to the depletion of nutrients, such as iron and proteins. Iron is necessary for hemoglobin synthesis. Both absolute and relative iron deficiency results in compromised hemoglobin synthesis, and since hemoglobin concentration determines the cessation of cell division, iron-deficient erythrocytes undergo more cell divisions, resulting in microcytes. Hypochromia may also be present.

11. Serum iron concentration alone is an unreliable reflection of body iron stores. Diagnosing absolute iron deficiency depends on a combination of tests, including transferrin saturation, and ferritin levels, as well as the evaluation of stainable iron in bone marrow aspirates.

DIAGNOSIS

2. FeLV infection is associated with a variety of neoplastic and non-neoplastic hematologic diseases. Bone marrow suppression by the virus, myelodysplasia, anemia of chronic disease, and hemolytic regenerative anemia have been reported. Understanding the correct pathogenetic mechanism of FeLV-associated anemia could be useful for both treatment and prognostic aims. In myelodysplasia, macrocytosis seems to be caused by a FeLV-induced genetic defect in cell division during erythropoiesis.

5. The replacement of hematopoietic tissue by abnormal tissue (myelophthisis) is likely to result in pancytopenia. Both primary and metastatic tumors may proliferate in the marrow, causing destruction of the normal hematopoietic cells and alteration of the marrow microenvironment. Generalized bone marrow involvement is more common with acute and chronic lymphoid or myeloid leukemia, stage 5 lymphoma, multiple myeloma, histiocytic sarcoma, and mast cell tumors.

6. Precursor-targeted immune-mediated anemia (PIMA) should be suspected in dogs with non-regenerative anemia. In this condition, different erythroid precursors are targeted for

immune-mediated destruction, and bone marrow findings vary from erythroid hyperplasia to pure red cell aplasia. The phagocytosis of erythroid precursors by macrophages, as well as lymphoplasmacytosis and secondary myelofibrosis, are observed in PIMA.

8. Anemia of chronic inflammatory disease is the most common cause of non-regenerative anemia. It is typically mild to moderate and normocytic-normochromic. This condition has multifactorial pathogenesis (decreased iron availability, known as relative iron deficiency, downstream effects of inflammatory cytokines, and decreased erythrocyte half-life). The diagnosis of a hormonally silent adrenal mass can only be established by excluding the above-mentioned differential diagnoses.

TREATMENT

4. In the absence of a known inciting agent in bone marrow aplasia, given the suspicion of an immune-mediated etiology, trial treatment with immunosuppressive drugs has been recommended. Prednisone (not for cats) or prednisolone at an initial PO dose of 2-3 mg/kg/day (or 50 mg/m^2/day for dogs >25 kg), is described as first-line immunosuppressive therapy. A second immunosuppressive drug, such as cyclosporine (5 mg/kg PO q12h), mycophenolate mofetil (8-12 mg/kg PO q12h), or leflunomide (2 mg/kg dogs or 10 mg/cat q24h), may be introduced in animals with a life-threatening disease, or as "steroid-sparing" combination therapy. Bone marrow stimulants, such as eltrombopag (an orally available synthetic mimetic of thrombopoietin), found to have bi- and tri-lineage bone marrow stimulatory effects in human patients, may be empirically added in dogs (at 1.25/mg/kg PO q 24h).

7. In CKD patients, the presence of symptomatic anemia (or an HCT value < 22% for dogs, and an HCT value <18% for cats) could be treated with darbepoetin alpha, administered at 0.45-2.0 µg/kg weekly SC. Supplementation with oral ferrous sulfate (100-300 mg/day for dogs and 50-100 mg/day for cats), is recommended due to the high demand for iron associated with stimulated erythropoiesis.

9. The treatment of anemia in inflammatory disease involves addressing the underlying disease. Iron supplementation is generally not necessary. In functional iron deficiency, total body iron stores are normal or increased: however, iron is relatively unavailable for heme synthesis. The use of erythropoiesis-stimulating agents, such as erythropoietin, is usually not recommended since patients with this condition seem to have a decreased response to both its endogen and exogen form.

SUGGESTED READINGS
-   Green CE (editor). Infectious Diseases of the Dog and Cat. St. Louis, Elsevier Saunders, 2011.
-   Grimes CN, Fry MM. Nonregenerative anemia: mechanisms of decreased or ineffective erythropoiesis. *Vet Pathol* 52:298-311, 2015.
-   Harvey JW (editor). Veterinary Hematology: a Diagnostic Guide and Color Atlas. St. Louis, Elsevier, 2012.
-   Kelly D, Lamb V, Juvet F. Eltrombopag treatment of a dog with idiopathic aplastic pancytopenia. *J Vet Intern Med* 34:890-892, 2020.
-   Lucidi CA, de Rezende CLE, Jutkowitz LA, et al. Histologic and cytologic bone marrow findings in dogs with suspected precursor-targeted immune-mediated anemia and associated phagocytosis of erythroid precursors. *Vet Clin Pathol* 46:401-415, 2017.

ANEMIA: REGENERATIVE

Chiara Agnoli

Anemia is a common laboratory finding in critically sick dogs and cats, defined as a reduction in the oxygen-carrying capacity of blood resulting from decreases in hemoglobin (Hb) concentration and red blood cells (RBCs).

Diagnosing anemia usually starts with a complete blood count (CBC), including reticulocyte evaluation, erythrocyte indices, and blood smear evaluation. A thorough history, physical examination, and supplementary clinical and clinicopathological investigations are generally helpful in defining the underlying cause. One of the most useful approaches in classifying anemia is determining whether a bone marrow response to the anemia is present. The anemia is classified as regenerative if the absolute number of peripheral blood reticulocytes is adequate for the severity of the anemia. Healthy dogs and cats usually release aggregate reticulocytes from the bone marrow in low numbers. As anemia develops and its severity increases, in the absence of primary or secondary bone marrow dysfunction, an increased number of reticulocytes is formed from nucleated erythrocyte precursors. Reticulocytes need time to reach the expected peak. This usually occurs around 4-5 days after the onset of the anemia since it takes time for the erythropoietin response to stimulate the bone marrow release of immature red blood cells.

Moreover, it is essential to remember that mild anemias may have minimally increased reticulocyte counts; therefore, some authors have considered an absolute aggregate reticulocyte count of ≥60.000/µL for cats and ≥80.000/µL for dogs to be already suggestive of regeneration.

Marked to moderately regenerative anemias are usually hemolytic and posthemorrhagic.

Hemolytic anemia seems to stimulate the most intense regenerative response, which could be partly due to the great availability of iron typical of these medical conditions. The erythrocyte indices, mean corpuscular volume (MCV), and mean corpuscular hemoglobin concentration (MCHC) can also be useful in characterizing regenerative anemia since immature red blood cells are commonly hypochromic and macrocytic.

ANEMIA: REGENERATIVE

PCV/HCT, RBC, and Hb below RI
Absolute reticulocyte count ≥150 × 10³/μL

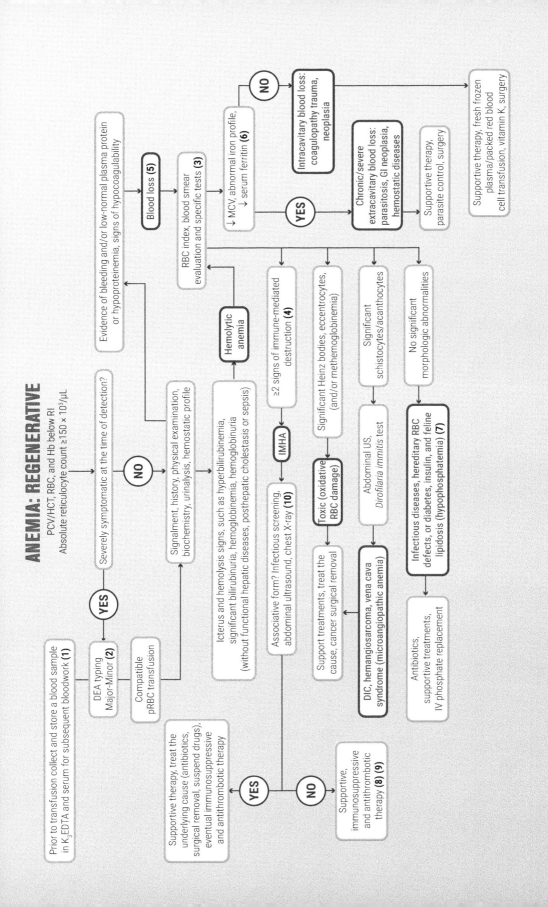

Prior to transfusion collect and store a blood sample in K₃EDTA and serum for subsequent bloodwork **(1)**

YES

DEA typing Major-Minor **(2)**

Compatible pRBC transfusion

Severely symptomatic at the time of detection?

NO

Evidence of bleeding and/or low-normal plasma protein or hypoproteinemia, signs of hypocoagulability

Blood loss (5)

RBC index, blood smear evaluation and specific tests **(3)**

↓ MCV, abnormal iron profile, → serum ferritin **(6)**

NO

Intracavitary blood loss: coagulopathy trauma, neoplasia

YES

Chronic/severe extracavitary blood loss: parasitosis, GI neoplasia, hemostatic diseases

Supportive therapy, parasite control, surgery

Supportive therapy, fresh frozen plasma/packed red blood cell transfusion, vitamin K, surgery

Signalment, history, physical examination, biochemistry, urinalysis, hemostatic profile

Icterus and hemolysis signs, such as hyperbilirubinemia, significant bilirubinuria, hemoglobinemia, hemoglobinuria (without functional hepatic diseases, posthepatic cholestasis or sepsis)

Hemolytic anemia

≥2 signs of immune-mediated destruction **(4)**

IMHA

Significant Heinz bodies, eccentocytes, (and/or methemoglobinemia)

Toxic (oxidative RBC damage)

Significant schistocytes/acanthocytes

Abdominal US, *Dirofilaria immitis* test

No significant morphologic abnormalities

Infectious diseases, hereditary RBC defects, or diabetes, insulin, and feline lipidosis (hypophosphatemia) **(7)**

Antibiotics, supportive treatments, IV phosphate replacement

DIC, hemangiosarcoma, vena cava syndrome (microangiopathic anemia)

Support treatments, treat the cause, cancer surgical removal

Associative form? Infectious screening, abdominal ultrasound, chest X-ray **(10)**

YES

Supportive therapy, treat the underlying cause (antibiotics, surgical removal, suspend drugs), eventual immunosuppressive and antithrombotic therapy

NO

Supportive, immunosuppressive and antithrombotic therapy **(8) (9)**

DIAGNOSTIC PROTOCOL

1. Whenever possible, appropriate blood samples (EDTA blood, serum, and citrate plasma) should be collected before any therapeutic intervention, especially before immunosuppressive, antibiotic, and transfusion treatments. This could also help in reaching a definitive diagnosis for the anemia after the first life-saving procedures and could improve the overall management of the patient.

2. Before transfusion, all canine and feline blood recipients should be typed for Dog Erythrocyte Antigen (DEA) 1 and AB blood group, respectively. Blood from dogs previously transfused should also be crossmatched (Major-Minor) before receiving another transfusion treatment, while cats should always be crossmatched because of the presence of possible alloantibodies (e.g., anti-Mik antibodies).

3. Blood smear evaluation is a crucial part of classifying anemia; recognizing RBC morphologic defects may be helpful. Some examples include the identification of blood parasites or Heinz bodies (slightly pale, round aggregates of Hb, often protruding from the RBC surface), that are suggestive of oxidative RBC damage. Schistocytes indicate excessive shear or turbulence in the circulation as it can happen during disseminated intravascular coagulation (DIC), or they can be associated with diseases such as hemangiosarcoma and heartworm disease.

4. Based on the recent American College of Veterinary Internal Medicine (ACVIM) Consensus statement regarding the diagnosis of the immune-mediated hemolytic anemia (IMHA), the hallmarks of immune-mediated RBC destruction include a significant number of spherocytes in the blood smear evaluation, a positive saline agglutination test (SAT), a positive direct antiglobulin test (DAT) and/or the detection of anti-erythrocyte antibodies using flow cytometry (FC). When diagnosing IMHA, the patient should present at least two of the above-mentioned criteria or, alternatively, a positive SAT, which persists with washing. At least one sign of hemolysis should also be present for a definite diagnosis of IMHA. Variations on this model would allow a supportive or only a suspicious diagnosis.

6. Microcytic (low MCV) hypochromic (low MCHC) anemia indicates iron deficiency. This form of anemia varies from moderately regenerative to non-regenerative. Both the MCV and the MCHC tend to be decreased in iron deficiency; however, the MCHC may be normal in some cases, and only a mildly decreased MCV is present.

10. Any infection with different evidence levels can trigger an immune-mediated disease. *Babesia* spp., *Anaplasma* spp., *Ehrlichia* spp., *Leishmania infantum*, *Leptospira* spp., and *Dirofilaria immitis* have been reported in dogs. *Mycoplasma haemofelis*, *Babesia felis*, *Cytauxzoon felis*, feline leukemia virus (FeLV), feline immunodeficiency virus (FIV), and feline infectious peritonitis (FIP) are reported in cats.

DIAGNOSIS

5. The absence of overt blood loss does not rule out hemorrhagic anemia. Gastrointestinal blood loss may not be noted by owners, or it may not clearly change fecal characteristics. Reductions in serum protein or elevations in blood urea nitrogen (BUN) may be indicative of bleeding.

Diagnostic imaging may also be indicated to search for cavitary bleeding or bleeding lesions.

7. Severe hypophosphatemia with depletion of total body stores can cause detrimental clinical consequences, including hemolytic anemia, decreasing the erythrocyte glycolytic rate, and resulting in a reduced RBC adenosine triphosphate (ATP) concentration.

TREATMENT

8. Prednisone (in dogs) or prednisolone (in dogs and cats) at an initial PO dose of 2-3 mg/kg/day (or 50 mg/m^2/day for dogs >25 kg) is recommended as first-line immunosuppressive therapy. A second immunosuppressive drug, such as cyclosporine (5 mg/kg PO q12h), mycophenolate mofetil (8-12 mg/kg PO q12h), or leflunomide (2 mg/kg dogs or 10 mg/cat q24h) may be introduced in animals with a life-threatening disease, or as "steroid-sparing" combination therapy.

9. Thrombotic events are the most common cause of mortality in IMHA dogs; however, they are rarely reported in cats. Antiplatelet drugs should be provided for all dogs with IMHA (except for those with severe thrombocytopenia). Clopidogrel (1-2 mg/kg PO q24h) should be administered starting from the time of diagnosis and continued until clinical remission. A therapeutic regimen incorporating anticoagulants may also be desirable (subcutaneous unfractionated heparin at 150-300 U/kg q6h or dalteparin at 150-175 U/kg q8h) in the acute phase of the disease in dogs.

SUGGESTED READINGS

- Garden OA, Kidd L, Mexas A, et al. ACVIM consensus statement on the diagnosis of immune-mediated hemolytic anemia in dogs and cats. *J Vet Intern Med* 33:313-334, 2019.
- Harvey JW. Veterinary Hematology. A Diagnostic Guide and Color Atlas. St. Louis, Elsevier Saunders, 2012.
- Swann JW, Garden OA, Fellman CL, et al. ACVIM consensus statement on the treatment of immune-mediated hemolytic anemia in dogs. *J Vet Intern Med* 33:1141-1172, 2019.
- Weiss DJ, Wardrop KJ. Schalm's Veterinary Hematology. Ames, Iowa, Blackwell Publishing, 2010.

ANOREXIA
DECREASED APPETITE

Andrea Corsini

Decreased appetite is a non-specific finding and a common reason for the owner to seek medical care for their pets. A complete lack of appetite is referred to as anorexia, while the term hyporexia better identifies a partial decrease in appetite. Decreased appetite must be differentiated from the inability to eat, as seen in diseases causing pain at the opening of the mouth or in oral dysphagia. This difference is crucial but not always apparent to the owner.

Regulating food intake involves many internal and external stimuli, such as sensory signals (e.g., olfaction, physical attributes of food, flavor), metabolic signals (e.g., orexigenic and anorexigenic factors), environmental signals (e.g., timing and location of meals, ambient noise level, the person offering the food, previous negative or positive associations), and previously learned behavior. Consequently, many diseases or conditions can negatively impact appetite. Patients with organ failure, neoplasia, inflammatory disease, and fever usually have increased circulation of anorexigenic factors (e.g., inflammatory cytokines, uremic toxins, or other substances generally metabolized by the organs affected). Both pain and nausea, common in abdominal and GI diseases, result in anorexia/hyporexia.

The resolution of anorexia/hyporexia depends on the effective treatment of its etiology, which can sometimes be easily achieved. Anorexia/hyporexia due to chronic conditions or untreatable diseases is usually challenging and more critical for the negative consequences of prolonged decreased food intake. However, even a few days of anorexia can significantly impact a patient's condition, especially in cats. For example, protein and fat catabolism markedly increase since both are used for gluconeogenesis in place of carbohydrates, which are depleted. This leads to immune system suppression, muscle and weight loss, and secondary organ dysfunction (e.g., hepatic lipidosis in cats), which in turn worsen anorexia/hyporexia. When anorexia/hyporexia is not resolved promptly, appetite stimulants or assisted feeding are warranted to counteract the negative impact of prolonged decreased food intake.

ANOREXIA – DECREASED APPETITE

```
History ─── Physical exam
  │
  ├── Interested in food
  │     ├── Environmental stress ── Treat accordingly
  │     └── Dietary changes ── Diet change
  │
  └── Not interested in food
        └── Medications affecting appetite? (1)
              ├── YES ── Possible drug-induced anorexia
              │           └── Consider drug discontinuation (if possible), or appetite stimulants (10)
              └── NO
```

Physical exam branches:

- Abnormal oral, nasal or cranial findings
  → Consider appropriate diagnostic: endoscopy, fluoroscopy, radiology or CT, cytology, infectious diseases testing
  → Oral/nasal disease (2) ── Treat accordingly
  → Neuromuscular disease (3) ── Treat accordingly

- Respiratory distress
  → Consider appropriate diagnostic: chest X-rays, chest US, echocardiography
  → Cardiac disease / Pulmonary/thoracic disease ── Treat accordingly

- Signs and/or history of chronic pain, neck pain, swollen joints, lameness, fever
  → Orthopedic and/or neurological evaluation
  → CBC, chemistry, UA, X-rays, joint tap, CSF tap, serology, advanced imaging
  → Orthopedic or neurologic disease (4)
  → Consider pain management and appropriate treatment

- Abnormal mentation, vestibular signs (head tilt, ataxia, nystagmus)
  → Neurological evaluation

- Unremarkable or specific signs
  → CBC, chemistry, UA, abdominal US, chest X-rays (if indicated)

CBC, chemistry, UA, abdominal US, chest X-rays (if indicated) branches:

- Moderate to severe azotemia, hyperphosphatemia, USG <1.030 ± proteinuria
  → Renal disease (5) ── Treat accordingly

- Hyperlipasemia, suggestive US findings
  → Pancreatic disease ── Treat accordingly

- Increased liver enzymes, hyperbilirubinemia, suggestive US findings
  → Hepatobiliary disease ── Appropriate diagnostic workup (6)

- Suggestive clinical signs, GI abnormalities on US
  → Primary GI disease ── Appropriate diagnostic workup (7)

- Hyperkalemia, hyponatremia, hypercalcemia, lack of stress leukogram
  → ACTH stimulation test (8)
  → Addison's disease ── Start appropriate treatment

- Hyperglycemia, glucosuria, ketonuria
  → Venous blood gas analysis, ketonemia
  → Diabetic ketoacidosis ── Appropriate diagnostic workup

- Moderate to severe anemia with or without signs of hemolysis
  → Blood loss / Hemolytic anemia / Ineffective erythropoiesis ── Treat accordingly

- No clear reason for anorexia identified
  → Further testing (9)
  → Is the cause of anorexia identified?
        ├── YES ── Treat accordingly
        └── NO ── Consider trial with appetite stimulants (10)
```
```

DIAGNOSTIC PROTOCOL

1. Non-steroidal anti-inflammatory drugs, opioid analgesics, proton pump inhibitors, antibiotics (beta-lactams, erythromycin, sulphonamides), chemotherapeutic agents, cardiac glycosides, penicillamine, and ferrous sulfate are some medications that can affect appetite.

6. Liver function is evaluated by measuring serum bile acids and ammonia. Computed tomography angiography helps identify macroscopic vascular anomalies. Liver cytology is an easy and inexpensive method for evaluating hepatic lipidosis or some neoplasias (e.g., round-cell neoplasia). Percutaneous ultrasound-guided cholecystocentesis with bile culture and cytology is warranted whenever a bacterial infection is suspected. A liver biopsy must be performed to confirm chronic hepatitis and to gain information regarding etiology. It also allows differentiation between neutrophilic cholangitis, lymphocytic cholangitis, or small cell lymphoma in cats.

7. Chronic enteropathies (CEs) are common both in dogs and cats. A fecal exam and determination of serum folate and cobalamin concentrations should always be carried out. Serum basal cortisol or adrenocorticotropic hormone (ACTH) stimulation tests should be considered. Upper and lower GI endoscopy with biopsies are indicated for patients who fail to respond to diet trials or when gastrointestinal neoplasia is strongly suspected. Focal intestinal lesions should be evaluated performing full thickness biopsies.

8. Hypoadrenocorticism can present with normal potassium and sodium serum concentrations (eunatremic, eukalemic hypoadrenocorticism), and an ACTH stimulation test should be considered in patients with suggestive clinical signs, even in the absence of hyperkalemia or hyponatremia. To avoid false-positive results, the animal's history must be carefully assessed for exogenous glucocorticoid administration; concurrent endogenous ACTH measurement should be considered.

9. Additional testing should be considered based on history and physical examination findings if the cause of anorexia is not apparent at this point. Lymph node cytology must be performed if lymphadenomegaly is present to assess the possibility of neoplasia (e.g., lymphoma) or infectious diseases (e.g., leishmaniasis). Tests for infectious diseases should be conducted based on clinical suspicion and epidemiological exposure. Total and ionized calcium concentrations should be measured since both hypocalcemia and hypercalcemia can decrease appetite (see hypocalcemia and hypercalcemia). Advanced diagnostic imaging can help to identify a neoplasia that is not apparent (e.g., intracranial neoplasia). Bone marrow aspiration is indicated if peripheral cytopenias are present or hematopoietic neoplasia (e.g., multiple myeloma) is suspected. Prostatic disease (e.g., prostatitis) in male dogs and uterine disease in females should be ruled out.

DIAGNOSIS

2. A broad spectrum of diseases involving the oral cavity, skull, or nose can lead to anorexia. Common diseases to rule out are stomatitis, dental/periodontal disease, foreign bodies, neoplasia, fracture, osteomyelitis, temporomandibular joint problems, retrobulbar abscess, and sinonasal aspergillosis. In cats, any nasal disease affecting the ability to smell food can decrease the appetite.

3. Masticatory myositis, trigeminal neuritis, and cranial nerve neoplasia affect the opening of the mouth and swallowing, thus reducing food intake.

4. The most common orthopedic diseases are osteoarthritis, panosteitis, septic arthritis, and immune-mediated polyarthritis. The most common neurological diseases are intervertebral disk disease, steroid-responsive meningoarteritis, meningoencephalitis of unknown etiology, discospondylitis, vestibular diseases, and brain neoplasia.

5. Renal diseases tend to cause anorexia when uremia or complications (e.g., nephrotic syndrome, metabolic acidosis) develop. Acute kidney injury, advanced chronic kidney disease (CKD) (IRIS stage 3 or 4), acute pyelonephritis, and severe glomerulopathies commonly cause anorexia, while appetite is usually unaffected in early CKD or in chronic pyelonephritis.

TREATMENT

10. A trial with appetite stimulants can be considered when an extensive workup has failed to provide a clear reason for decreased appetite. Mirtazapine (¼ of a 7.5 mg tablet PO q48h or 2 mg/cat of the transdermal ointment applied to the inner pinna q24h) is commonly used in cats, with the additional benefit of its antiemetic activity. Adverse effects (e.g., vocalization, restlessness, ataxia, tremors, hypersalivation, tachycardia, tachypnea) are reported to be associated with higher dosages. Cyproheptadine (0.2 mg/kg PO q12h) is suitable for use in dogs. A reason for anorexia is almost always identifiable after a thorough assessment, and appetite stimulants should never substitute the effort to reach a diagnosis.

SUGGESTED READINGS

-   Batchelor DJ, German AJ. Anorexia and hyporexia. In Hall EJ, Williams DA, Kathrani A (editors). BSAVA Manual of Canine and Feline Gastroenterology 3rd edition. Gloucestershire, British Small Animal Veterinary Association, 2019.
-   Forman MA. Anorexia. In Ettinger SJ, Feldman EC, Côté E (editors). Textbook of Veterinary Internal Medicine 8th edition. St. Louis, Elsevier, 2017.
-   Michel KE. Anorexia. In Washabau RJ, Day MJ (editors). Canine and Feline Gastroenterology 1st edition. St. Louis, Elsevier, 2013.

ARRHYTHMIA:
SUPRAVENTRICULAR TACHYCARDIAS

Roberto Santilli and Manuela Perego

Supraventricular tachycardias (SVTs) are rhythm disturbances, the substrate of which includes at least one supraventricular anatomical structure.

Supraventricular tachycardias typically present heart rates >180 beats per minute (bpm) in adult dogs and >220 bpm in puppies and cats and are characterized by normal ventricular activation, resulting in QRS complexes of normal duration.

Supraventricular tachycardias can be classified as sinus tachycardia, junctional tachycardia (JT), tachycardias mediated by accessory patway, focal atrial tachycardia (FAT), atrial flutter (Afl), and atrial fibrillation (AFib).

Sinus tachycardia is characterized by an increase in the sinus node discharging rate in response to physiological or pathological stimuli.

Junctional tachycardias originate from the atrioventricular junction area from enhanced automaticity or triggered activity and include focal and non-paroxysmal JTs. Focal JT is more common in young Labradors and manifests as an incessant rhythm, which can worsen preexisting systolic dysfunction.

Tachycardias mediated by atrioventricular accessory patway are dependent on the presence of a congenital muscular bundle, which electrically connects the atria to the ventricles bypassing the atrioventricular node. They include orthodromic atrioventricular reciprocating tachycardia (OAVRT) and permanent junctional reciprocating tachycardia (PJRT). In dogs, accessory pathways are usually located around the tricuspid valve annulus; the most common correlated arrhythmia is OAVRT.

Focal atrial tachycardias originate from ectopic foci located in the atria or in the veins (venae cave and pulmonary veins). The arrhythmogenic mechanisms include enhanced abnormal automaticity, triggered activity, and micro-reentry. Although FATs can occur in dogs with a normal heart, it is commonly associated with underlying cardiac diseases.

Atrial flutter is correlated with an anatomical circuit usually located at the level of the right atrium. Two types of Afl have been described in dogs: anatomical (typical/atypical) and functional.

Atrial fibrillation is characterized by rapid and mechanically uncoordinated atrial activity with loss of atrial contraction; it is dependent on functional micro-reentrant circuits. Atrial fibrillation is more common in medium-sized/large/giant breed dogs.

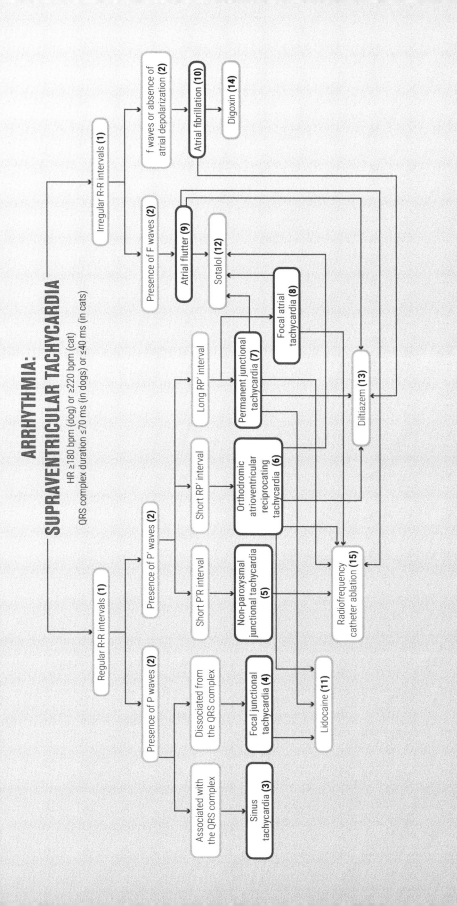

DIAGNOSTIC PROTOCOL

1. Supraventricular tachycardias can present regular R-R intervals (the intervals between two consecutive R waves are exactly equal) or irregular R-R intervals (the distance between two consecutive R waves is always different).

2. Analysis of the atrial deflection and its relationship with the QRS complex is crucial. Atrial deflections are classified as P waves (atrial deflections arising from the sinus node), P' waves (atrial deflections originating somewhere other than the sinus node), F waves (correlated with the presence of AFl), f waves (correlated with the presence of AFib).

DIAGNOSIS

3. Sinus tachycardia: P waves (positive in leads II, III, and aVF, negative in aVR, and positive or isodiphasic in lead I) associated with QRS complexes presenting normal and constant PQ intervals.

4. Focal JT (100-160 bpm): P waves dissociated from QRS complexes with variable PQ intervals (type I synchronization) or short and fixed P'Q intervals (type II synchronization).

5. Non-paroxysmal JT (60-130 bpm): P' waves with an inferior-to-superior axis and concentric atrial activation (negative in leads II, III, and aVF, and equally positive in aVR and aVL) associated with QRS complexes by short but constant PQ intervals.

6. Orthodromic atrioventricular reciprocating tachycardia (190-300 bpm): P' waves with an inferior-to-superior axis (negative in leads II, III, and aVF, and positive in aVR and aVL) and short RP' intervals (< 50% of the R-R interval), and often electrical alternans.

7. Permanent junctional reciprocating tachycardia (230-250 bpm): P' waves with an inferior-to-superior axis (negative in leads II, III, and aVF, and positive in aVR and aVL) and a long RP'.

8. Focal atrial tachycardia (210-330 bpm): P' wave morphology is dependent on the localization of the ectopic focus but usually presents a superior-to-inferior axis (P' wave positive in leads II, III, and aVF, and negative in aVR) since canine FAT commonly arises from the crista terminalis.

9. Atrial flutter (280-350 bpm): F waves, which can show different atrioventricular conduction ratios (usually from 1:1 to 6:1). In anatomical AFl (Wells type I), F waves have a saw-tooth pattern typical of atrial flutter, while the presence of positive F waves in leads II, III, and aVF and segments of the isoelectric line is associated with typical reverse (or atypical) AFl. Functional AFl (Wells type II) usually presents F waves with variable morphology and rapid, unstable atrial depolarization.

10. Atrial fibrillation (130-260 bpm): f waves of variable morphology and amplitude with an atrial rate of 400-600 bpm. In long-standing atrial fibrillation, f waves may not be visible.

TREATMENT

11. Lidocaine (Na+ channel blocker) can be used in the case of OAVRT (dogs: 2 mg/kg IV bolus given slowly, up to 8 mg/kg, followed by CRI 25-100 ug/kg/min; cats: 0.25-0.5 mg/kg IV bolus given slowly, repeatable at 0.15-0.25 mg/kg in 5-20 min, followed by CRI 10-20 µg/kg/min).

12. Sotalol (K+ channel blocker with beta-blocker properties) is used for OAVRT, FAT, and Afl (dogs and cats: 0.5-2 mg/kg PO q12h).

13. Diltiazem (Ca^{2+} channel blocker) is suggested at 2-3 mg/kg PO q12h (retard formulation both in dogs and cats). Diltiazem can be used to reduce the ventricular response in the case of AFib or to restore sinus rhythm in the case of OAVRT.

14. Digoxin (a vagotonic drug that blocks M2 receptors at the atrioventricular node) is used to reduce the ventricular response in AFib (dogs: 0.005-0.01 mg/kg PO q12h; cats: 0.007 mg/kg PO q48h).

15. The therapy of choice for OAVRT, FAT, and Afl is radiofrequency catheter ablation of the arrhythmic substrate.

SUGGESTED READINGS

- Battaia S, Perego M, Santilli R. Radiofrequency catheter ablation of cranial vena cava flutter in four dogs. *J Vet Cardiol* 36:123-130, 2021.
- Santilli R, Moise NS, Pariaut R, Perego M. Electrocardiography of the dog and the cat 2nd edition. Milan, Edra, 2018.
- Santilli RA, Mateos Pañero M, Porteiro Vázquez DM, et al. Radiofrequency catheter ablation of accessory pathways in the dog: the Italian experience (2008-2016). *J Vet Cardiol* 20:384-397, 2018.
- Santilli RA, Perego M, Crosara S, et al. Utility of 12-lead electrocardiogram for differentiating paroxysmal supraventricular tachycardias in dogs. *J Vet Intern Med* 22:915-923, 2008.
- Santilli RA, Perego M, Perini A, et al. Electrophysiologic characteristics and topographic distribution of focal atrial tachycardias in dogs. *J Vet Intern Med* 24:539-545, 2010.

ARRHYTHMIA: VENTRICULAR TACHYCARDIAS

Roberto Santilli and Manuela Perego

Ventricular tachycardias (VTs) are considered rhythm disturbances, the substrate of which includes structures distal to the bundle of His.

Ventricular tachycardias typically present heart rates >180 beats per minute (bpm) in adult dogs and >220 bpm in puppies and cats and are characterized by abnormal ventricular activation, which results in a QRS complex of increased duration.

There are different types of VT, namely monomorphic VT, polymorphic VT, bidirectional VT, and ventricular fibrillation.

Monomorphic VTs are characterized by a single QRS complex morphology and are usually associated with cardiostructural heart diseases inducing reentrant circuits at the level of the ventricular myocardium.

Polymorphic VTs present a beat-to-beat variation of the QRS complex morphology, which reflects a continuous change in the depolarization sequence of the ventricular myocardium. These forms are usually associated with functional reentrant circuits correlated with channelopathies. *Torsades de pointes* is a specific type of polymorphic VT associated with a prolonged QT interval during sinus rhythm. It is characterized by QRS complexes which seem to rotate around the baseline.

Bidirectional VTs are characterized by a beat-to-beat polarity switch of the QRS complex. These VTs are often correlated with digitalis toxicity.

Ventricular fibrillation is rapid and disorganized electrical activity in the ventricles. The ventricular myocardium is depolarized by a high number and continuously changing depolarization wavefronts, which cause the complete loss of organized ventricular contraction. Ventricular fibrillation is characterized by the absence of an identifiable QRS complex, which is replaced by irregular oscillations of the isoelectric line. It is correlated with rapid loss of consciousness and death within minutes if left untreated.

Ventricular tachycardias, beyond the morphology of the QRS complex, can be described by their clinical behavior and classified as: non-sustained VT (lasting <30 seconds), sustained VT (lasting >30 seconds, or inducing hemodinamic signs), permanent or incessant VT (sustained forms for more than 12 hour per day), repetitive VT (runs of non-sustained VT interspersed with sinus beats), and ventricular storm (hemodynamically unstable VT).

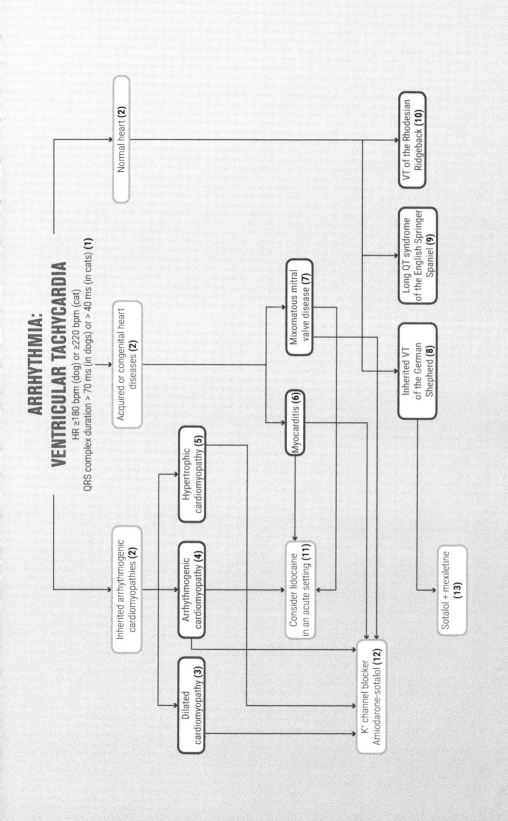

ARRHYTHMIA: VENTRICULAR TACHYCARDIA

HR ≥180 bpm (dog) or ≥220 bpm (cat)
QRS complex duration > 70 ms (in dogs) or > 40 ms (in cats) **(1)**

Normal heart **(2)**

Acquired or congenital heart diseases **(2)**

Inherited arrhythmogenic cardiomyopathies **(2)**

Hypertrophic cardiomyopathy **(5)**

Arrhythmogenic cardiomyopathy **(4)**

Dilated cardiomyopathy **(3)**

Mixomatous mitral valve disease **(7)**

Myocarditis **(6)**

VT of the Rhodesian Ridgeback **(10)**

Long QT syndrome of the English Springer Spaniel **(9)**

Inherited VT of the German Shepherd **(8)**

Consider lidocaine in an acute setting **(11)**

K⁺ channel blocker Amiodarone-sotalol **(12)**

Sotalol + mexiletine **(13)**

1. Ventricular tachycardias are characterized by an increased heart rate (dogs: >180 bpm; cats: >220 bpm) and wide QRS complexes.

2. Ventricular tachycardias can often be associated with inherited arrhythmogenic cardiomyopathies, acquired or congenital heart diseases, or can be present in patients with a normal heart.

DIAGNOSIS

3. Familial dilated cardiomyopathy is a myocardial disorder characterized by left ventricular systolic dysfunction in Dobermans and Great Danes. Ventricular tachycardias are usually sustained and monomorphic. The QRS complex presents negative polarity in leads II, III, and aVF and positive polarity in aVR and aVL.

4. Arrhythmogenic cardiomyopathy is a familial myocardial disease mainly affecting the right ventricle in Boxers and English Bulldogs, resulting in progressive myocardial replacement with fibro-fatty tissue. Ventricular tachycardias are usually non-sustained, repetitive, and monomorphic. The QRS complex presents positive polarity in leads II, III, and aVF and negative polarity in aVR and aVL.

5. Hypertrophic cardiomyopathy is a familial feline myocardial disease characterized by left ventricular concentric hypertrophy in the absence of increased afterload. VTs are usually monomorphic. The QRS complex presents negative polarity in leads II, III, and aVF and positive polarity in aVR and aVL.

6. Myocarditis is commonly associated with both the acute and chronic phases of VT. Although the correct diagnosis of myocarditis is verified by endomyocardial biopsy, the use of troponin-I can greatly facilitate the diagnosis in the presence of VT.

7. Myxomatous mitral valve disease is the most common canine cardiostructural disease and can be associated with premature ventricular ectopic beats/VT correlated with left ventricular remodeling. The QRS complex usually presents negative polarity in leads II, III, and aVF and positive polarity in aVR and aVL.

8. Inherited VTs of the German Shepherd are associated with abnormal sympathetic innervation of the myocardium. Its onset is usually at approximately 12 weeks of age, the VT tends to worsen until 24-30 weeks of age, and then the VT tends to decline until its disappearance by the age of 18 months. The affected dogs classically present non-sustained, repetitive, polymorphic VT with a high risk of sudden death.

9. Long QT syndrome is a familial channelopathy that has been described in the English Springer Spaniel. The affected dogs present an abnormal repolarization phase due to the mutation of the KCNQ1 gene encoding for the K^+ channels. The affected dogs classically present polymorphic VT, also called *torsades de pointes*, with a high risk of sudden death.

10. Familial VTs are described in Rhodesian Ridgebacks. The mutation of a variant in the Q1l1 gene results in mitochondrial cardiomyopathy characterized by cardiac arrhythmias correlated with sudden cardiac death in dogs of 7-12 months of age.

TREATMENT

11. Lidocaine (Na$^+$ channel blocker) can be used for the acute treatment of VT (dogs: 2 mg/kg IV bolus given slowly, up to 8 mg/kg followed by CRI 25-100 ug/kg/min; cats: 0.25-0.5 mg/kg IV bolus given slowly, can repeat at 0.15-0.25 mg/kg in 5-20 min, followed by CRI 10-20 ug/kg/min).

12. Sotalol (K$^+$ channel blocker with beta-blocker properties) is used at 0.5-2 mg/kg PO q12h both in dogs and cats. Amiodarone (K$^+$ channel blocker) can be used at a loading dose (10-25 mg/kg PO q12-24h for 48h) followed by a maintenance dose (7.5 mg/kg PO q12h in dogs, and 12.5/kg PO q24h in cats).

13. The association between sotalol (2 mg/kg PO q12h) and mexiletine (4-6 mg/kg PO q12h) is effective in German Shepherd-inherited VT.

SUGGESTED READINGS

- Meurs KM, Weidman JA, Rosenthal SL, et al. Ventricular arrhythmias in Rhodesian Ridgebacks with a family history of sudden death and results of a pedigree analysis for potential inheritance patterns. *J Am Vet Med Assoc* 248:1135-1138, 2016.
- Moise NS, Meyers-Wallen V, Flahive WJ. Inherited ventricular arrhythmias and sudden death in German Shepherd dogs. *J Am Coll Cardiol* 24:233-243, 1994.
- Santilli R, Moise NS, Pariaut R, Perego M. Electrocardiography of the dog and the cat 2nd edition. Milan, Edra, 2018.
- Ware WA, Reina-Doreste Y, Stern JA, et al. Sudden death associated with QT interval prolongation and KCNQ1 gene mutation in a family of English Springer Spaniels. *J Vet Intern Med* 29:561-568, 2015.
- Wess G, Domenech O, Dukes-McEwan J, et al. European Society of Veterinary Cardiology screening guidelines for dilated cardiomyopathy in Doberman Pinschers. *J Vet Cardiol* 19:405-415, 2017.

ATAXIA

Gualtiero Gandini

Ataxia defines a deficit in the sensory function and consists of the inability to perform normal, coordinated movements not being caused by weakness or musculoskeletal disorders. According to the neurological structure involved, three different types of ataxia can be distinguished: cerebellar, vestibular, and proprioceptive.

Cerebellar ataxia is caused by disorders of the cerebellum or, more rarely, lesions that selectively affect the spinocerebellar tracts. This type of ataxia is characterized by the inability to regulate the force and range of movements with consequent dysmetria, most often detected as hypermetria (an exaggerated elevation and protraction of the step). This type of ataxia can be associated with other cerebellar symptoms, such as a broad-based stance and intention tremors. Cerebellar ataxia, unlike proprioceptive ataxia, is never associated with paresis.

Vestibular ataxia, associated with a unilateral vestibular lesion, is characterized by a tendency to sheer, fall, or roll to one side (usually ipsilateral to that of the lesion). This type of ataxia is associated with vestibular signs, such as head tilt, resting nystagmus, positional strabismus, and a tendency to circle.

Proprioceptive ataxia results from lesions of the nervous structures involved in controlling general proprioception (sensory fibers of the peripheral nerves, dorsal nerve roots, spinal cord, brainstem, forebrain). In clinical practice, proprioceptive ataxia is more commonly found to be associated with spinal cord disorders. This type of ataxia is characterized by a loss of awareness of the spatial position of the body and, in particular, of the limbs (kinesthesia). The severity of the ataxia depends on the extent of the lesion and can range from just perceptible changes to obvious deficits. In the latter cases, the limbs are excessively abducted and/or adducted during walking; they cross, touch the other limb, and there is sometimes a tendency to stand on the dorsum of the foot ("knuckling"). It is important to remember that neuroanatomically, the proprioceptive and motor pathways are intimately related throughout the spinal cord and caudal brainstem; proprioceptive ataxia is, therefore, quite often associated with paresis. Proprioceptive ataxia can affect the hindlimbs (due to spinal lesions caudal to the T2 spinal cord segment) or all four limbs (due to spinal lesions cranial to the T2 spinal cord segment).

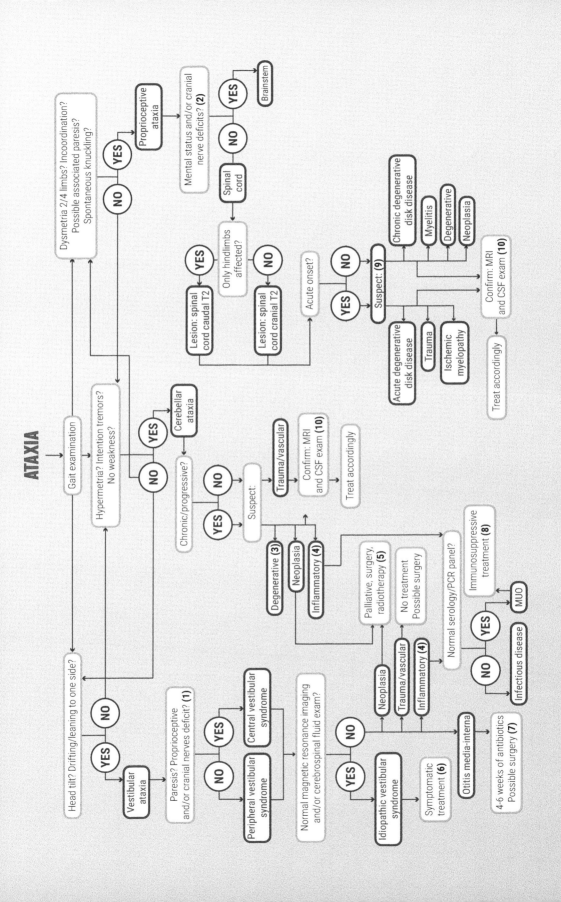

1. In the presence of vestibular ataxia, it is imperative to attempt to clinically distinguish the involvement of the peripheral or central part of the vestibular system. Differentiating peripheral from central vestibular syndrome is crucial for the different prognoses involved. Central vestibular syndrome results from damage to the vestibular nuclei located in the medulla oblongata, the caudal part of the most important part of the brain, the brainstem. The involvement of this region usually carries a guarded to poor prognosis while peripheral vestibular syndrome, despite much more severe presenting clinical signs, has a better outcome. Great attention should be paid to detecting signs of paresis, proprioceptive abnormalities and/or cranial nerve dysfunction.

2. Proprioceptive ataxia can result from either a spinal cord or a brainstem lesion. Therefore, it is important to be able to properly localize the lesion, paying attention to the possible involvement of the intracranial structures.

10. Magnetic resonance imaging is the gold standard for detecting spinal cord lesions. It is preferred to computed tomography due to its superior soft tissue resolution. Cerebrospinal fluid examination is recommended, especially when the differential diagnosis includes inflammatory diseases.

DIAGNOSIS

3. The cerebellum represents one of the targets of degenerative nervous diseases, including cerebellar cortical degeneration and spinocerebellar ataxia. These diseases have an inherited basis and are characterized by an insidious onset and a very slow-progressing evolution, which can last months to years.

4. Inflammatory central nervous system (CNS) disorders in dogs are mainly due to non-infectious disorders, most of them grouped under the umbrella term of meningoencephalomyelitis of unknown origin (MUO). The workup of an inflammatory disorder includes magnetic resonance imaging (MRI), cerebrospinal fluid (CSF) examination, and a PCR panel to exclude the most important infectious diseases. In cats, the situation is the opposite; infectious diseases are more frequently represented, and feline infectious peritonitis (FIP) is still one of the most important causes of CNS dysfunction.

9. Differential diagnoses of spinal cord disorders producing proprioceptive ataxia can be listed according to the onset. Acute-onset diseases include intervertebral disk disease, ischemic myelopathy, and trauma. It is mandatory for patients affected by acute-onset spinal cord disease to differentiate between non-compressive and compressive disorders. In the latter case, decompressive surgery is warranted.

5. Caudal fossa neoplasia is very difficult to treat surgically, and, in many instances, the treatment is symptomatic, using prednisolone at 0.5 mg/kg q24h. Radiotherapy can be

an option according to the size and location of the tumor and the availability of proper radiotherapy instruments.

6. Patients affected by idiopathic vestibular syndrome recover rapidly. In the initial period, symptomatic treatment with the aim of reducing the hyperexcitability (if hospitalized, midazolam 0.06-0.3 mg/kg/h CRI) or nausea and vomiting (maropitant 1-2 mg/kg q24h SC or orally) can be useful.

7. In many instances, otitis media interna is treated in the absence of an antibiogram. Treatment should be prolonged for 4-6 weeks using broad-spectrum antibiotics, including quinolones and/or first-generation cephalosporins. In the case of a recurrence and persistence of the empyema of the bulla, a bulla osteotomy may be required.

8. Meningoencephalomyelitis of unknown origin (MUO) requires prolonged immunosuppressive treatment. Glucocorticoids are the drugs of choice, more specifically prednisolone. The initial dosage is between 2-4 mg/day orally, slowly tapered off after at least 4-6 months. Other immunosuppressant drugs used in the treatment of MUO include cytosine-arabinoside, cyclosporine, mofetil mycophenolate, and azathioprine.

SUGGESTED READINGS

- da Costa R. Ataxia, paresis, paralysis. In Ettinger SJ, Feldman EC, Côté E (editors). Textbook of Veterinary Internal Medicine 8th edition. St. Louis, Elsevier, 2017, pp 554-559.
- de Lahunta A, Glass E, Kent M (editors). De Lahunta's Veterinary Neuroanatomy and Clinical Neurology 5th edition. St. Louis, Elsevier, 2020.
- Dewey C, da Costa R (editors). Practical guide to canine and feline neurology 3rd edition. Ames, Wiley Blackwell, 2015.

AZOTEMIA

Francesco Dondi

Azotemia is defined as the increase in urea and/or creatinine concentration measured as part of the non-protein nitrogenous compounds in the blood. In most cases, azotemia indicates a severe reduction in the glomerular filtration rate (GFR), associated or not with parenchymal renal disease. Azotemia is rarely associated with nonrenal conditions or excess dietary protein intake.

Urea and creatinine only correlate tardively with a significant decrease in renal function (nephron loss >50%). Early renal damage can occur without azotemia and, in these cases, the presence of renal injury or mild renal dysfunction can only be detected by using urinary biomarkers or measuring the GFR.

Both serum creatinine (sCr) and urea can easily assess renal function in veterinary laboratories using colorimetric methods, and these analytes are quite stable in a refrigerated sera.

When azotemia is detected, clinicians should consider two main differential diagnoses: acute kidney injury (AKI) or chronic kidney disease (CKD). Differentiating between these syndromes requires a careful evaluation of signalment, history, and clinical signs, including systolic blood pressure measurement (SBP) and complete bloodwork associated with urinalysis and urine chemistry. Urine specific gravity (USG) is extremely useful when approaching these patients. Imaging evaluation (abdominal ultrasound and/or radiology) is also mandatory. Infectious diseases and urinary tract infections should be ruled out in many cases.

Urinary output (UO) and response to fluid therapy are helpful in approaching azotemic patients. In AKI, volume responsive forms of renal damage are characterized by a progressive reduction in azotemia (<48h) and an increased UO following appropriate fluid therapy. However, in some AKI cases, UO does not strictly correlate with the GFR, and azotemia can persist or even worsen despite an increase in UO.

Severe azotemia (creatinine >5 mg/dL) alone is not consistently related to the presence of CKD or with a bad prognosis in renal-diseased patients. Etiological diagnosis, specific therapy, and supportive care remain the cornerstone of medical management in azotemic patients.

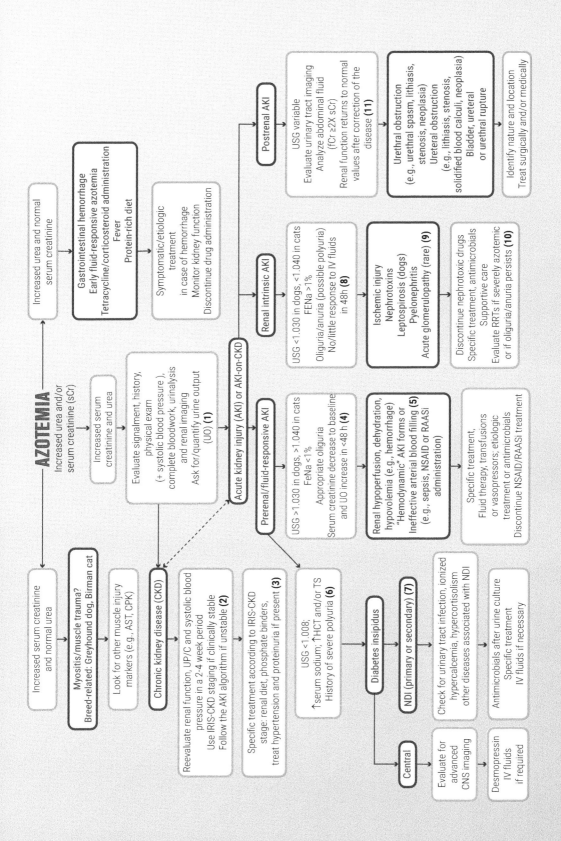

AZOTEMIA — Increased urea and/or serum creatinine (sCr)

Increased serum creatinine and normal urea
- Myositis/muscle trauma? Breed-related: Greyhound dog, Birman cat
- Look for other muscle injury markers (e.g., AST, CPK)

Increased serum creatinine and urea
- Evaluate signalment, history, physical exam (+ systolic blood pressure), complete bloodwork, urinalysis and renal imaging. Ask for/quantify urine output (UO) (1)

Increased urea and normal serum creatinine
- Gastrointestinal hemorrhage, Early fluid-responsive azotemia, Tetracycline/corticosteroid administration, Fever, Protein-rich diet
- Symptomatic/etiologic treatment in case of hemorrhage, Monitor kidney function, Discontinue drug administration

Chronic kidney disease (CKD)
- Reevaluate renal function, UP/C and systolic blood pressure in a 2-4 week period. Use IRIS-CKD staging if clinically stable. Follow the AKI algorithm if unstable (2)
- Specific treatment according to IRIS-CKD stage: renal diet, phosphate binders, treat hypertension and proteinuria if present (3)

Acute kidney injury (AKI) or AKI-on-CKD

Prerenal/fluid-responsive AKI
- USG >1.030 in dogs, >1.040 in cats. FENa <1%. Appropriate oliguria. Serum creatinine decrease to baseline and UO increase in <48 h (4)
- Renal hypoperfusion, dehydration, hypovolemia (e.g., hemorrhage) "Hemodynamic" AKI forms or Ineffective arterial blood filling (5) (e.g., sepsis, NSAID or RAASi administration)
- Specific treatment, Fluid therapy, transfusions or vasopressors; etiologic treatment or antimicrobials. Discontinue NSAID/RAASi treatment

- USG <1.008; ↑serum sodium; ↑HCT and/or TS. History of severe polyuria (6)

Diabetes insipidus

NDI (primary or secondary) (7)
- Check for urinary tract infection, ionized hypercalcemia, hypercortisolism, other diseases associated with NDI
- Antimicrobials after urine culture, Specific treatment, IV fluids if necessary

Central
- Evaluate for advanced CNS imaging
- Desmopressin, IV fluids if required

Renal intrinsic AKI
- USG <1.030 in dogs, <1.040 in cats. FENa >1%. Oliguria/anuria (possible polyuria). No/little response to IV fluids in 48 h (8)
- Ischemic injury, Nephrotoxins, Leptospirosis (dogs), Pyelonephritis, Acute glomerulopathy (rare) (9)
- Discontinue nephrotoxic drugs, Specific treatment, antimicrobials, Supportive care. Evaluate RRTs if severely azotemic or if oliguria/anuria persists (10)

Postrenal AKI
- USG variable. Evaluate urinary tract imaging. Analyze abdominal fluid (fCr ≥2X sCr). Renal function returns to normal values after correction of the disease (11)
- Urethral obstruction (e.g., urethral spasm, lithiasis, stenosis, neoplasia). Ureteral obstruction (e.g., lithiasis, stenosis, solidified blood calculi, neoplasia). Bladder, ureteral or urethral rupture
- Identify nature and location. Treat surgically and/or medically

DIAGNOSTIC PROTOCOL

1. When azotemia is detected, the diagnostic protocol should be extended to include urinalysis and renal/urinary tract imaging, and the clinical data should be carefully reevaluated. Urinary specific gravity is extremely useful for additional nephrological characterization. Polyuria/polydipsia, reduced appetite, weight loss, and vomiting are common in patients with azotemic CKD. Acute kidney injury patients can be exposed to specific historical risk factors (e.g., toxin exposure, infections) and frequently present a sudden worsening of their clinical signs. Urine volume should be almost approximatively quantified or measured.

2. When CKD is suspected, the patient should be reevaluated following current recommendations (see IRIS-CKD guidelines), including the urine protein to creatine (UPC) ratio quantification and SBP measurement. Chronic kidney disease staging should be performed only in clinically stable patients and after the correction of prerenal or postrenal factors (e.g., dehydration) and the treatment of comorbidities (e.g., urinary tract infection). Serum creatinine can be underestimated when muscle mass reduction or poor body condition are present. The evaluation of symmetric-dimethyl-arginine (SDMA) can occasionally be useful in staging these patients.

4. Prerenal AKI is typically characterized by highly concentrated urine (in animals not previously "renal diseased") associated with physiological/appropriate oliguria. Renal urine concentrating ability can be "sub-maximal" in CKD patients (near the appropriate concentration thresholds of 1.030 in dogs and 1.035-1.040 in cats). Fractional excretion of sodium (FeNa) is frequently reduced to below 1% in dogs with prerenal AKI; however, some overlap exists between pre-renal and renal-parenchymal AKI forms. Prerenal AKI (or volume responsive AKI) is also characterized by increasing urinary output and decreasing serum creatinine concentration within 24-48 hours after fluid resuscitation/therapy.

6. Prerenal AKI can be associated with severe polyuria. When the USG is <1.008, diabetes insipidus should be suspected (rare in cats). Signs of hemoconcentration, with an increased hematocrit value (HCT), increased total solids (TS), and hypernatremia can be present, especially when access to water is limited or when other fluid losses (e.g., vomiting/diarrhea) are reported.

8. Intrinsic AKI is usually characterized by persistent azotemia. Oliguria/anuria are more frequently detected. However, some AKI patients can present polyuria (e.g., leptospirosis). Severe polyuria can appear during the course of the disease (recovery phase). Severe abnormalities in the FeNA (usually >1%) and urine chemistry are reported in dogs.

11. The chemical composition of the abdominal fluid combined with urinary tract imaging can be useful when uroabdomen is suspected. In these cases, fluid creatinine (fCr) is increased more than twofold when compared to sCr.

DIAGNOSIS

5. Non-steroidal anti-inflammatory drugs (NSAIDs) and renin-angiotensin-aldosterone inhibitors (RAASi) can reversibly decrease the GFR and reduce renal function; however, these drugs can also predispose to ischemic tubular damage.

7. Secondary forms of nephrogenic diabetes insipidus (NDI) are frequently reported in dogs. Specific diagnostic protocols and treatments are required (e.g., Cushing's syndrome in dogs, urinary tract infections).

9. Leptospirosis should be ruled out in AKI dogs. A combination of serology (microagglutination test upon admission and after 7-14 days) and PCR on urine and/or blood is considered the gold standard.

TREATMENT

3. Starting a renal diet is indicated beginning with IRIS-CKD stage 2. Phosphate concentration should be maintained below CKD-specific thresholds. Metabolic acidosis should be diagnosed and managed with supplementation of alkali. Hypokalemia is a frequent finding in cats and should be treated appropriately. Gastroprotectant agents, antiemetics, appetite stimulants (e.g., mirtazapine in cats), or enteral feeding tubes should be considered in selected patients.

10. Fluid therapy should be used judiciously, avoiding any degree of fluid overload. Parenteral beta-lactam antimicrobials followed by doxycycline are recommended for canine leptospirosis. There are no standard guidelines aimed at identifying when renal replacement therapies (RRTs) should be started.

SUGGESTED READINGS

- http://www.iris-kidney.com/pdf/IRIS_Staging_of_CKD_modified_2019.pdf
- http://www.iris-kidney.com/pdf/4_ldc-revised-grading-of-acute-kidney-injury.pdf
- Dunaevich A, Chen H, Musseri D, et al. Acute on chronic kidney disease in dogs: etiology, clinical and clinicopathologic findings, prognostic markers, and survival. *J Vet Intern Med* 34:2507-2515, 2020.
- Troìa R, Gruarin M, Grisetti C, et al. Fractional excretion of electrolytes in volume-responsive and intrinsic acute kidney injury in dogs: diagnostic and prognostic implications. *J Vet Intern Med* 32:1372-1382, 2018.

BLEEDING

Andrea Zoia

Following vascular and endothelial injury, vasoconstriction limits hemorrhage and causes turbulent blood flow, allowing the interaction of platelets, subendothelial collagen, and coagulation factors.

In the "cellular model of hemostasis", coagulation factors (F) are activated (a) in three sequential phases on fibroblast and activated platelet surfaces: initiation, amplification, and propagation. During initiation, the surface of the subendothelial cells, expressing tissue factor (FIIIa) to the bloodstream, causes the formation of a small amount of FIXa and thrombin (FIIa). Thrombin detaches from the subendothelial cells to adhere to the adjacent platelet plug, which is formed by means of platelet adhesion and aggregation at the site of the vascular injury via specific receptors and the subendothelial von Willebrand factor (vWF). The amplification phase is then triggered with thrombin-mediated platelet activation (with the release of their granules and further platelet aggregation) and thrombin-mediated FV, FVIII, and FXI activation.

Thus, activation of secondary hemostasis further primary hemostasis since these phenomena are intrinsically and temporally linked. Finally, in the propagation phase, the coagulation factors generated by the two previous phases assemble on the procoagulant surface of the activated platelets, forming the "intrinsic tenase" (FVIIIa-FIXa complex), leading to the formation of FXa on the platelet surface. The prothrombinase complex (FVa-FXa complex) causes a burst of thrombin formation directly on the platelet surface, transforming the fibrinogen (FI) into a fibrin network stabilizing the platelet plug. In the "waterfall-cascade model", coagulation factors are sequentially activated in the intrinsic pathways (i.e., FXII, FXI, FIX, and FVIII), in the extrinsic pathway (i.e., FVII), and in the common pathways (i.e., FX, FV, FII, FI, and FXIII). High molecular weight kininogen, prekallikrein, Ca^{2+}, and platelet phospholipids also participate in the extrinsic pathway, while FIIIa and Ca^{2+} are required for the intrinsic pathway. While obsolete for explaining coagulation *in vivo*, this model is still useful for explaining the coagulation test results. Tertiary hemostasis (i.e., fibrinolysis) starts with the production of tissue plasminogen activator (tPA) by the endothelial cells adjacent to the injury site.

The tPA transforms plasminogen into plasmin, which has fibrin/fibrinogenolytic activity. Plasmin activity, under physiological conditions, is directed towards fibrin clots and not towards plasma fibrinogen. This localized action avoids generalized fibrinogenolysis, which would lead to bleeding diathesis. Finally, inhibitory systems for blood coagulation (e.g., antithrombin, protein C system, tissue factor pathway inhibitor [TFPI]) and fibrinolysis (e.g., plasminogen activator inhibitor [PAI-1]) also have a regulating role in clot formation and lysis.

Trauma, decreased platelet function or number, decreased clotting factors, increased fibrinolysis, or a combination of these conditions can lead to bleeding.

BLEEDING

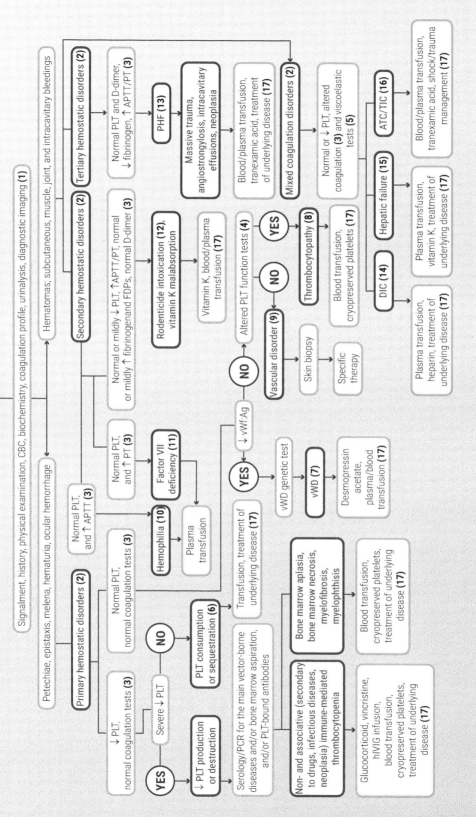

Signalment, history, physical examination, CBC, biochemistry, coagulation profile, urinalysis, diagnostic imaging **(1)**

Petechiae, epistaxis, melena, hematuria, ocular hemorrhage

Hematomas; subcutaneous, muscle, joint, and intracavitary bleedings

Primary hemostatic disorders (2)

Secondary hemostatic disorders (2)

Tertiary hemostatic disorders (2)

↓ PLT, normal coagulation tests **(3)**

Normal PLT, normal coagulation tests **(3)**

YES → ↓ PLT production or destruction

Severe ↓ PLT

NO → PLT consumption or sequestration **(6)**

Serology/PCR for the main vector-borne diseases and/or bone marrow aspiration, and/or PLT-bound antibodies

Non- and associative (secondary to drugs, infectious diseases, neoplasia) immune-mediated thrombocytopenia

Glucocorticoid, vincristine, hIVIG infusion, blood transfusion, cryopreserved platelets, treatment of underlying disease **(17)**

Bone marrow aplasia, bone marrow necrosis, myelofibrosis, myelophthisis

Blood transfusion, cryopreserved platelets, treatment of underlying disease **(17)**

Transfusion, treatment of underlying disease **(17)**

Normal PLT, and ↑ APTT **(3)**

Hemophilia (10)

Plasma transfusion

Normal PLT, and ↑ PT **(3)**

Factor VII deficiency (11)

Normal or mildly ↓ PLT, ↑APTT/PT, normal or mildly ↑ fibrinogen and FDPs, normal D-dimer **(3)**

Rodenticide intoxication (12), vitamin K malabsorption

Vitamin K, blood/plasma transfusion **(17)**

↓ vWf:Ag

YES → **vWD (7)**

vWD genetic test

Desmopressin acetate, plasma/blood transfusion **(17)**

NO → **Vascular disorder (9)**

Skin biopsy

Specific therapy

Altered PLT function tests **(4)**

NO

YES → **Thrombocytopathy (8)**

Blood transfusion, cryopreserved platelets **(17)**

Normal PLT and D-dimer, ↓ fibrinogen, ↑ APTT/PT **(3)**

PHF (13)

Massive trauma, angiostrongylosis, intracavitary effusions, neoplasia

Blood/plasma transfusion, tranexamic acid, treatment of underlying disease **(17)**

Mixed coagulation disorders (2)

Normal or ↓ PLT, altered coagulation **(3)** and viscoelastic tests **(5)**

DIC (14)

Plasma transfusion, heparin, treatment of underlying disease **(17)**

Hepatic failure (15)

Plasma transfusion, vitamin K, treatment of underlying disease **(17)**

ATC/TIC (16)

Blood/plasma transfusion, tranexamic acid, shock/trauma management **(17)**

DIAGNOSTIC PROTOCOL

1. Familial history of bleeding and young age suggest an inherited disorder. Adult animals with concurrent comorbidities likely have an acquired coagulation disorder.

3. Activated partial thromboplastin time (APTT) evaluates the intrinsic and common coagulation pathways. Factor deficiency/inhibition of these pathways will prolong this test. Prothrombin time (PT) evaluates the extrinsic and common coagulation pathways. Factor deficiency/inhibition of these pathways will prolong the PT. Thrombin time (TT) evaluates part of the common coagulation pathway (FII, FXII, and fibrinogen). Deficiency/inhibition of these factors, elevation in fibrin degradation products (FDPs), and hypoalbuminemia will prolong the TT. Fibrinogen defects can be qualitative (dysfibrinogenemia) or quantitative (hypo- or afibrinogenemia) and either acquired (i.e., consumption, decreased hepatic synthesis, or inhibitory antibodies) or congenital. FDPs and D-dimer are markers of fibrinolysis. Fibrinolysis causes the formation of FDPs and D-dimer, while fibrinogenolysis produces only FDPs.

4. Buccal mucosal bleeding time (BMBT) detects platelet dysfunction, abnormalities in vascular integrity, and vW disease (vWD); however, it lacks standardization and reproducibility. Platelet function analyzers, such as PFA-100, platelet aggregometer, or rotational thromboelastometry (ROTEM) platelet assays are preferred.

5. Viscoelastic instrumentations such as thromboelastography (TEG) and ROTEM provide global assessments of coagulation *in vitro*, from the initiation of a fibrin clot to its dissolution. In human medicine, their major application is in the emergency and critical care of bleeding patients (e.g., patients with acute traumatic coagulopathy [ATC] and trauma-induced coagulopathy [TIC]).

DIAGNOSIS

2. Primary hemostatic disorders are characterized by mucosal bleeding, petechiae, and bruising; it is frequently observed in patients with a platelet (PLT) count <20,000/µL. Secondary, tertiary, and mixed hemostatic disorders may also result in larger bleeding, such as hematomas and intracavitary hemorrhage.

6. Platelet consumption can occur with disseminated intravascular coagulation (DIC), acute traumatic coagulopathy (ATC) and trauma-induced coagulopathy (TIC), vasculitis, and severe acute bleeding. Platelet sequestration can occur with hepatomegaly, splenomegaly, hypotension, endotoxemia, and hypothermia.

7. Von Willebrand disease (vWD) is a hereditary platelet adhesion disorder resulting from quantitative (type I and III) or qualitative (type II) deficiency of the von Willebrand factor (vWF).

8. Platelet function defects can be inherited (e.g., Glanzmann thrombasthenia, Scott syndrome) or acquired secondary to rickettsial infections, hepatic diseases, uremia, neoplasia, and drugs.

9. Vascular disorders are mainly due to vasculitis, which can be immune-mediated or occur secondary to medications, infections, neoplastic conditions, and other diseases.

10. In animals with hemophilia A, B, and C (inherited FVIII, IX, and XI deficiencies, respectively),

bleeding is prolonged after trauma/surgery. In cats, FXII deficiency causes APTT prolongation without bleeding tendencies. Measurement of the coagulation factor activity and genetic tests (if available) are required for diagnosis.

11. Factor VII deficiency causes bleeding after trauma/surgery. Diagnosis requires FVII quantification and genetic tests.

12. Rodenticide intoxication causes bleeding due to inhibition of FIIa, FVIIa, FIXa, and FXa synthesis. Rodenticide determination in vomiting or blood strengthens the diagnosis.

13. Primary hyperfibrinolysis (PHF), named also hyperfibrinogenolysis, is due to an excess of free plasmin which degrades plasma fibrinogen.

14. Disseminated intravascular coagulation (DIC) results from systemic inflammatory or neoplastic diseases. In non-overt DIC (hypercoagulable phase), APTT is prolonged, FDPs and D-dimer are increased, PT is normal, and fibrinogen and platelet counts are normal to increased. In overt DIC, fibrinogen and platelet counts decrease while PT increases. Viscoelastic tests are also useful for DIC diagnosis.

15. Due to the central role of the liver in pro- and anticoagulant factor synthesis and in the regulation of fibrinolysis, hepatic failure is associated with both thrombosis and bleeding. Clotting abnormalities are similar to DIC.

16. Trauma and shock induce acute traumatic coagulopathy (ATC). Acute traumatic coagulopathy and resuscitation-associated coagulopathy involving hypothermia, acidosis, and dilutional coagulopathy cause trauma-induced coagulopathy (TIC). In ATC and TIC, the activation of coagulation and fibrinolysis can result in thrombosis or bleeding.

TREATMENT

17. Bleeding diatheses can be a primary problem or occur secondary to systemic diseases. Dosages for some of the drugs utilized are as follows: desmopressin acetate 1 µg/kg q24h SC for Von Willebrand disease (vWD); loading vitamin K dose 5 mg/kg q12h twice, followed by a 3-4-week maintenance dose of 2.5 mg/kg q12h PO for rodenticide intoxication; and tranexamic acid 10-20 mg/kg q8h PO/IV/SC until necessary to control primary hyperfibrinolytic states. Supportive plasma, blood transfusions, and treatment of the underlying disorders are also required to stop blood loss.

SUGGESTED READINGS

- Blois S. Hyper-and hypocoagulable states. In Ettinger SJ, Feldman EC, Côté E (editors). Textbook of Veterinary Internal Medicine 8th edition. St. Louis, Elsevier, 2017, pp 2062-2077.
- Herring J, McMichael M. Diagnostic approach to small animal bleeding disorders. *Top Companion Anim Med* 27:73-80, 2012.
- Kushimoto S, Kudo D, Kawazoe Y. Acute traumatic coagulopathy and trauma-induced coagulopathy: an overview. *J Intensive Care* 5:6, 2017.
- Stokol T. Disorder of haemostasis. In Villiers E, Ristić J (editors). BSAVA Manual of Canine and Feline Clinical Pathology 3rd edition. British Small Animal Veterinary Association, 2016, pp 94-122.
- Zoia A, Drigo M, Piek CJ, Calcini H, Caldin M, et al. Enhanced fibrinolysis detection in a naturally occurring canine model with intracavitary effusions: comparison and degree of agreement between thromboelastometry and FDPs, D-dimer and fibrinogen concentrations. *PLoS One* 14:e0225089, 2019.

BLINDNESS

Elsa Beltrán

Lesions affecting any structures involving visual perception can cause visual deficits: retina, optic nerve (optic neuropathy), optic chiasm, optic tract, lateral geniculate nucleus (LGN), optic radiation, and/or visual cortex (either unilaterally or bilaterally). Clear ocular media are required to allow vision; any opacity affecting the cornea, aqueous humor, lens, and/or vitreous can contribute to vision loss; these structures should be carefully assessed during the ophthalmologic examination.

If visual deficits are present, the fundus should be examined, followed by an electroretinogram if the fundus is normal. Pupillary light reflex (PLR) is useful for differentiating between cortical and subcortical lesions. The PLR is present in both eyes if the lesion affects only part of the optic tract, lateral geniculate nucleus, optic radiation, or visual cortex. If there is absent/decreased direct and consensual (indirect) PLR, the lesion is located either in the retina, optic nerve (ipsilateral to the absent direct PLR and visual deficits), or optic chiasm (bilaterally absent direct and indirect PLR and visual deficits). Severe iris muscle atrophy, extensive posterior synechiae, and atropinization can lead to a decreased to absent PLR without representing a dysfunction of the neurological pathways.

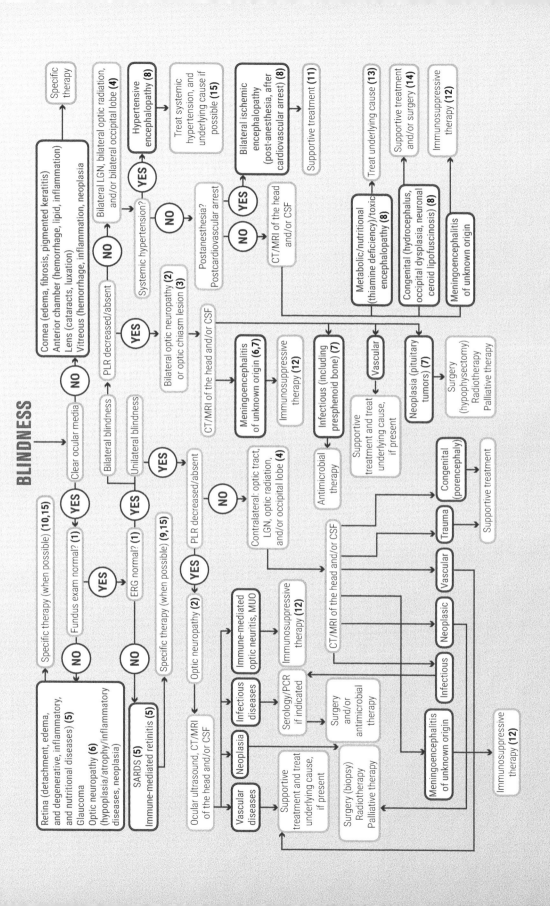

1. Retinal diseases: ophthalmologic examination (increased tapetal reflectivity could suggest retinal degeneration as the cause of visual impairment) and electroretinography (ERG) are essential in cases with visual deficits in order to differentiate lesions affecting the retina from post-retinal structures. Systemic blood pressure should be evaluated in cases with retinal detachment.

2. Optic neuropathy: the main neurologic signs of optic neuropathy include visual deficits, and a decreased to absent direct and consensual pupillary light reflex (PLR). Fundus examination may identify a normal, swollen, or pale optic disc, peripapillary vascular attenuation, prominence of the lamina cribrosa, and/or proliferation of the neural tissue within/from the optic nerve head. An acute onset of visual deficits is usually seen as a result of inflammatory, vascular (mainly ischemic), and traumatic causes. A chronic course of visual impairment is usually caused by compressive, neoplastic, and degenerative disorders. With a normal fundus examination, advanced diagnostic imaging provides a vital tool for studying structural changes in the optic nerve and, hence, guiding clinical decision-making.

3. Optic chiasm lesions: an optic chiasm lesion can result in bilateral vision loss and bilateral decreased to absent PLRs. The visual loss may present with acute onset despite the slow development of the underlying disease process. Advanced diagnostic imaging provides a vital tool to study structural changes in the optic chiasm and hence guides clinical decision-making.

4. Lesions affecting the optic tract, lateral geniculate nucleus (LGN), optic radiation, and/or visual cortex. Unilateral lesions cause contralateral vision loss. Dogs and cats with a lesion affecting the thalamocortex are likely to show other clinical signs in addition to vision loss, including altered mentation/level of consciousness, abnormal behavior, head turn, circling, postural reaction deficits, hemi-inattention syndrome, and seizures. Advanced diagnostic imaging is the optimal imaging modality for diagnosing disorders involving the thalamic area and visual cortex, and also for delineating the extent of the lesion. Cerebrospinal fluid analysis may contribute to the diagnosis in the case of inflammatory/infectious diseases and neoplasias (such as lymphoma). Transient vision loss (cortical blindness) of variable duration might occur after an epileptic seizure. Hypoxia associated with cardiorespiratory arrest can lead to transient or permanent dysfunction of the bilateral occipital cortex.

DIAGNOSIS

5. Retinal diseases: sudden acquired retinal degeneration syndrome (SARDS), progressive retinal atrophy (PRA), retinal pigment epithelial dystrophy (vitamin E deficiency), retinal detachment, retinal toxicity (frequently enrofloxacin in cats and ivermectin in dogs), chorioretinitis (inflammatory, infectious, neoplastic), immune-mediated retinitis (IMR), IMR-cancer-associated retinopathy (CAR), and inborn error of metabolism.

6. Optic neuropathy. Optic nerve hypoplasia is the most common congenital optic neuropathy. Other congenital abnormalities include optic disc coloboma. Acquired optic neuropathies mainly involve immune-mediated optic neuritis, meningoencephalitis of unknown origin (MUO), infectious optic neuritis, neoplasia (meningioma, glial cell tumor, ependymoma),

and vascular, compressive, degenerative, traumatic, and toxic disorders.

7. Optic chiasm lesions. Intracranial extension of orbital lesions (neoplasia or inflammation), disease of the sphenoid bones, traumatic brain injury, central nervous system (CNS) diseases (neoplasia, inflammatory or congenital), and tumors of the pituitary area which extend rostrally cause damage to the optic chiasm (e.g., adenocarcinoma, meningioma).

8. Lesions affecting the optic tract, lateral geniculate nucleus, optic radiation, and/or visual cortex. Canine distemper virus can cause demyelination of both optic tracts with vision loss. Trauma, and vascular, inflammatory (MUO), congenital, metabolic, and neoplastic diseases can also affect these structures. The neuronal cell bodies in the lateral geniculate nucleus and the visual cortex are particularly vulnerable to storage diseases (degenerative), developmental abnormalities, vitamin B_1 (thiamine) deficiency, and hypoxia. Hypertensive encephalopathy causes bilaterally symmetrical edema of the cerebral white matter with vision loss. Vision loss (temporary and permanent) has been reported in cats following general anesthesia, usually after an oral procedure when the mouth is held open by a gag.

TREATMENT

9. There is currently no effective treatment for SARDS and PRA.

10. Supplementation with vitamin E might prevent the progression of retinal pigment epithelial dystrophy.

11. Vascular encephalopathy is treated with supportive treatment and treating the underlying cause, if present.

12. Immunosuppressive therapy for cases with optic neuritis/MUO.

13. Thiamine deficiency: 10-25 mg/kg IM q24h for several days until the signs are resolved; then, 10 mg/kg PO q24h for 21 days.

14. Congenital malformation should be treated with supportive treatment; in some cases (e.g., congenital hydrocephalus), surgery might be indicated.

15. Retinal detachment due to systemic hypertension and hypertensive encephalopathy requires normalization of blood pressure with amlodipine, either alone or in combination with enalapril, and treating the underlying cause, if present (refer to the chapter on "hypertension").

SUGGESTED READINGS

- Martin-Flores M, Scrivani PV, Loew E, et al. Maximal and submaximal mouth opening with mouth gags in cats: implications for maxillary artery blood flow. *Vet J* 200:60-64, 2014.
- Meekins JM. Acute blindness. *Top Companion Anim Med* 30:118-125, 2015.
- O'Neill J, Kent M, Glass EN, Platt SR. Clinicopathologic and MRI characteristics of presumptive hypertensive encephalopathy in two cats and two dogs. *J Am Anim Hosp Assoc* 49:412-420, 2013.
- Palus V, Penderis J, Jakovljevic S, et al. Thiamine deficiency in a cat: resolution of MRI abnormalities following thiamine supplementation. *J Feline Med Surg* 12:807-810, 2010.
- Palus V, Penderis J, Jakovljevic S, Cherubini GB. Thiamine deficiency in a cat: resolution of MRI abnormalities following thiamine supplementation. *J Feline Med Surg* 12:807-810, 2010.

BRADYARRHYTHMIAS

Federica Marchesotti

Bradyarrhythmias are defined as cardiac rhythms resulting in a reduction in the heart rate (HR), which appears out of proportion to the animal's signalment or level of activity or stress.

A HR <60 bpm in hospitalized dogs and <140 bpm in hospitalized cats should usually be investigated, especially if the animals are unsedated and awake and the HR does not increase with stimulation.

Based on the cause, bradyarrhythmias can be classified as
   a) physiologic, due to increasing vagal tone;
   b) pharmacological, due to drug overdose (e.g., β-blockers, calcium channel blockers) or as a consequence of the use of sedative/anesthetic agents;
   c) pathological, due to extracardiac diseases (e.g., electrolyte disturbances, hypothermia, central nervous system diseases), or cardiac diseases involving the conduction system, such as degenerative (e.g., fibrous or fibrous-fatty replacement), infiltrative (e.g., cardiac neoplastic infiltration) and inflammatory processes (e.g., myocarditis).

The most frequent bradyarrhythmias in dogs include sinus bradycardia, atrioventricular conduction disturbances, sinus arrest, sinus standstill, sinoatrial block, sinus node (SN) dysfunction (which can also be called sick sinus syndrome if symptomatic), sinoventricular rhythm and atrial standstill (which has also been called atrioventricular muscular dystrophy).

The development of clinical signs depends on many factors, including the rate and duration of the bradyarrhythmia, the abruptness of rate variation, the temporal relationship between atrial and ventricular activation, the animal's overall health, and the severity of the underlying cardiac disease. Typical clinical signs include lethargy, exercise intolerance, and syncope. In some animals, congestive heart failure can also develop, leading to tachypnea/dyspnea and/or ascites. However, it should be noted that some animals may not exhibit overt clinical signs at the time of physical examination.

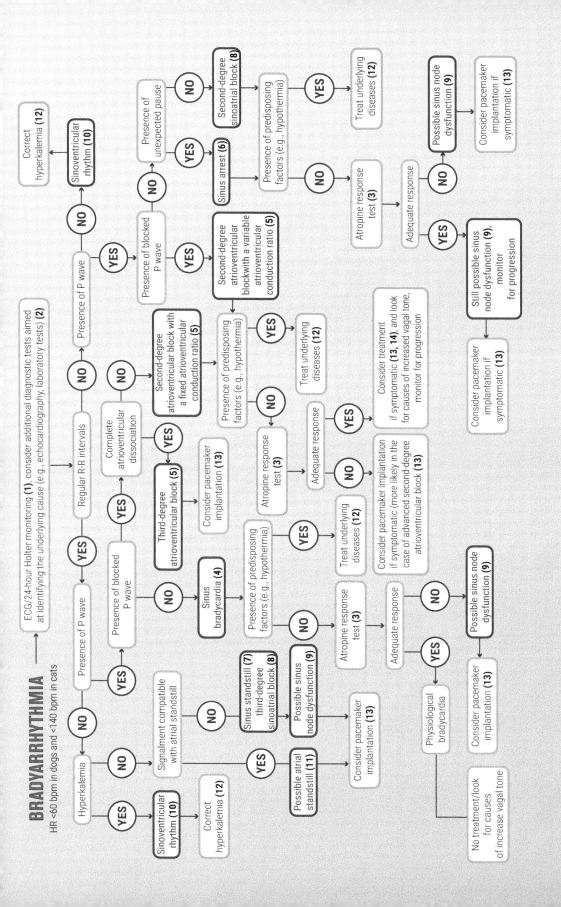

1. When bradyarrhythmia is suspected, a 6-/12-lead electrocardiogram (ECG) is mandatory; in some cases, 24-hour Holter monitoring should also be performed.

2. Based on the results of the electrocardiography, the following diagnostic protocol should be considered: echocardiography (cardiac infiltrative/inflammatory diseases, cardiomyopathies, valvular diseases); cardiac troponin I (cardiac inflammatory diseases); CBC, biochemistry, electrolytes (extracardiac/metabolic disorders, such as electrolyte disturbances or hypothyroidism); thoracic and abdominal imaging, such as radiography and ultrasonography (neoplasia, systemic diseases).

3. Atropine response test: it is used to help differentiate intrinsic SN disease from vagally-mediated bradyarrhythmias if no causes for the bradyarrhythmias are evident (e.g., hypothermia). An adequate response usually suggests vagally-mediated bradyarrhythmia, whereas an incomplete/absent response supports the diagnosis of nodal diseases. However, a positive response may sometimes be documented in patients with abnormal SN function. The most common indications include inappropriate sinus bradycardia, sinus arrest, second-degree sinoatrial block, and second-degree atrioventricular block (AVB).

DIAGNOSIS

4. Sinus bradycardia: regular rhythm, with a HR <60 bpm in dogs and <140 bpm in cats, and normal atrioventricular association.

5. Atrioventricular blocks: the common AVBs inducing bradyarrhythmia are second-degree, consisting of regular/irregular rhythm depending on the regularity of the sinus rhythm and the atrioventricular conduction ratio, with the presence of non-conducted P waves, and third-degree AVB. It can be characterized either by gradual prolongation of the PQ interval (Mobitz type I) or by a sudden loss of atrioventricular conduction without antecedent PQ interval prolongation (Mobitz type II). Other types of second-degree AVB are 2:1 block (one blocked P wave alternates with one conducted P wave) and advanced second-degree AVB (>2 non-conducted P waves). The third-degree block is a regular rhythm with the presence of P waves but complete atrioventricular dissociation. An escape junctional/ventricular rhythm is also present.

6. Sinus arrest: unexpected pause of the underlying sinus rhythm, which is longer than twice and not a multiple of the preceding P-P interval.

7. Sinus standstill: persistent/prolonged sinus arrest with the absence of P waves, regular R-R intervals, and the presence of an escape junctional/ventricular rhythm. It cannot be differentiated from third-degree sinoatrial block and atrial standstill.

8. Sinoatrial block: the second-degree is characterized by a regularly irregular rhythm with the absence of a P wave during the pause and P-P intervals, which include the pause, longer than twice and a multiple of the preceding P-P interval. The third-degree is a regular rhythm with the absence of a P wave and the presence of an escape junctional/ventricular rhythm.

9. Sinus node dysfunction: common ECG findings include sinus bradycardia, sinus arrest, sinus standstill, sinoatrial block and/or supraventricular tachycardias.

10. Sinoventricular rhythm: caused by severe hyperkalemia and characterized by the absence of P waves and a QRS with normal morphology. The regularity of the R-R intervals and the HR depends on the SN discharge rate.

11. Atrial standstill: diagnosable even in young dogs and characterized by the absence of P waves, regular R-R intervals, and the presence of an escape junctional/ventricular rhythm.

TREATMENT

12. Treat the underlying disease, if possible (e.g., therapeutic warming for hypothermia).

13. The definitive therapy for most pathological bradyarrhythmias is permanent pacemaker implantation, especially if symptoms are present.

14. Pharmacological therapy may be attempted if the animal has comorbid medical conditions that preclude pacemaker implantation if the owner declines pacemaker implantation or while awaiting pacemaker implantation.

The following drugs may be prescribed for bradyarrhythmias. Sympathomimetics: terbutaline (0.14 mg/kg PO q8-12h in dogs, 0.1-0.2 mg/kg PO q12h in cats); isoproterenol (0.04-0.08 µg/kg/min IV in dogs and cats); methylxanthines: theophylline (10 mg/kg PO q12h in dogs and 4 mg/kg PO q8-12h in cats). Anticholinergics: propantheline (0.25-0.5 mg/kg PO q8-12h in dogs, 0.8-1.6 mg/kg PO q8h in cats). Unfortunately, medical therapy is rarely effective and is not intended as long-term therapy.

SUGGESTED READINGS

- Bonagura JD, Twedt DC. Bradyarrhythmias. In Bonagura JD (editor). Kirk's Current Veterinary Therapy XV 15th edition. St. Louis, Elsevier, 2014.
- Estrada AH. Cardiac pacing. In Ettinger SJ, Feldman EC, Côté E (editors). Textbook of Veterinary Internal Medicine 8th edition. St. Louis, Elsevier, 2017, pp 1200-1206.
- Santilli R, Moïse SN, Pariaut R, et al. Bradyarrhythmias. In Electrocardiography of the dog and cat 2nd edition. Milan, Edra, 2018, pp 239-258.
- Santilli R, Moïse SN, Pariaut R, et al. Conduction disorders. In Electrocardiography of the dog and cat 2nd edition. Milan, Edra, 2018, pp 259-292.
- Willis R, Oliveira P, Mavropoulou A. Bradyarrhythmias and conduction disturbances. In Guide to Canine and Feline Electrocardiography 1st edition. Wiley Blackwell, 2018.

COUGH

Luca Ferasin

Cough is an important defensive physiological mechanism that the body activates to prevent the aspiration of harmful material, such as inhaled foreign particles, pathogens, or excessive bronchial secretions, to maintain the normal health and function of the respiratory system. Cough is induced by stimulation of coughing receptors localized in the larynx, trachea, or bronchi, whereas irritation of bronchioles and alveoli does not elicit coughing. The typical coughing reflex (CR), also known as "tracheobronchial cough", is characterized by an initial deep inspiration, followed by a forceful expiration against a closed glottis and blocked nasopharynx. When the glottis eventually opens, the expiratory air rapidly flows through the mouth producing a distinctive loud sound originating from the vibration of the vocal cords.

Another form of cough, called "laryngeal cough" or expiration reflex (ER), is induced by the stimulation of the larynx or trachea and consists of a forced expiratory effort against a closed glottis but not preceded by a deep inspiration, producing a characteristic "huff" sound. These two reflexes have different physiological functions: tracheobronchial cough provides airway clearance and maintenance of the mucociliary clearance, while laryngeal cough protects the airways from aspiration of potentially noxious material. Therefore, when tracheobronchial cough is observed, clinical investigations should focus on potential bronchial diseases (e.g., chronic bronchitis), whereas laryngeal cough is more commonly associated with upper airway irritation, like acute laryngotracheitis (e.g., kennel cough).

Isolated cough is frequently observed in healthy individuals and does not have any clinical relevance. However, persistent cough can affect a pet's quality of life by interfering with sleeping, breathing, eating, drinking, and exercising. Furthermore, many coughing pets can keep their owners awake at night, especially when they sleep in the same bedroom, prompting a visit to their veterinarian. Occasionally, cough can also cause syncope, urinary and fecal incontinence, muscle pain, and exhaustion.

The frequent and noticeable presentation of coughing makes this sign a widespread complaint reported to veterinarians worldwide.

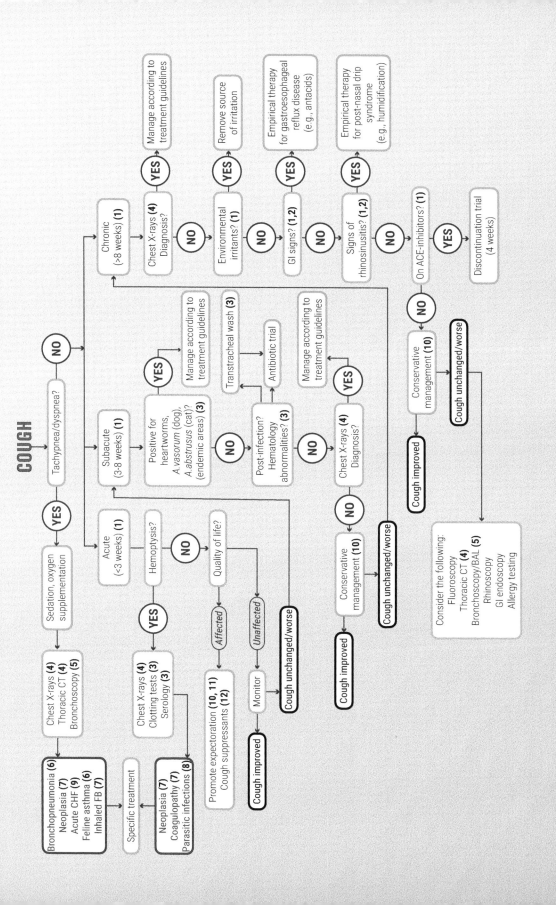

COUGH

Tachypnea/dyspnea?

YES → Sedation, oxygen supplementation → Chest X-rays **(4)**, Thoracic CT **(4)**, Bronchoscopy **(5)** → Bronchopneumonia **(6)**, Neoplasia **(7)**, Acute CHF **(9)**, Feline asthma **(6)**, Inhaled FB **(7)**

NO → Chronic (>8 weeks) **(1)**

Acute (<3 weeks) **(1)** → Hemoptysis?
- **YES** → Chest X-rays **(4)**, Clotting tests **(3)**, Serology **(3)** → Specific treatment → Neoplasia **(7)**, Coagulopathy **(7)**, Parasitic infections **(8)**
- **NO** → Quality of life?
  - *Affected* → Promote expectoration **(10, 11)**, Cough suppressants **(12)** → Monitor → **Cough improved**
  - *Unaffected* → Monitor → **Cough unchanged/worse**

Subacute (3-8 weeks) **(1)** → Positive for heartworms, *A. vasorum* (dog), *A. abstrusus* (cat)? (endemic areas) **(3)**
- **YES** → Manage according to treatment guidelines
- **NO** → Transtracheal wash **(3)** → Post-infection? Hematology abnormalities? **(3)**
  - **YES** → Antibiotic trial
  - **NO** → Chest X-rays **(4)** Diagnosis?
    - **YES** → Manage according to treatment guidelines
    - **NO** → Conservative management **(10)**
      - → **Cough improved**
      - → **Cough unchanged/worse**

Chronic (>8 weeks) **(1)** → Chest X-rays **(4)** Diagnosis?
- **YES** → Manage according to treatment guidelines
- **NO** → Environmental irritants? **(1)**
  - **YES** → Remove source of irritation
  - **NO** → GI signs? **(1,2)**
    - **YES** → Empirical therapy for gastroesophageal reflux disease (e.g., antacids)
    - **NO** → Signs of rhinosinusitis? **(1,2)**
      - **YES** → Empirical therapy for post-nasal drip syndrome (e.g., humidification)
      - **NO** → On ACE-inhibitors? **(1)**
        - **YES** → Discontinuation trial (4 weeks)
        - **NO** → Conservative management **(10)**
          - → **Cough improved**
          - → **Cough unchanged/worse** → Consider the following: Fluoroscopy, Thoracic CT **(4)**, Bronchoscopy/BAL **(5)**, Rhinoscopy, GI endoscopy, Allergy testing

DIAGNOSTIC PROTOCOL

1. History alone does not offer sufficient clinical information to determine the origin of coughing. However, the duration of coughing may help differentiate between acute (<3 weeks), subacute (3-8 weeks), and chronic (>8 weeks) cough to decide the most appropriate diagnostic approach. Cough is often classified as "productive" when it is associated with expectoration of mucus or "dry" when there is little production of phlegm. However, some pets can display both types of cough at the same time, showing productive cough, followed by dry cough after expectoration. Therefore, the timing and character of the cough are not diagnostically helpful since the diagnostic approach is almost identical. Persistent coughing is usually associated with respiratory diseases, but it can also be related to other underlying conditions not necessarily associated with typical airway pathologies, like inhalation of irritants, post-nasal drip syndrome (PNDS), gastroesophageal reflux disease (GORD), neurological conditions, passive smoke, and administration of ACE inhibitors.

2. Clinical examination may uncover a potential underlying cause. Nasal and ocular discharge accompanied by frequent licking and swallowing could indicate rhinosinusitis associated with PNDS. Cough associated with regurgitation, halitosis, and change in bark could raise the suspicion of GORD. Auscultation of stridors, rhonchi, crackles, and wheezes indicate the presence of an airway disease at different levels in the respiratory tract. Chest percussion can reveal a horizontal line of dullness in pets with pleural effusion, often associated with cough, or focal dullness in case of thoracic masses, which can cause mechanical compression of the airways and cough.

3. Laboratory tests can offer valuable diagnostic information. Hematology, for example, may reveal neutrophilia in inflammatory conditions or eosinophilia and basophilia associated with parasitic or fungal infections. Fecal Baermann test can identify lungworms and serological tests are available for detection of *Dirofilaria immitis* (heartworm disease, HWD) and *Angiostrongylus vasorum*. Clotting tests should be considered for suspected coagulopathies. Transtracheal wash (TTW) allows blind sampling of the larger airways for cytologic and culture analysis.

4. Thoracic radiography should be performed before invasive diagnostics, despite its limited sensitivity in identifying dynamic airway collapse, infectious tracheobronchitis, or parasitic infections. A more sensitive radiographic investigation can be achieved with thoracic CT scanning.

5. Bronchoscopy should only be considered in selected cases, such as removing inhaled foreign bodies, identifying airway collapse, or airway sampling (mucosal biopsy or bronchoalveolar lavage). Transtracheal wash represents an alternative sampling technique but with lower diagnostic yield.

DIAGNOSIS

6. Acute inflammatory airway disease (e.g., kennel cough, cat flu) are common causes of coughing in pets, which rarely require diagnostic tests. Conversely, bronchopneumonia requires dedicated diagnostic tests, supportive therapy (cage rest, oxygen, sedation),

and often, antibiotic cover. Chronic bronchitis represents the most common chronic inflammatory condition in dogs, while asthma is commonly recognized in cats but not in dogs. Laryngeal paralysis and tracheobronchomalacia are relatively common degenerative airway conditions in the dog.

7. Neoplastic lesions of the respiratory tract, coagulopathies, and inhaled foreign bodies (FB) are the most common causes of hemoptysis.

8. Parasitic infections (e.g., lungworms, *Angiostrongylus vasorum* (dogs), *Aelurostrongylus abstrusus* [cats], *Dirofilaria immitis*) should always be ruled out in endemic areas. Confirmed infections should be treated accordingly.

9. Pulmonary edema in congestive heart failure (CHF), despite several inaccurate reports and opinions, does not cause coughing. However, cardiomegaly can exacerbate a preexisting cause of coughing in advanced cardiac disease.

TREATMENT

10. Therapy is not always necessary since many causes of cough are self-limiting, and a conservative approach is often sufficient to relieve airway obstruction and reduce the source of irritation. Such interventions include avoidance of potential irritants (e.g., cigarette smoke, dust, spray cleaners), light exercise to enhance dislodgement of bronchial secretions, use of a harness instead of a collar when dogs are walked on a lead, weight reduction, and environmental humidification, ideally with ultrasound humidifiers. Inhaled steroids (e.g., fluticasone, beclomethasone) can be considered if conservative management alone is not sufficient.

11. Mucolytics (e.g., acetylcysteine, bromhexine) can reduce mucus viscosity, improving the efficiency of cough to remove bronchial secretions (expectoration).

12. Cough suppressants (e.g., butorphanol, codeine, dextromethorphan) are centrally acting antitussives, which inhibit the cough reflex by acting on the medullary cough center. Bronchodilators (salbutamol/albuterol, theophylline, terbutaline) are only useful during bronchospasm, such as in cats with asthma, while naturally occurring bronchospasm has not been demonstrated in dogs. Neuromodulating medications (e.g., gabapentin) can reduce cough frequency and severity of chronic cough secondary to laryngeal neuropathy.

SUGGESTED READINGS

-   Chung KF. The clinical and pathophysiological challenge of cough. In Chung KF, Widdicombe JG, Boushey HA (editors). Cough: Causes, Mechanisms and Therapy. Malden, Massachusetts, Blackwell Publishing, 2003, pp 3-10.
-   Ferasin L, Crews L, Biller DS, et al. Risk factors for coughing in dogs with naturally acquired myxomatous mitral valve disease. *J Vet Intern Med* 27:286-292, 2013.
-   Ferasin, L. Coughing. In Ettinger SJ, Feldman EC, Côté E (editors). Textbook of Veterinary Internal Medicine 8th edition. St. Louis, Elsevier, 2017, pp 107-111.
-   Ferasin L, Linney C. Coughing in dogs: what is the evidence for and against a cardiac cough? *J Small Anim Pract* 60:139-145, 2019.

CYANOSIS

Giovanni Romito

The term cyanosis (from the Greek "cyanós" = blue) describes the abnormal bluish discoloration of the skin and/or mucous membranes. All conditions that increase the levels of deoxygenated hemoglobin (or its derivatives) circulating within the superficial dermal capillaries and subpapillary venous plexus, regardless of the mechanism, can cause cyanosis. The peculiar color change depends on the different light-absorbing properties of the two hemoglobin conformations since the oxygenated conformation reflects more red wavelengths of light (contributing to the physiological skin/mucous membrane color), while the deoxygenated conformation reflects more blue wavelengths of light (contributing to the cyanotic hue).

Physiologically, cyanosis occurrence depends on the state of the capillary circulation, the total amount of hemoglobin in the blood, and the degree of hemoglobin saturation in the arterial blood (SaO_2). The SaO_2, in turn, is related to the partial pressure of oxygen dissolved in the plasma phase of arterial blood (PaO_2), which mainly depends on the pressure of inhaled oxygen and the lung architecture/function. From a classification point of view, cyanosis can be classified as central, peripheral, and differential. Central cyanosis is a generalized bluish discoloration due to arterial deoxygenation (hypoxemia). It is due to conditions leading to increased deoxygenated hemoglobin (including central nervous system disorders causing depression of the respiratory drive, respiratory system disorders causing hypoventilation, ventilation-perfusion mismatch or impaired oxygen diffusion, and cardiovascular disorders causing intracardiac right-to-left shunts [R-Ls]), or abnormal hemoglobin (congenital/acquired).

Peripheral cyanosis is the bluish discoloration of the distal extremities due to inadequate oxygenation of peripheral capillary blood. It is caused by desaturation of the hemoglobin in the arterial blood supply (conditions leading to central cyanosis) and peripheral circulatory problems (local hypoperfusion/vasoconstriction/stasis/occlusion). Differential cyanosis refers to the appearance of cyanosis limited to the caudal part of the body. It is caused by cardiovascular diseases resulting in extracardiac right-to-left shunts.

Considering the numerous potential causes of cyanosis, a multidisciplinary diagnostic approach is often needed to identify the underlying etiology and prescribe the proper therapy.

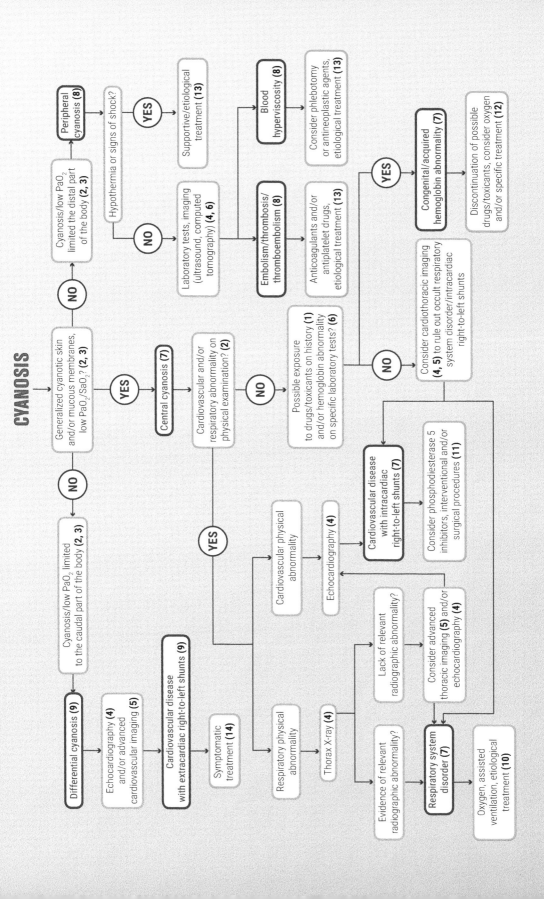

CYANOSIS

Generalized cyanotic skin and/or mucous membranes, low PaO_2/SaO_2? **(2, 3)**

NO → Cyanosis/low PaO_2 limited to the caudal part of the body **(2, 3)**

Differential cyanosis (9) → Echocardiography **(4)** and/or advanced cardiovascular imaging **(5)** → **Cardiovascular disease with extracardiac right-to-left shunts (9)** → Symptomatic treatment **(14)**

YES → Central cyanosis **(7)** → Cardiovascular and/or respiratory abnormality on physical examination? **(2)**

YES →

Respiratory physical abnormality → Thorax X-ray **(4)** → Evidence of relevant radiographic abnormality? → **Respiratory system disorder (7)** → Oxygen, assisted ventilation, etiological treatment **(10)**

Lack of relevant radiographic abnormality? → Consider advanced thoracic imaging **(5)** and/or echocardiography **(4)** → **Respiratory system disorder (7)**

Cardiovascular physical abnormality → Echocardiography **(4)** → **Cardiovascular disease with intracardiac right-to-left shunts (7)** → Consider phosphodiesterase 5 inhibitors, interventional and/or surgical procedures **(11)**

NO → Possible exposure to drugs/toxicants on history **(1)** and/or hemoglobin abnormality on specific laboratory tests? **(6)**

NO → Consider cardiothoracic imaging **(4, 5)** to rule out occult respiratory system disorder/intracardiac right-to-left shunts

YES → **Congenital/acquired hemoglobin abnormality (7)** → Discontinuation of possible drugs/toxicants, consider oxygen and/or specific treatment **(12)**

NO → Cyanosis/low PaO_2 limited the distal part of the body **(2, 3)** → **Peripheral cyanosis (8)** → Hypothermia or signs of shock?

YES → Supportive/etiological treatment **(13)**

NO → Laboratory tests, imaging (ultrasound, computed tomography) **(4, 6)**

→ Blood hyperviscosity **(8)** → Consider phlebotomy or antineoplastic agents, etiological treatment **(13)**

→ **Embolism/thrombosis/thromboembolism (8)** → Anticoagulants and/or antiplatelet drugs, etiological treatment **(13)**

1. Medical history may unveil possible exposure to drugs/toxicants capable of reducing the hemoglobin oxygen-carrying capacity (e.g., acetaminophen-induced methemoglobinemia).

2. Physical examination helps in classifying cyanosis as central (generalized bluish discoloration often associated with respiratory and/or cardiovascular physical abnormalities), peripheral (extremities bluish discoloration often associated with lameness, hypothermia and/or paresis of the affected limb), or differential (bluish discoloration of the caudal part of the body often associated with heart murmurs/heart failure signs since birth).

3. Arterial blood gas analysis and pulse oximetry are useful for non-invasively documenting PaO_2 and SaO_2 values (normal, approximately 97% and 80-110 mmHg, respectively; when the hemoglobin concentration is normal, cyanosis generally becomes evident at SaO_2 and PaO_2 values ≤75% and ≤45 mmHg, respectively).

4. The next diagnostic steps are aimed at diagnosing the underlying etiology. Non-invasive routine tests are usually initially performed: complete blood count (anemia, erythrocytosis, platelet abnormalities); serum biochemistry, urinalysis (prothrombotic metabolic disorders), coagulation profile (prothrombotic hemostatic disorders), abdominal/limb ultrasound (prothrombotic metabolic disorders, vascular occlusion detection); thoracic radiography (intrathoracic respiratory system diseases/masses, cardiomegaly, congestive heart failure); echocardiography with/without contrast agents (right-to-left shunts).

5. Advanced imaging tests may be needed for some respiratory disorders (endoscopy, computed tomography, scintigraphy) and extracardiac right-to-left shunts (computed tomography, angiography).

6. Specific laboratory tests may be needed for some hemoglobin abnormalities (e.g., quantification of the methemoglobin levels) and hyperviscosity syndrome (e.g., bone marrow aspiration/biopsy in polycythemia).

DIAGNOSIS

7. Central cyanosis: generalized bluish discoloration with decreased PaO_2 or high abnormal (nonfunctional) hemoglobin. Severe respiratory disorders (e.g., pulmonary edema, inflammation/infection, contusion/hemorrhage, thromboembolism) and intracardiac right-to-left shunts (e.g., tetralogy of Fallot, atrial/ventricular septal defect with severe pulmonic stenosis/pulmonary hypertension) represent the most common causes; diagnosis mainly relies on cardiothoracic imaging. Hemoglobin abnormalities are very rare (the most common is methemoglobinemia); specific laboratory tests are needed to document the diagnostic findings (e.g., high methemoglobin levels).

8. Peripheral cyanosis: bluish discoloration of the distal extremities typically with normal PaO_2. Local hypoperfusion (e.g., shock) and vasoconstriction (cold exposure/hypothermia) represent common causes; diagnosis is primarily based on a thorough physical examination.

Peripheral circulatory problems due to embolism/thrombosis/thromboembolism (usually due to metabolic disorders in dogs and cardiovascular disorders in cats) or blood hyperviscosity (e.g., erythrocytosis, polycythemia) represent less frequent causes; diagnosis mainly relies on laboratory and imaging tests.

9. Differential cyanosis: asymmetrical physical and /or arterial blood gas findings between the upper (normal color/normal PaO_2) and lower (cyanosis/decreased PaO_2) parts of the body due to extracardiac right-to-left shunts (e.g., "reversed" patent ductus arteriosus); diagnosis mainly relies on cardiovascular imaging.

TREATMENT

10. Central cyanosis due to respiratory system disorders: oxygen therapy helps stabilize patients before starting specific treatments according to the underlying etiology. Assisted ventilation may sometimes be necessary.

11. Central cyanosis due to intracardiac R-Ls: oxygen therapy is not resolutive since the amount of venous blood reaching the arterial blood is not decreased. Some medical (e.g., phosphodiesterase 5 inhibitors for severe pulmonary hypertension), interventional (e.g., balloon valvuloplasty for severe pulmonic stenosis) and/or surgical (e.g., Blalock-Taussig shunt procedure for tetralogy of Fallot) approaches may alleviate cyanosis.

12. Central cyanosis due to hemoglobin abnormalities: oxygen benefit is variable according to the type of abnormality (e.g., not resolutive in methemoglobinemia since methemoglobin does not bind oxygen). Drug/toxicant discontinuation is important in acquired abnormalities. Specific drugs can sometimes be useful (e.g., methylene blue in methemoglobinemia).

13. Peripheral cyanosis: treatment includes both supportive (e.g., warming for hypothermia) and etiological (e.g., antibiotics for septic shock) approaches. Anticoagulants/antiplatelet drugs are useful for embolism/thrombosis/thromboembolism. If erythrocytosis is present, phlebotomy and antineoplastic agents (e.g., hydroxyurea) may alleviate blood hyperviscosity.

14. Differential cyanosis: an interventional/surgical shunt closure is generally contraindicated, as extracardiac right-to-left shunts are typically associated with irreversible pulmonary hypertension. Therefore, treatment is usually focused on controlling complications (e.g., phlebotomy/hydroxyurea for secondary erythrocytosis).

SUGGESTED READINGS

- Beijerink NJ, Oyama MA, Bonagura JD. Congenital heart disease. In Ettinger SJ, Feldman EC, Côté E (editors). Textbook of Veterinary Internal Medicine 8th edition. St. Louis, Elsevier, 2017, pp 1207-1248.
- Haskins SC. Hypoxemia. In Silverstein DC, Hopper K (editors). Small Animal Critical Care Medicine 2nd edition. St. Louis, Elsevier, 2015, pp 81-86.
- McMullen SM, Patrick W. Cyanosis. *Am J Med* 126: 210-212, 2013.
- Tidholm A. Cyanosis. In Ettinger SJ, Feldman EC, Côté E (editors). Textbook of Veterinary Internal Medicine 8th edition. St. Louis, Elsevier, 2017, pp 210-213.

DIARRHEA: ACUTE

Andrea Boari and Paolo Emidio Crisi

Diarrhea can be defined as an increased frequency, fluidity, or volume of feces and is categorized as acute if it lasts for fewer than 14 days in a previously healthy patient. Acute diarrhea is a very common presenting complaint in companion animal practice, with dogs more represented than cats. In most cases, the diarrhea is mild and can resolve spontaneously in a few days or with minimum symptomatic/supportive therapy without a specific cause being discovered. Only a minority of animals have acute or even peracute severe life-threatening disease. A recent study has demonstrated that acute diarrhea in dogs is more often associated with lifestyle factors than with specific pathogens.

Although diarrhea is a classical sign of intestinal dysfunction, it can result from primary intestinal disease (dietary indiscretion/adverse food reaction, various inflammatory disorders, infectious problems, drugs and toxins, neoplasia) or extraintestinal diseases (e.g., hypoadrenocorticism, liver and kidney diseases, and pancreatitis).

Diarrhea is classified according to localization, pathophysiologic mechanism, and etiology. Unlike chronic diarrhea, localization to the small or large bowel may be less relevant in acute diarrhea as biopsies are less likely to be required, and symptomatic treatment may not differ. In regard to mechanisms, diarrhea can be secondary to increased osmotic activity of the gastrointestinal content or due to altered secretions, permeability, or motility of the gastrointestinal tract; it is very common that more than one of these mechanisms is involved.

Acute diarrhea can induce increased loss of water and electrolytes (sodium, chloride, potassium, bicarbonate); furthermore, dehydration, electrolytes, and acid-base abnormalities can occur when the losses are not adequately replaced.

Signalment, a thorough history, and accurate physical examination are crucial to differentiating between self-limiting or a potentially life-threatening problem. For the most part, the diagnostic workup should be aimed at evaluating whether the diarrhea is caused by a primary gastrointestinal disease or by an extragastrointestinal illness.

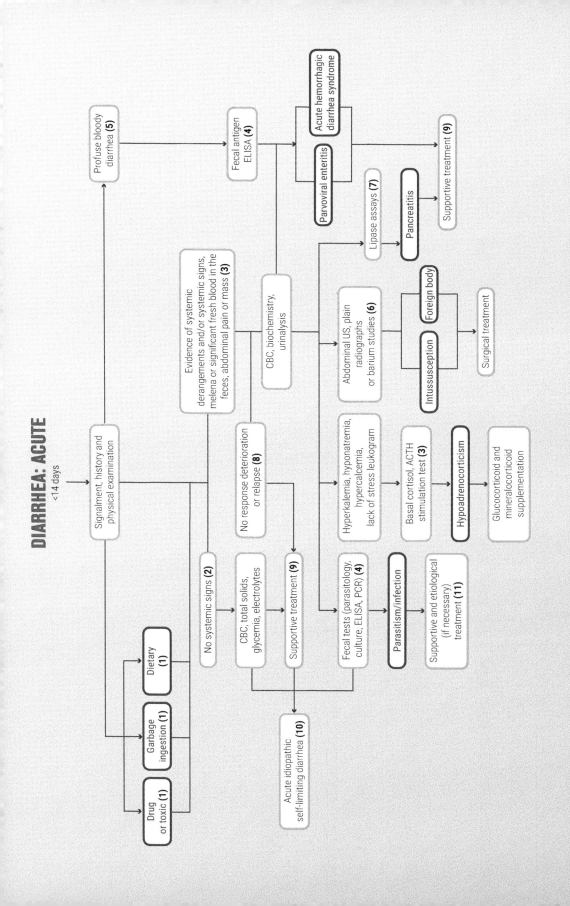

DIARRHEA: ACUTE
<14 days

DIAGNOSTIC PROTOCOL

2. The majority of animals presenting with acute diarrhea have a self-limiting problem not requiring extensive investigation or treatment. In these cases, hematocrit, total proteins, electrolytes, glycemia, blood smear for leukocyte evaluation, and copromicroscopy are required to assess the hydration status in order to ensure that systemic complications are not present (e.g., sepsis) and, in some cases, to suggest the presence of an underlying condition (e.g., hypoadrenocorticism when hyperkalemia and/or hyponatremia are detected). Because the eggs and cysts of parasites/worms are shed intermittently, samples collected over 3-5 days may need to be examined by copromicroscopy.

3. A potentially life-threatening problem should be suspected if one or more of the following signs are present: anorexia, frequent vomiting, polyuria/polydipsia, oliguria/anuria, abdominal pain, weakness, depression, melena or hematochezia, fever, lymphadenopathy, mucous membrane alterations, moderate to severe dehydration, ascites, the presence of organomegaly, an abdominal mass or dilated intestinal loops, tachysphygmia, bradysphygmia, arrhythmias or pulse deficit. The diagnostic protocol should include a complete blood count, serum chemistry, urinalysis, basal cortisol or ACTH stimulation test, pancreatic specific lipase assays (cPL and fPL), and abdominal diagnostic imaging. Basal cortisol >2 µg/dL excludes hypoadrenocorticism in dogs; unfortunately, the specificity of serum basal cortisol is low, and when a value <2 µg/dL is detected, an ACTH stimulation test should always be carried out.

4. Culture, toxin assay, PCR, or ELISA on feces are not routinely performed because pathogenic organisms (e.g., *Salmonella*, *Campylobacter*, *Escherichia coli*, *Clostridium perfringens*, and *Clostridium difficile*) may be found in the feces of healthy animals; the results should be interpreted with caution. These tests should be considered when there are signs of systemic involvement or a high suspicion of an infectious etiology. In inadequately vaccinated animals with compatible clinical signs, a diagnosis of parvovirosis can be obtained by demonstrating the antigen in the feces (ELISA and PCR) or with a better sensitivity and specificity on blood and pharynx (PCR).

5. Young vaccinated adults presenting with a large amount of fecal fresh blood, with high hematocrit values, the absence of leukopenia, normal total proteins, and negative for tests for parvoviral infection are likely to have an acute hemorrhagic diarrhea syndrome (AHDS). The acute onset of bloody diarrhea (resembling raspberry jam) is often preceded by vomiting and anorexia. Clostridial overgrowth and toxins might be responsible for AHDS; however, the diagnosis is still based on the exclusion of other causes of acute hemorrhagic diarrhea.

6. A suspicion of intestinal mechanical obstruction (intussusception, foreign bodies) can be made on the basis of history and physical examination. On simple radiography, a small intestinal external diameter at the level of L5 and a vertebral body ratio greater than 2 indicate a high probability of obstruction. Linear foreign bodies are characterized by one or more loops of bowel bunched or pleated together and wrinkled. Abdominal ultrasonography has greater accuracy and provides greater diagnostic confidence than radiography for diagnosing mechanical obstructions

7. A negative SNAP for canine pancreatic lipase immunoreactivity (cPL) or a lipase DGGR <130

U/L may exclude acute pancreatitis. In dogs with compatible clinical signs, the Spec cPL has high diagnostic performance. In cats, these assays are less sensible and specific.

8. Those animals with a mild clinical presentation that do not respond to supportive therapy, or experience worsening or relapse, should be managed as if they had a life-threatening problem. A chronic disease, initially presented acutely, should be suspected in these cases.

DIAGNOSIS

1. History may help identify dietary causes, such as rapid dietary change or the ingestion of garbage, exposure to drugs, or toxins. It is also important to assess the deworming/vaccination status and the conditions of every animal living in contact with the dog or cat with acute diarrhea.

TREATMENT

9. Very young animals, particularly those with profuse watery diarrhea and vomiting, can very quickly become severely dehydrated and/or hypoglycemic; intravenous fluid therapy and glucose administration should be instituted as soon as possible. Animals with life-threatening diarrhea should be approached with fluid and electrolyte therapy (crystalloids); colloids may be indicated in patients with hypoalbuminemia. Withdrawal of food could be detrimental; it should be considered only for those animals with severe vomiting. Small and frequent feedings of hyper digestible foods limit the amount of acid secreted at each meal, decreasing the amount of additional irritation. Recovery from AHDS is often rapid and complete with appropriate symptomatic treatment (e.g., IV fluid therapy), while complications, such as sepsis and hypoalbuminemia, rarely occur. Recent studies provide evidence that, in the absence of signs of life-threatening SIRS/sepsis (e.g., tachypnea, tachycardia, leukocytosis or leukopenia, and fever or hypothermia), antibiotics may not be indicated for the treatment of acute diarrhea, even if hemorrhagic.

10. Bright and alert animals with self-limiting diarrhea with no abnormalities on physical examination may require only symptomatic therapy. In some studies, probiotics have been shown to shorten the duration of acute, nonspecific diarrhea.

11. Identification of worms or their eggs in the feces of diarrheic animals is an indication for administration of an appropriate endoparasiticide (e.g., fenbendazole at the dose of 50 mg/kg orally once a day for 5 consecutive days). Protozoal infections are usually subclinical, and diarrhea may follow heavy infections, infections in young or immunocompromised animals, or infections together with other pathogens or concurrent disease.

SUGGESTED READINGS

- Boari A. Small intestine: acute disease. In Hall E, Williams DA, Kathrani A (editors). BSAVA Manual of Canine and Feline Gastroenterology 3rd edition. Quedgeley, British Small Animal Veterinary Association, 2019, pp 204-2012.
- Washabau RJ, Day MJ (editors). Canine and Feline Gastroenterology 1st edition. St. Louis, Elsevier, 2012.
- Willard MD. Diarrhea. In Ettinger SJ, Feldman EC, Côté E (editors). Textbook of Veterinary Internal Medicine 8th edition. St. Louis, Elsevier, 2017, pp 164-166.

DIARRHEA: CHRONIC

Marco Pietra

Chronic diarrhea indicates an increase in fecal water content, volume, and/or defecation frequency, associated or not with alteration of the characteristics of the stool (color, consistency, presence of mucus or blood), for almost three weeks. The condition is attributable to chronic enteropathy (CE), while extraintestinal diseases (including eukalemic/eunatremic hypoadrenocorticism, hepatic disease, and pancreatic failure), as well as parasitic, protozoal, neoplastic, and infectious intestinal diseases, should be ruled out. In dogs, CE has been classified in relation to the treatment response as food-responsive enteropathy (FRE), antibiotic-responsive enteropathy (ARE), immunosuppressant-responsive enteropathy (IRE), and non-responsive enteropathy (NRE). To reduce the antibiotic resistance risk, in a One-Health approach, the use of antimicrobials should be limited, and the above diagnostic steps should be reviewed. Thus, a new proposal of CE classification provides diagnosing FRE as a first step, followed by diagnosing dysbiotic enteropathy (DE), a clinical condition that responds to the administration of products capable of modifying the intestinal microbiota, then diagnosing ARE after the use of immunosuppressants (IRE), or by using antibiotics when there are systemic signs of disease or sepsis, leaving the diagnosis of NRE as the last step.

Moreover, protein-losing enteropathy (PLE) is a condition associated with a higher degree of mortality; it is a syndrome characterized by an abnormal loss of serum proteins into the gastrointestinal lumen due to severe IRE, intestinal lymphoma, or lymphangiectasia, developing severe hypoalbuminemia, hypocholesterolemia, lymphopenia, or thrombocytosis. In cats, the differential diagnosis for CE, characterized by weight loss, vomiting, diarrhea, and anorexia, are FRE, inflammatory bowel disease (IBD), and low-grade intestinal T-cell lymphoma (LGITL).

History and physical examination, biomarkers, endoscopic and histological examination of gastroenteric biopsies alone are not capable of efficiently differentiating CE categories; thus, a treatment trial is necessary.

DIARRHEA: CHRONIC

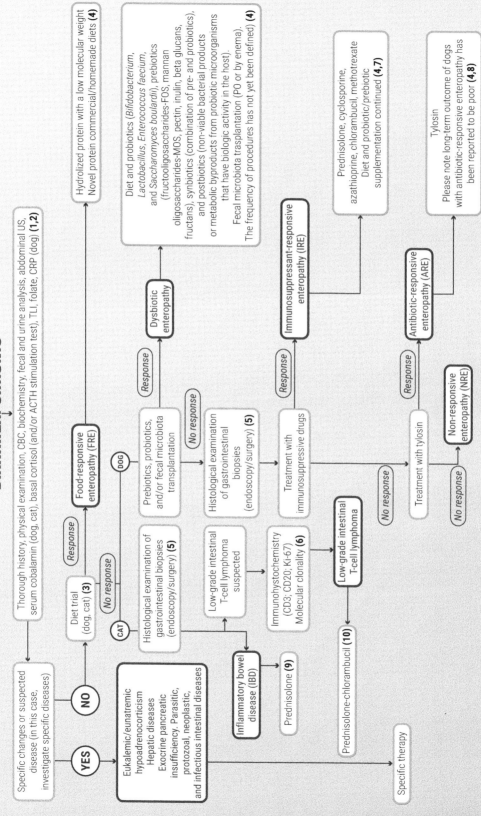

Thorough history, physical examination, CBC, biochemistry, fecal and urine analysis, abdominal US, serum cobalamin (dog, cat), basal cortisol (and/or ACTH stimulation test), TLI, folate, CRP (dog) **(1,2)**

Specific changes or suspected disease (in this case, investigate specific diseases)

NO

YES

Eukalemic/eunatremic hypoadrenocorticism
Hepatic diseases
Exocrine pancreatic insufficiency. Parasitic, protozoal, neoplastic, and infectious intestinal diseases

Diet trial (dog, cat) **(3)**

Response

Food-responsive enteropathy (FRE)

Hydrolized protein with a low molecular weight
Novel protein commercial/homemade diets **(4)**

No response

DOG

CAT

Prebiotics, probiotics, and/or fecal microbiota transplantation

Response

Dysbiotic enteropathy

Diet and probiotics (*Bifidobacterium, Lactobacillus, Enterococcus faecium,* and *Saccharomyces boulardii*), prebiotics (fructooligosaccharides-FOS, mannan oligosaccharides-MOS, pectin, inulin, beta glucans, fructans), synbiotics (combination of pre- and probiotics), and postbiotics (non-viable bacterial products or metabolic byproducts from probiotic microorganisms that have biologic activity in the host).
Fecal microbiota trasplantation (PO or by enema).
The frequency of procedures has not yet been defined) **(4)**

No response

Histological examination of gastrointestinal biopsies (endoscopy/surgery) **(5)**

Treatment with immunosuppressive drugs

Response

Immunosuppressant-responsive enteropathy (IRE)

Prednisolone, cyclosporine, azathioprine, chlorambucil, methotrexate
Diet and probiotic/prebiotic supplementation continued **(4,7)**

No response

Treatment with tylosin

Response

Antibiotic-responsive enteropathy (ARE)

Tylosin
Please note long-term outcome of dogs with antibiotic-responsive enteropathy has been reported to be poor **(4,8)**

No response

Non-responsive enteropathy (NRE)

Histological examination of gastrointestinal biopsies (endoscopy/surgery) **(5)**

Low-grade intestinal T-cell lymphoma suspected

Immunohystochemistry (CD3; CD20; Ki-67)
Molecular clonality **(6)**

Low-grade intestinal T-cell lymphoma

Prednisolone-chlorambucil **(10)**

Inflammatory bowel disease (IBD)

Prednisolone **(9)**

Specific therapy

DIAGNOSTIC PROTOCOL

1. Clinical pathology: fecal parasite examination using a three-day sample to exclude enteric parasitism (dog/cat); baseline serum cortisol concentration and/or an ACTH stimulation test, to exclude a diagnosis of eukalemic/eunatremic hypoadrenocorticism (basal or post-adrenocorticotropic hormone (ACTH) cortisol >2 µg/dL excludes hypoadrenocorticism); serum albumin concentration (2.75-3.85 g/dL [dogs]; 2.60-4.0 g/dL [cats]): in addition to protein-losing enteropathy (in severe IRE, intestinal lymphoma, lymphangiectasia), hypoalbuminemia may result from malnutrition, protein-losing nephropathy, weeping of proteinaceous fluid from burns, and decreased production because of hepatic failure; serum cholesterol concentration (123-345 mg/dL [dogs]; 59-230 mg/dL [cats]): hypocholesterolemia can depend on protein-losing enteropathy and/or hepatic failure; C-reactive protein (0-0.85 mg/dL [dogs]): a non-specific index of inflammation, serum concentration can increase in acute and chronic enteropathy; serum trypsin-like immunoreactivity (TLI) (4-35 µg/L [dogs]; 12-42 µg/L [cats]): values below 2.5 µg/L and 8.0 µg/L (dogs and cats, respectively) indicate exocrine pancreatic insufficiency; serum cobalamin (250-730 ng/L [dogs]; 290-1500 ng/L [cats]): hypocobalaminemia reflects distal small intestinal malabsorption, small intestinal dysbiosis, and exocrine pancreatic insufficiency; serum folate [(6.5-11.5 µg/L [dogs]; 9.5-21.5 µg/L [cats]): hyperfolatemia is suggestive of bacterial dysbiosis, and hypofolatemia can indicate upper small intestine malabsorption (dogs); fecal dysbiosis index: it identifies the bowel microbiota composition, values >2 log DNA/gram of feces suggests a dysbiosis condition, common in dogs with IRE.

2. Abdominal ultrasound examination is useful for excluding extraenteric diseases, focal or diffuse enteric lesions, and evaluating abdominal lymph nodes. In CE, ultrasound can show mucosal striations/speckling and muscular layer thickening, with a muscularis-to-submucosa ratio of greater than 1; unfortunately, in cats, it cannot differentiate IBD from LGITL.

3. A diet trial for two weeks with hydrolyzed protein having a low molecular weight, or commercial/home-prepared diets with a novel protein, can confirm/exclude food-responsive enteropathy (dogs/cats).

5. Gastroenteric biopsies (stomach, duodenum, jejunum/ileum, and colon) should be carried out by endoscopy or, in patients weighing less than 2-3 kg, by surgery (dogs, cats).

6. Immunophenotypic evaluation of the lymphocyte infiltrate of gastroenteric biopsies (CD3, CD20, and Ki-67); molecular clonality is applied if LGITL is suspected. Clinical signs or gross appearance of the enteric mucosal surface are not sufficient for differentiating between IBD and intestinal lymphoma (cats).

TREATMENT

4. In the case of serum cobalamin values ≤200 ng/L (dogs) and ≤400 ng/L (cats), weekly subcutaneous cobalamin injections (250 -1500 µg [dogs]; 250 µg [cats]) are recommended for 6 weeks, then one dose one month later in order to re-check the serum cobalamin concentration one month after the last dose. Otherwise, oral daily supplementation at the same dosage for 12 weeks, with a re-check of the serum cobalamin concentration one week following the last administration, is recommended. Oral folic acid supplementation (10 µg/kg

or 200-400 µg/dog PO q24h for 30 days) is recommended in dogs with hypofolatemia.

7. Treatment of canine immunosuppressant-responsive enteropathy provides prednisolone (1-2 mg/kg PO q24h for 2 weeks, then slowly tapering over 6 weeks). Alternatively (in dogs with body weight over 20 kg, or in the case of a non-adequate therapeutic response), cyclosporine (5 mg/kg PO q24h), azathioprine (2 mg/kg PO q24h for 2 weeks, then 2 mg/kg every other day for 2-4 weeks, then 1 mg/kg PO every other day), or chlorambucil (0.1-0.2 mg/Kg PO q24h), either alone or in combination with low doses of prednisolone, or methotrexate (2.5 mg/m^2 PO q24h).

8. To reduce antibiotic resistance risk, the use of antimicrobials (tylosin at 10 mg/kg PO q12h) should be limited.

9. Treatment of feline IBD involves prednisolone at 2 mg/kg PO q24h (or 1 mg/kg PO q12h), associated, or not, with a hypoallergenic diet. The corticosteroid dose is tapered off by 50% every 3 to 4 weeks until the lowest effective dose is identified.

10. The treatment protocol for LGITL in cats includes prednisolone and chlorambucil (2 mg per cat PO, every 48h to every 72h, or by using a pulse-dose protocol, at 20 mg/m^2 every 2 weeks).

SUGGESTED READINGS

- Dandrieux JRS, Mansfield CS. Chronic enteropathy in canines: prevalence, impact and management strategies. *Vet Med* 10:203-214, 2019.
- Marsilio S. Differentiating inflammatory bowel disease from alimentary lymphoma in cats: does it matter? *Vet Clin North Am Small Anim Pract* 51: 93-109, 2021.
- Ziese A-L, Suchodolski JS. Impact of changes in gastrointestinal microbiota in canine and feline digestive diseases. *Vet Clin North Am Small Anim Pract* 51:155-169, 2021.

DYSPHAGIA

Harry Swales

In veterinary medicine, dysphagia is defined as any abnormality of the phases of swallowing. The phases of swallowing can be separated into (1) oral preparatory – taking food/liquid into the mouth, chewing and lubrication, (2) oral – moving the bolus to the pharynx, (3) pharyngeal – initiation of the swallow reflex and movement of the bolus through the upper esophageal sphincter, and (4) esophageal – movement of the bolus down the esophagus, through the lower esophageal sphincter, and into the stomach. Observing an animal's ability to consume foods/liquids of different consistency can help narrow differential diagnoses by separating into the broad categories of oropharyngeal and esophageal dysphagia. Examples of clinical signs associated with oropharyngeal dysphagia include difficulty prehending or chewing food/liquids, gagging or retching, frequent attempts at swallowing, and dropping food from the mouth. Esophageal dysphagia more commonly presents as regurgitation (see vomiting and regurgitation chapters); however, there can be a crossover between the two phases. Another helpful differentiation is between functional and structural dysphagia. Structural dysphagia typically occurs with more solid food, whereas functional dysphagia typically occurs with both solids and liquids.

Aspects of the clinical history such as a recent transition from liquid to solid food or previous trauma/radiotherapy may help narrow differential diagnoses. Examples of breed predispositions include Golden Retrievers (pharyngeal weakness), Bouvier des Flanders (muscular dystrophy), Collies (dermatomyositis), as well as English Springer Spaniels, Cocker Spaniels, and, in this author's experience, Cockapoos (cricopharyngeal achalasia).

A standardized videofluoroscopic swallowing study (VFSS) is the cornerstone of the investigation into dysphagia and helps localize the area(s) of dysphagia to oropharyngeal/esophageal. VFSS may also help discern whether functional or structural dysphagia is present. Causes of structural dysphagia can often be identified on radiography, CT angiography, or endoscopy. However, causes of functional dysphagia typically involve ruling out potential primary causes, the list of which can often prove extensive. An MRI scan and CSF analysis may take precedence over other tests if cranial nerve or brainstem lesions are suspected.

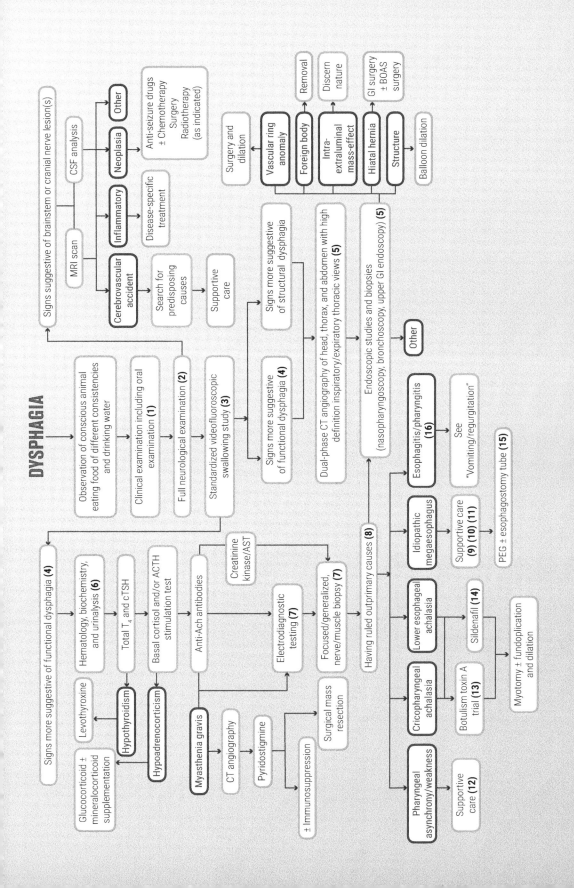

1. An oral examination should also be repeated under anesthetic, looking for lesions such as soft/hard palate defects, periodontal disease, and pharyngitis. As α2-agonists may mask pharyngeal hyperemia, their use is best avoided until after examination of the pharynx. Laryngeal function should be assessed, and doxapram (0.25-0.5 mg/kg IV) may help reduce false-positive diagnoses of laryngeal dysfunction.

2. If a neurological examination reveals signs suggestive of cranial nerve defects or brainstem lesions, an MRI ± CSF analysis takes precedence over other investigations.

3. A standardized VFSS protocol can be found in the references. Although a 12-hour fast (if appropriate) may encourage consumption of the test food, this author has found capromorelin (3 mg/kg PO) to be of benefit, although any effects on swallowing are unknown.

4. Investigations into functional dysphagia may follow these two pathways sequentially or simultaneously.

5. Pulmonary changes, especially those in the cranioventral lung field, may be suggestive of recurrent aspiration episodes, potentially as part of an aerodigestive disorder. More proximal changes documented on bronchoscopy may also support this. Although a barium swallow and radiographs may detect structural lesions, their utility is limited for functional dysphagia and may increase the risk of aspiration.

6. Serum testing for lead should be considered depending on the likelihood of exposure. Anti-nuclear antibodies can also be measured to investigate the likelihood of systemic lupus erythematosus (SLE); however, given the low specificity, other criteria will need to be present to diagnose SLE.

7. Electrodiagnostic tests and nerve biopsies may yield potential causes of dysphagia, the discussion of which is beyond the scope of this chapter.

8. Although VFSS may confirm the presence of megaesophagus or endoscopy may have diagnosed esophagitis, it is important to rule out potential underlying causes before reaching a presumed diagnosis. For functional causes of dysphagia, this may be an extensive list of investigations.

DIAGNOSIS

16. In cats, the presence of chronic gingivostomatitis must be considered.

9. General supportive treatment typically involves postural feeding and dietary alterations. Postural feeding, during and following eating/drinking, may result in an improvement in some causes of dysphagia. Food consistency may be best guided by the VFSS, although

methods such as "little and often feeding" or feeding of "meatballs" may prove effective in some animals. Thickening powders may also help the ability to consume fluids.

10. Although prokinetics such as cisapride (0.1-0.5 mg/kg PO q8-12h) may be of benefit in gastroesophageal regurgitation by increasing lower esophageal sphincter tone, they may be detrimental in cases with esophageal dysphagia. The empirical use of other prokinetic medications such as sildenafil remains controversial.

11. Ampicillin or cephalosporin antimicrobials may be indicated in cases of aspiration pneumonia without systemic involvement.

12. Treatment of pharyngeal weakness is generally supportive. Food consistency may be best dictated by the VFSS; however, gastrostomy tube placement may be required if calorie, electrolyte, and water requirements cannot be met. Myotomy may worsen clinical signs.

13. Injections of *Clostridium botulinum* toxin A into the upper esophageal sphincter or lower esophageal sphincter may temporarily relieve signs of cricopharyngeal or lower esophageal sphincter achalasia, respectively, although the effect may only last 3-6 months. A positive response to treatment may predict response to surgical myotomy, balloon dilation, and fundoplication.

14. A previous study showed an improvement in radiographic features of megaesophagus with sildenafil (1 mg/kg PO q12h); however, it was unknown if any cases had lower esophageal sphincter achalasia. It remains controversial whether sildenafil should be used without confirmation of lower esophageal sphincter achalasia.

15. Placement of a gastrostomy tube will ensure calorie, electrolyte, and water requirements can be met. Concurrent placement of an esophagostomy tube allows removal of esophageal fluid and may improve survival.

SUGGESTED READINGS

- Harris RA, Grobman ME, Allen MJ, et al. Standardization of a videofluoroscopic swallow study protocol to investigate dysphagia in dogs. *J Vet Intern Med* 31:383-393, 2017.
- Lappin MR, Blondeau J, Boothe D, et al. Antimicrobial use guidelines for treatment of respiratory tract disease in dogs and cats: Antimicrobial Guidelines Working Group of the International Society of Companion Animal Infectious Disease. *JJ Vet Intern Med* 31:79-294, 2017.
- Manning K, Birkenheuer AJ, Briley J, et al. Intermittent at-home suctioning of esophageal content for prevention of recurrent aspiration pneumonia in 4 dogs with megaesophagus. *J Vet Intern Med* 30:1715-1719, 2016.
- Quintavalla F, Menozzi A, Pozzoli C, et al. Sildenafil improves clinical signs and radiographic features in dogs with congenital idiopathic megaoesophagus: a randomized control trial. *Vet Rec* 180:1-4, 2017.

EPILEPTIC SEIZURES

Federica Balducci

Epileptic seizures are a common neurological disorder in dogs. They are defined by the International Veterinary Epilepsy Task Force (IVETF) as a manifestation of excessive synchronous, usually self-limiting, epileptic activity of neurons in the brain. This results in a transient occurrence of different clinical signs, such as generalized or focal motor, autonomic or behavioral features, due to abnormal activity of the neurons in the cerebral cortex. Epileptic seizures are classified based on underlying etiology and semiology. Based on etiology, epileptic seizures are defined as reactive seizures, idiopathic epilepsy, and structural epilepsy.

This classification is of paramount importance as it affects the diagnostic protocol and the therapy. Reactive seizures are a natural response from the normal brain to a transient disturbance in function, usually caused by a metabolic or nutritional disorder or exogenous toxin exposure. This type of seizure is reversible when the underlying disorder is resolved; in this case, the term epilepsy is incorrect. Epilepsy is a disease of the brain characterized by an enduring predisposition to generate epileptic seizures (at least two epileptic seizures >24h apart). Idiopathic epilepsy (IE) is defined as a disease "by itself" and can be subclassified into genetic epilepsy, suspected genetic epilepsy, and epilepsy of unknown cause. Structural epilepsy (SE) refers to epileptic seizures caused by a structural lesion of the forebrain, such as vascular, inflammatory/infectious, traumatic, anomalous/developmental, neoplastic, and degenerative diseases.

Based on semiology, epileptic seizures are classified into focal, generalized, and focal with secondary generalization. In focal epileptic seizures, characterized by lateralized or regional signs, the origin of the abnormal electrical activity is within one cerebral hemisphere or in a subcortical structure. Generalized epileptic seizures are characterized by bilateral involvement of the cerebral hemispheres. In focal epileptic seizures with secondary generalization, the abnormal electrical activity starts in one hemisphere (lateralized signs) and then spreads into bilateral cerebral involvement. This is the most common seizure type described in dogs.

EPILEPTIC SEIZURES

Excessive synchronous, self-limiting epileptic activity of neurons in the brain

Signalment and history **(1)**

Interictal neurological examination **(2)**

CBC, biochemistry, urinalysis, pre- and postprandial bile acids

Brain MRI/CT CSF analysis **(4)**

Structural epilepsy

Abnormal/normal

Abnormal

Abnormal/normal

Abnormal/normal

Abnormal

Abnormal/normal

Normal

Idiopathic epilepsy **(5)**

Vascular disease (ischemic/hemorrhagic)
Inflammatory-infectious diseases
(i.e., meningoencephalitis of unknown origin;
distemper (in dogs), toxoplasmosis, FIP (in cats)
Traumatic brain injury
Anomalous/developmental diseases
(i.e., hydrocephalus, porencephaly)
Neoplastic diseases
(meningioma, glioma, lymphoma)
Degenerative diseases
(lysosomal storage disease, Lafora) (in dogs)

Antiepileptic drugs and therapy for the specific diseases **(9)**

Phenobarbital (PB) 2.5 mg/kg bid (in dogs), 2 mg/kg bid (in cats) or imepitoin 10-30 mg/kg bid **(6)**

Test serum PB 14 days after starting treatment or after a change in PB dose **(7)**

Adequate seizure control

NO

YES

CBC, biochemistry, serum PB level at 3 months then every 6-12 months

If PB serum level <30 mg/L, increase PB
If PB serum level 30-35 mg/L, add second antiepileptic drug if the patient has seizures
If PB serum level >35 mg/L, reduce PB and second antiepileptic drug

Toxin ingestion
Weakness
Abnormal behavior after eating
Anuria/oliguria
Anorexia
Vomiting/diarrhea

Reactive seizures

US abdomen, possible angio-CT **(3)**

Intoxication
Hypoglycemia
Electrolyte disorders
Hepatic encephalopathy
Renal-associated encephalopathy
Thiamine deficiency

Benzodiazepine 0.5 mg/kg, levetiracetam 20 mg/kg q8h if the patient has seizures at presentation, and specific therapy **(8)**

DIAGNOSTIC PROTOCOL

1. A detailed history and signalment are the cornerstones of diagnosis. Some breeds are predisposed to idiopathic epilepsy (i.e., Border Collie, Labrador Retriever, Australian Shepherd, Lagotto Romagnolo, Italian Spinone). Age at epileptic seizure onset is critical in differentiating between IE and secondary epilepsy (for the diagnosis of IE, the onset of the first seizure should be between 6 months and 6 years of age). Ask the client to describe or videotape the event to differentiate epileptic seizures from other paroxysmal events (paroxysmal dyskinesia, syncope, vestibular attack). Ask if other family members of the dog suffer from epilepsy as well as information regarding vaccination status, diet, significant previous injury or severe diseases, potential toxin exposure, and presence of interictal abnormalities (e.g., abnormal mental status and behavior, abnormal gait).

2. In the first 48 hours after an epileptic seizure, the neurological examination may be abnormal due to the post-ictal phase. Re-examine the patient after this to point out the presence of neurological deficits. Take into account the previous administration of antiepileptic drugs.

3. Abdominal US and angio-CT are suggested in the case of suspected reactive seizures in order to investigate causes of hypoglycemia, hepatic failure, portosystemic shunt, renal failure, or other systemic diseases capable of causing seizures.

4. Magnetic resonance imaging (MRI) of the brain is rarely performed in the case of reactive seizures due to the underlying etiology. When performed, they are usually normal, with some exceptions: thiamine deficiency and portosystemic shunt. Magnetic resonance imaging of the brain and cerebrospinal fluid (CSF) analysis are highly recommended when the age at epileptic seizure onset is <6 months or >6 years; the interictal neurological examination is abnormal, suggesting an intracranial localization; in the case of cluster seizures or status epilepticus and when a patient with presumptive idiopathic epilepsy is refractory to an antiepileptic drug titrated to the highest tolerable dose.

DIAGNOSIS

5. The Tier I confidence level for diagnosing IE included a history of two or more unprovoked epileptic seizures occurring at least 24 hours apart, epileptic seizure onset between 6 months and 6 years of age, unremarkable interictal physical and neurological examination, unremarkable minimum database blood test, fasting bile acids and urinalysis. The Tier II confidence level for diagnosing IE includes factors listed for Tier I, unremarkable fasting and post-prandial bile acids, MRI of the brain, and CSF analysis. The Tier III confidence level for diagnosing IE includes factors listed for Tier II and the electroencephalogram abnormalities characteristic of seizure disorders.

TREATMENT

6. Therapy for IE is recommended in the case of two or more epileptic seizures within a 6-month period; status epilepticus or cluster seizures; severe or prolonged (more than 24h) post-ictal phase; increasing frequency, and severity or duration of the epileptic seizures over

three interictal periods. There are no evidence-based guidelines regarding the selection of antiepileptic drugs (AEDs) in dogs and cats. Phenobarbital and imepitoin are the two most recommended AEDs to treat epilepsy.

7. The phenobarbital therapeutic range reported for dogs is 15-35 mg/L, although efficacy can be seen at lower concentrations. For this reason, when the dose of phenobarbital serum is <15 mg/L but the seizures are under control, it is not necessary to increase the dose.

8. In the case of reactive seizures, chronic antiepileptic therapy is not usually necessary. One exception is a portosystemic shunt; in that case, consider levetiracetam at 20 mg/kg tid, especially before and after surgical treatment.

9. In the case of structural epilepsy, the therapy must be started as soon as possible, even if the patient has had only one epileptic seizure.

SUGGESTED READINGS

-   Berendt M, Farquhar RG, Mandigers PJJ, et al. International veterinary epilepsy task force consensus report on epilepsy definition, classification and terminology in companion animals. *BMC Vet Res* 11:182, 2015.
-   Bhatti SFM, De Risio L, Munana K, et al. International veterinary epilepsy task force consensus proposal: medical treatment of canine epilepsy in Europe. *BMC Vet Res* 11:176, 2015.
-   De Risio L, Muñana K (editors). A practical guide to seizure disorders in dogs and cats. Edra Publishing, 2022.
-   Podell M, Volk HA, Berendt M, et al. 2015 ACVIM Small animal consensus statement on seizures management in dogs. *J Vet Intern Med* 30:477-490, 2016.
-   De Risio L, Bhatti SFM, Munana K, et al. International veterinary epilepsy task force consensus proposal: diagnostic approach to epilepsy in dogs. *BMC Vet Res* 11:148, 2015.

EQUILIBRIUM DISORDERS

Teresa Gagliardo

Equilibrium disorders are a common neurological problem in dogs and cats due to dysfunction of the vestibular system. This system is the most important in the maintenance of the body's equilibrium, antigravitational extensor posture, and coordination of the eyes' position according to the movement of the head.

The vestibular system is traditionally divided into peripheral and central. The peripheral component includes the receptors located in the membranous labyrinth of the inner ear and the vestibular portion of the VIII cranial nerve. The central part is located in the brainstem (vestibular nuclei) and the cerebellum (flocculonodular lobe and fastigial nucleus). Signs of vestibular disease are usually manifested as unilateral asymmetric ataxia. Depending on the severity of the disease, the animal may show leaning, falling, or rolling movements towards the lesion. Vestibular ataxia is due to the loss of the ipsilateral extensor tone and hypertonicity of the contralateral extensor muscle.

One characteristic sign of a unilateral vestibular syndrome (VS) is the head tilt, which in most cases is ipsilateral to the side of the lesion. Head tilt results from the decreased tone of the ipsilateral antigravitational muscles of the neck. This abnormal head posture is characterized by rotation of the midline plane of the head, resulting in the lower carriage of the ear of the affected side. Other clinical signs of VS include pathological nystagmus, vestibular strabismus, and sometimes nausea and vomiting due to motion sickness.

The above-mentioned signs may be present both in peripheral and central VS. For the clinician, determining whether the lesion affects the central or peripheral vestibular structures is of fundamental importance for the prognostic implications. In the case of peripheral VS, the prognosis is generally good, while in the case of central involvement prognosis is worse.

Alteration of mental status, tetraparesis, proprioceptive deficits, and cranial nerves dysfunction could be observed in central VS. Facial nerve paralysis and/or Horner's syndrome are highly suggestive of peripheral vestibular disease.

EQUILIBRIUM DISORDERS

Head tilt, vestibular ataxia, nystagmus, vestibular strabismus

Abnormal mentation, postural reaction deficits, paresis, vertical or variable nystagmus, involvement of CNS other than CN VII or VIII or cerebellar signs?

YES → Probably central vestibular syndrome

NO → Probably peripheral vestibular syndrome

NO branch (peripheral vestibular syndrome)

Investigate for ototoxic drugs administration **(7)**

- **YES** → Discontinue drugs
- **NO** → Otoscopic examination **(1)**

Otoscopic examination **(1)**:

- **Abnormal** → Miringotomy, cytology, culture
  - No bacteria
    - Mass → CT/MRI + biopsy → Inner ear polyp/neoplasia → Surgical removal
  - Bacterial suppurative inflammation → Otitis **(5)** → Antibiotics **(11)**
- **Normal**
  - Puppy **(dog)** → Normal MRI and CSF analysis **(4)** → Congenital vestibular syndrome **(9)** → No treatment
  - Adult → CBC and biochemistry: increased cholesterol, triglycerides **(2)** → Thyroid profile **(3)**
    - Abnormal (e.g., high TSH and low TT₄) → Hypothyroidism (Dog) **(8)** → Thyroid hormone supplementation **(12)**
    - Normal → MRI and CSF analysis **(4)**
      - Normal → Idiopathic vestibular syndrome **(6)** → Spontaneous resolution **(13)**

YES branch (central vestibular syndrome)

Metronidazole administration?

- **YES** → Discontinue the drug + diazepam **(14)**
- **NO** → Signalment and history
  - Chronic or acute onset/progressive → Possible thiamine deficiency, inflammatory, neoplastic **(10)** → Confirm suspicion
  - Acute onset/non progressive → Possible vascular, anomalous, traumatic → Confirm suspicion

Confirm suspicion → CBC, biochemistry profile; MRI; CSF analysis, infectious diseases test **(4)** → Supportive treatment, antiemetic therapy, specific treatment according to the final diagnosis

DIAGNOSTIC PROTOCOL

1. A careful examination of the ear structures, including otoscopy, should always be carried out to verify the presence of lesions.

2. If normocytic, normochromic regenerative anemia, and hypercholesterolemia are present, thyroid dysfunction should be suspected.

3. A thyroid panel (TSH, T_4, ± free T_4) is recommended, especially in cases with other clinical signs of hypothyroidism (e.g., dermatological changes) and high serum cholesterol concentration. In doubtful cases (e.g., when TSH is not increased), and rhTSH stimulation test or thyroid scintigraphy should be considered.

4. Advanced diagnostic imaging such as computed tomography (CT) or magnetic resonance imaging (MRI) is essential to obtain a diagnosis. MRI is the "gold standard"; it has greater sensitivity than CT in the visualization of soft tissues and the caudal fossa. The presence of the beam hardening artifact produced in the caudal fossa where central vestibular structures are located limits the use of this diagnostic technique in the diagnosis of central VS. Cerebrospinal fluid (CSF) examination and specific tests for infectious diseases (e.g., distemper, *Toxoplasma*, *Neospora*) should be considered when a central VS of inflammatory/infectious origin is suspected.

7. Other causes of peripheral VS include the administration of ototoxic agents such as aminoglycoside, loop diuretics, or ear canal cleaners containing iodophors and chlorhexidine. Both parenteral and topical administration can result in ototoxicity. The diagnosis is based on history.

DIAGNOSIS

5. The diagnosis of otitis media/interna is based on clinical signs, otoscopic examination, and, especially, advanced diagnostic imaging findings. The visualization of the intact eardrum by otoscopy does not rule out a diagnosis of otitis media/interna. In the case of otitis media/interna myringotomy with associated cytology of the exudate, antimicrobial culture and antibiogram should be carried out after MRI confirmation to establish the proper treatment regimen.

6. Idiopathic vestibular syndrome is one of the most common causes of peripheral vestibular dysfunction occurring both in dogs and cats. Dogs usually have advanced age; therefore, the disease is usually referred to as idiopathic geriatric vestibular disease. In cats, it could appear at any age. The onset of vestibular signs is peracute/acute, and the course may be progressive during the first 24-48 hours. The recovery is spontaneous and usually occurs in 2-3 weeks. The diagnosis is based on the exclusion of other causes.

8. Hypothyroidism has been associated with peripheral and central vestibular disease. The exact pathogenesis related to polyneuropathy during hypothyroidism is unknown. It is likely due to the deposition of myxomatous material compressing the cranial nerves as they exit from the skull foramina. The diagnosis is based on the measurement of low T_4, free T_4, and elevated TSH concentration in animals with consistent clinical signs.

9. Congenital vestibular syndrome has been reported in several breeds such as German Shepherd, Doberman Pinscher, Akita Inu, English Cocker Spaniel, and Burmese. Clinical signs are present from birth but can improve in time due to a compensation mechanism. Head tilt and deafness may persist.

10. Several disorders are associated with central vestibular disease. Tumors of the caudal fossa and inflammatory/infective diseases are the two most common causes of central VS. Both primary and metastatic tumors can affect the brainstem and the cerebellum. The most common primary tumor causing central VS are meningiomas and choroid plexus tumors. The inflammatory or infectious disorders often responsible for central VS include distemper, feline infectious peritonitis (FIP), and otogenic brain abscesses. Non-infectious inflammatory disorders such as meningoencephalitis of unknown etiology are also frequent. Toxic and metabolic conditions, such as metronidazole intoxication or thiamine deficiency, should also be considered as causes of central VS.

TREATMENT

11. In the case of otitis media/interna, antibiotic treatment should be initiated according to the antibiogram result. In the absence of an etiological diagnosis, broad-spectrum antibiotics should be chosen based on bony penetration (e.g., amoxicillin/clavulanate, cephalosporin, or fluoroquinolones).

12. Levothyroxine supplementation (10 µg/kg, PO bid) is recommended in dogs with hypothyroidism.

13. In dogs and cats with idiopathic vestibular syndrome, there is no specific treatment. To control nausea and vomiting, antiemetics (maropitant 1 mg/kg q24h SC or IV; ondansetron 0.5 mg/kg q24h IV) should be used.

14. The treatment of metronidazole intoxication consists of supportive care, drug withdrawal, and administration of diazepam (0.5 mg/kg IV once; then 0.5 mg/kg by mouth q8h for 3 days).

SUGGESTED READINGS

- de Lahunta A, Kent M, Glass E. Vestibular system: special proprioception. In de Lahunta A, Kent M, Glass E (editors). de Lahunta's Veterinary Neuroanatomy and Clinical Neurology 4th edition. St. Louis, Elsevier, 2015, pp 338-367.
- Grapes NJ, Taylor-Brown FE, Volk HA, et al. Clinical reasoning in feline vestibular syndrome which presenting features are the most important? *J Feline Med and Surg* 23:669-678, 2021.
- Kent M, Platt SR, Schatzberg SJ. The neurology of balance: function and dysfunction of the vestibular system in dogs and cats. *Vet J* 185:247-258, 2010.
- Rossmeisl JH. Vestibular disease in dogs and cats. *Vet Clin North Am Small Anim Pract* 40:81-100, 2010.

ERYTHROCYTOSIS

Michele Tumbarello

Erythrocytosis refers to an increase in the red blood cell (RBC) count, hemoglobin (Hb) concentration, and hematocrit (HCT) above the reference intervals. The terms erythrocytosis and polycythemia are often used interchangeably; however, if the increase affects only red blood cells, the term erythrocytosis is more appropriate. Based on pathogenesis, erythrocytosis can be either relative or absolute. In relative erythrocytosis, the increase in HCT does not reflect an expansion of the RBC mass but rather develops from diminished plasma volume due to water loss.

Absolute erythrocytosis, defined as a true increase in RBC mass, may develop secondary to increased erythropoietin (EPO) production (secondary erythrocytosis) or in disorders with normal or low EPO concentrations (primary erythrocytosis). Primary erythrocytosis is a chronic myeloproliferative neoplasm resulting from the clonal expansion of erythroid progenitor cells; mutations of JAK2 appear to be involved in the pathogenesis. Secondary erythrocytosis can be appropriate, in which the increase in EPO production occurs in response to hypoxemia, or inappropriate, with an increase in EPO production without hypoxemia.

The latter is caused by EPO-secreting tumors or renal disorders, which cause regional hypoxia. A specific type of inappropriate secondary erythrocytosis (usually mild erythrocytosis) is related to some endocrinopathies; thyroxine, growth hormone, and cortisol could induce a stimulatory effect on the erythropoiesis. Appropriate secondary erythrocytosis is due to pulmonary disease resulting in dyspnea from impaired oxygen transfer or congenital heart anomalies resulting in right-to-left shunting with blood bypassing the lungs. The latter condition causes delivery of poorly oxygenated blood to the systemic circulation and the stimulation of EPO production.

The clinical signs of erythrocytosis include erythema of the mucous membranes, hemorrhage, polyuria/polydipsia, and neurological clinical manifestations related to hyperviscosity, ocular manifestations caused by hypervolemia, and clinical signs due to the underlying disease.

The goal of the therapy is to treat any causes of secondary erythrocytosis and to reduce and maintain the HCT within the reference intervals. The optimal treatment for primary erythrocytosis is unknown.

In dogs and cats, absolute erythrocytosis is usually managed with phlebotomy, alone or in combination with myelosuppressive agents.

ERYTHROCYTOSIS

HCT, Hb, RBC increase

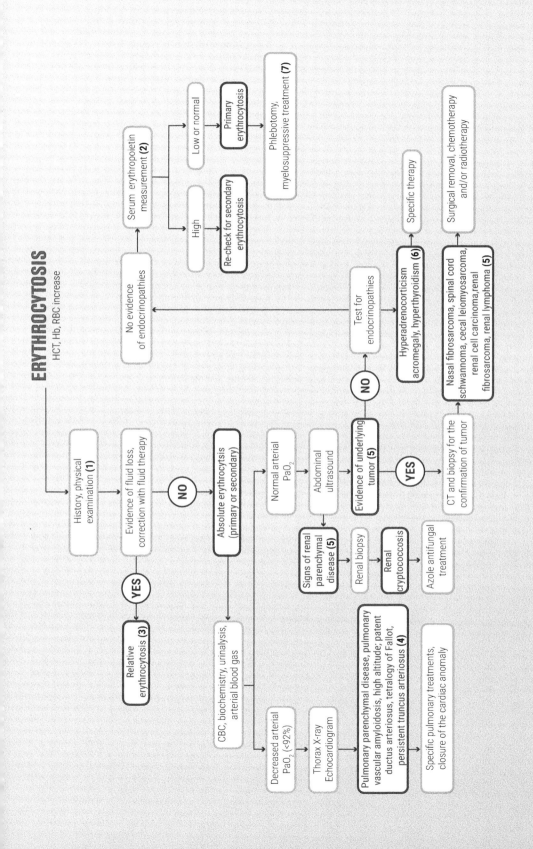

1. Before a complete diagnostic workup, it must be kept in mind that many sighthound breeds, such as Greyhounds, Whippets, Salukis, and some non-sighthound breeds, such as Poodles, German Shepherds, Boxers, Beagles, Dachshunds, and Chihuahuas, can normally have mild erythrocytosis when compared to standard canine reference intervals.

2. Erythropoietin determination should only be included in a complete diagnostic protocol intended to identify the cause of absolute erythrocytosis. Although most dogs and cats with primary erythrocytosis have low or normal EPO concentrations, and some animals with secondary erythrocytosis have higher EPO values, results outside these expected ranges have been encountered. In fact, the overlap in EPO production reported among normal animals, dogs, and cats with primary erythrocytosis and animals with secondary erythrocytosis suggests that erythropoietin values must be interpreted cautiously. Finally, the current availability of validated EPO assays for dogs and cats is limited.

DIAGNOSIS

3. In dogs and cats suspected of having relative erythrocytosis due to diminished plasma volume and hemoconcentration due to fluid loss, treatment with intravenous fluids and resolution of the erythrocytosis confirm the diagnosis.

4. Arterial oxygen saturation below 92% suggests hypoxia. In these cases, erythrocytosis is defined as "secondary appropriate erythrocytosis" and is commonly caused by congenital heart diseases with a right-to-left shunt (e.g., patent ductus arteriosus); this condition causes the introduction of poorly oxygenated blood into the systemic arterial circulation with consequent EPO production and erythrocytosis.

5. In the absence of systemic hypoxia, EPO stimulation can cause erythrocytosis; EPO production can be the result of regional renal hypoxia caused by renal cryptococcosis or renal tumors or can be due to other EPO-secreting neoplasia. Paraneoplastic erythrocytosis, due to EPO production by neoplasia, has been reported in dogs having a variety of renal tumors (e.g., carcinoma, lymphoma, fibrosarcoma).

6. Hormones, such as growth hormone, cortisol, androgen, and thyroxine, may induce a stimulation of erythropoiesis. Adrenal hyperactivity in dogs with hypercortisolism or an increase in androgen concentrations can produce an increase in the RBC count. Moreover, mild erythrocytosis has been reported in feline hyperthyroidism and is secondary to an excess of growth hormone in acromegalic cats. Erythrocytosis associated with endocrine disorders is rare and usually mild.

7. When the disease-causing secondary erythrocytosis is not treatable, or in the case of primary erythrocytosis, the following therapeutic management is recommended: phlebotomy (10-20 mL/kg whole blood); this procedure is performed to control clinical signs

and prevent any potential thrombotic and hemorrhagic complications of erythrocytosis by a rapid reduction in the HCT of up to 58-65%, and by volume replacement using colloids or crystalloids. Long-term repeated phlebotomies can lead to complications (e.g., iron deficiency). Myelosuppressive therapy is indicated when phlebotomy is not feasible due to hyperviscosity, other complications, or in long-term management. Hydroxyurea (50 mg/kg q48h or 30 mg/kg daily for 7 days, followed by a maintenance dosage of 12.5-15 mg/kg q24 h) is the most commonly used antineoplastic drug for dogs and cats. Serial complete blood counts to monitor the possible development of cytopenias are recommended.

SUGGESTED READINGS

- Hohenhaus AE. Primary polycythemia and erythrocytosis. In Ettinger SJ, Feldman EC, Côté E (editors). Textbook of Veterinary Internal Medicine 8th edition. St. Louis, Elsevier, 2017, pp. 2113-2119.
- Randolph JF, Peterson ME, Stokol T. Erythrocytosis and polycythemia. In Weiss DJ, Wardrop KJ (editors). Schalm's Veterinary Hematology 6th edition. Ames, Wiley Blackwell, 2010, pp 162-166.

EXERCISE INTOLERANCE

Gualtiero Gandini

Exercise intolerance is defined as the inability or decreased ability of an animal to perform physical activity considered normal in relation to the animal's age, type, and physical condition. In other words, exercise intolerance can also be defined as early and excessive fatigue following normal exercise.

Exercise intolerance can be the consequence of neurologic or non-neurologic disorders. Non-neurologic causes include anemia, cardiovascular, and respiratory disorders. On physical examination, special attention should be paid to recognizing the presence of pale mucous membranes, respiratory distress, coughing, abnormal pulse, peripheral edema, all possible signs of an underlying hematological, cardiac, or respiratory disease.

Exercise intolerance associated with neurological disorders is a specific type of paresis. Paresis (weakness), defined as the partial loss of the ability to perform a voluntary movement, results from a disturbance of the motor (descending) function. Paresis can be the consequence of an upper motor neuron (UMN) or a lower motor neuron (LMN) lesion. Neurologic exercise intolerance is the consequence of disorders affecting the neuromuscular system (LMNs), including myasthenia gravis, poly(radiculo)neuropathies, and polymyopathies. Unlike UMN paresis, neuromuscular exercise intolerance is not associated with proprioceptive ataxia.

In neuromuscular disorders, gait analysis identifies a patient initially showing a normal gait and quickly progressing to hypometry, a short strided gait, hyperflexion of the joints, dragging of the limbs, and rubbing the nails on the ground, associated with a lowered tail and neck ventroflexion. Exercise intolerance is characterized by the progressive inability of the animal to support its weight; the animal is forced to recumbency to rest and recover the strength needed to walk again. Rest usually improves the condition, which will reoccur every time the patient is forced to exercise. Progressively worsening generalized tremors, indicative of weakness, may also be noted during walking.

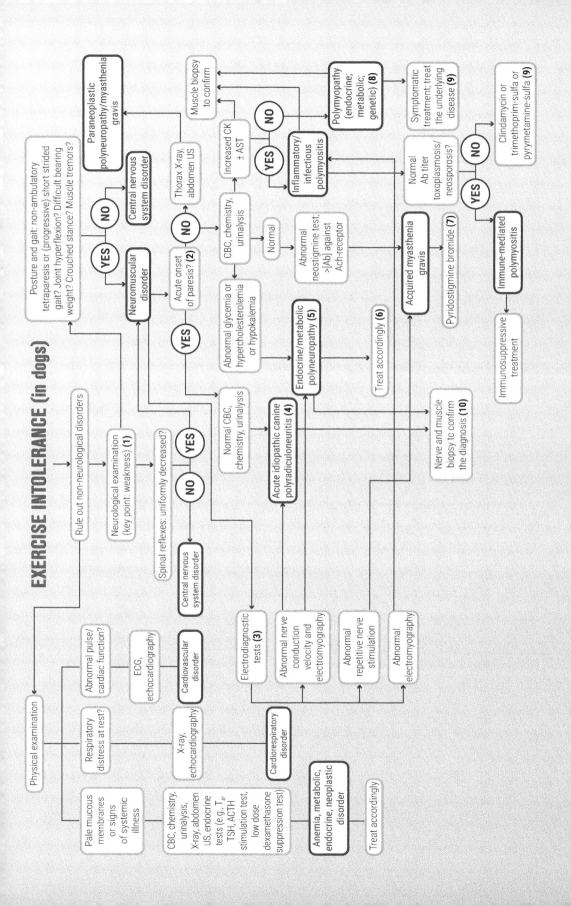

EXERCISE INTOLERANCE (in dogs)

Physical examination

Rule out non-neurological disorders

Pale mucous membranes or signs of systemic illness
→ CBC, chemistry, urinalysis, X-ray; abdomen US, endocrine tests (e.g., T₄, TSH, ACTH stimulation test, low dose dexamethasone suppression test)
→ **Anemia, metabolic, endocrine, neoplastic disorder**
→ Treat accordingly

Respiratory distress at rest?
→ X-ray, echocardiography
→ **Cardiorespiratory disorder**

Abnormal pulse/cardiac function?
→ ECG, echocardiography
→ **Cardiovascular disorder**

Posture and gait: non-ambulatory tetraparesis or (progressive) short strided gait? Joint hyperflexion? Difficult bearing weight? Crouched stance? Muscle tremors?
→ YES → **Neuromuscular disorder**
→ NO → **Central nervous system disorder**

Neurological examination (key point: weakness) (1)
→ **Spinal reflexes: uniformly decreased?**
→ NO → **Central nervous system disorder**
→ YES → Electrodiagnostic tests **(3)**

Acute onset of paresis? (2)
→ YES → Normal CBC, chemistry, urinalysis
→ NO → Thorax X-ray, abdomen US

Abnormal glycemia or hypercholesterolemia or hypokalemia → **Endocrine/metabolic polyneuropathy (5)** → Treat accordingly **(6)**

CBC, chemistry, urinalysis → Increased CK ± AST

Electrodiagnostic tests (3)
- Abnormal nerve conduction velocity and electromyography → **Acute idiopathic canine polyradiculoneuritis (4)**
- Abnormal repetitive nerve stimulation → **Acquired myasthenia gravis** → Pyridostigmine bromide **(7)**
- Abnormal electromyography → **Immune-mediated polymyositis** → Immunosuppressive treatment

Normal → Abnormal neostigmine test; >[Ab] against Ach-receptor → **Acquired myasthenia gravis**

Increased CK ± AST → YES / NO
- YES → **Inflammatory/infectious polymyositis**
- NO → **Polymyopathy (endocrine; metabolic; genetic) (8)** → Symptomatic treatment; treat the underlying disease **(9)**

Inflammatory/infectious polymyositis → Normal Ab titer toxoplasmosis/neosporosis?
- YES → **Immune-mediated polymyositis**
- NO → Clindamycin or trimethoprim-sulfa or pyrimetamine-sulfa **(9)**

Muscle biopsy to confirm

Nerve and muscle biopsy to confirm the diagnosis **(10)**

Paraneoplastic polyneuropathy/myasthenia gravis

Central nervous system disorder

DIAGNOSTIC PROTOCOL

1. Weakness is the key point of the neurological examination of the patient with neuromuscular (NM) problems. Weakness can be observed in the gait, spinal reflexes, and examination of the cranial nerves. Typically, NM patients do not show primary ataxia. Proprioceptive and postural reactions can be affected due to weakness.

2. Most neuromuscular disorders have an insidious onset and a progressive course. Very few diseases have an acute onset, the most important being acute idiopathic canine polyradiculoneuritis (AICP). Less common acute-onset neuromuscular disorders include acute fulminant myasthenia gravis, botulism, and tick paralysis.

3. Electrodiagnostic tests (electromyography, nerve conduction velocity, repetitive nerve stimulation) are useful for confirming the localization, assessing the most affected areas, and differentiating between primary myopathy and neuropathy. Unfortunately, electrodiagnostic tests are rarely able to produce an etiological diagnosis.

10. Muscle and nerve biopsies are useful for confirming the diagnosis, even if they rarely contribute to clarifying the etiological diagnosis. This is particularly true for neuropathies, due to the relatively paucity of modalities expressing the nerve pathology consequent to different neuropathic disorders. Muscle biopsy is more precise in differentiating primary myopathies. Due to its specificity, it is important to point out the necessity of sending the specimens to qualified laboratories.

DIAGNOSIS

4. Acute idiopathic canine polyradiculoneuritis (AICP) is probably the best known polyneuropathy in dogs. It predominantly affects the ventral roots of the nerves. Pathophysiology is immune-mediated, and the diagnostic protocol is often frustrating since blood results are normal, and electrodiagnostic tests and muscle and nerve biopsies only show generic signs of abnormality. The disease has a spontaneous benign course and requires symptomatic treatment, including physiotherapy and general care.

5. Endocrine/metabolic polyneuropathies represent an important group of neuromuscular diseases, including diabetic and hypothyroid neuropathy and hypercortisolism. A diagnosis is reached based on the blood results of the biochemical profile and specific blood tests. Electrodiagnostic and muscle/nerve biopsies are of little value in establishing the diagnosis, providing only generic signs of nerve/muscle dysfunction.

8. Many non-inflammatory polymyopathies are inherited degenerative disorders. The most important include centronuclear myopathy, muscular dystrophy, and myotonia congenita. Metabolic myopathies include hypokalemic myopathy in cats, a relatively common disorder associated with chronic renal disturbances and, more recently reported, hyperaldosteronism. Metabolic myopathy, characterized by type II fiber atrophy, is a well-documented result of spontaneous or iatrogenic Cushing's Syndrome, the latter due to chronic glucocorticoid treatment.

TREATMENT

6.   Therapy for endocrine/metabolic polyneuropathies is aimed at treating the underlying disease. Recovery of the muscle/nerve dysfunction accompanies the recovery of the endocrinopathy, usually in 4-12 weeks.

7.   Therapy with pyridostigmine bromide, an anticholinesterase drug, the dosage of which ranges from 0.5 to 3 mg/kg in dogs, should be started using the lower dose administered orally q8h or q12h. Anticholinesterase treatment should be associated with supportive treatment, including nutritional support oriented to prevent regurgitation and gastro- and esophageal protection. Great care should be taken regarding the early detection of aspiration pneumonia, the most frequent complication in myasthenic dogs.

9.   Except for centronuclear myopathy, inherited degenerative myopathies usually have a poor prognosis. Therapy is symptomatic, using a combination of L-carnitine, coenzyme Q, and B-vitamins. Metabolic myopathies, such as hypothyroid and hyperadrenocorticoid myopathy, are generally resolved in a few weeks by treating the underlying disease. Hypokalemic myopathy may require continuous oral potassium supplementation.

SUGGESTED READINGS

-   de Lahunta A, Glass E, Kent M. Lower motor neuron: spinal nerve, general somatic efferent system. In de Lahunta A, Glass E, Kent M (editors). De Lahunta's Veterinary Neuroanatomy and Clinical Neurology 5th edition. St Louis, Elsevier, 2020, pp. 106-165.
-   Dewey C, da Costa R (editors). Practical Guide to Canine and Feline Neurology 3rd edition. Ames, Wiley Blackwell, 2015.
-   Glass E, Kent M. The clinical examination for neuromuscular disease. *Vet Clin North Am Small Anim Pract* 32:1-29, 2002.

FAILURE TO GROW

Dolores Pérez Alenza

Failure to grow is defined as not growing at the expected rate; it is a common complaint from kitten and puppy owners. Dogs and cats grow rapidly over the first 6 to 9 months of life; abnormal growth can be caused by non-endocrine and endocrine disorders. Non-endocrine causes include constitutional/familial-related disorders, malnutrition, infection, inflammation, severe chronic diseases, congenital cardiac disorders, swallowing disorders, gastrointestinal and pancreatic disorders, hepatic, renal, immunological, and central nervous system disorders, bone growth abnormalities, and mucopolysaccharidosis. Endocrine disorders include hyposomatotropism (growth hormone and insulin-like growth factor-1 deficiency), congenital hypothyroidism, diabetes mellitus, hypoadrenocorticism, and glucocorticoid excess. Considering the endocrine causes in dogs, the most common are juvenile diabetes mellitus, hyposomatotropism, and congenital hypothyroidism. In cats, the most common endocrine cause is congenital hypothyroidism. Small size in a puppy or a kitten can be familial or constitutional, or it might be secondary to an inadequate diet. Therefore, familial information and a dietary history must be carefully evaluated. A complete history including deworming and vaccination protocols, information on littermates, treatments or supplements, and the presence of additional clinical signs must be obtained.

Treatment is based on the underlying cause. Many of the non-endocrine causes can be medically managed, while others might need surgical resolution. Endocrine causes, such as diabetes mellitus, hypoadrenocorticism, and hypothyroidism should be managed with lifelong administration of the deficient hormones. Diabetes mellitus needs to be treated with lente insulin or protamine zinc insulin (PZI). Dietary management is also needed, a puppy diet must be given until the dog or cat is 12 months, with a high fiber low-fat diet (dogs) or low carbohydrate diet (cats) afterward.

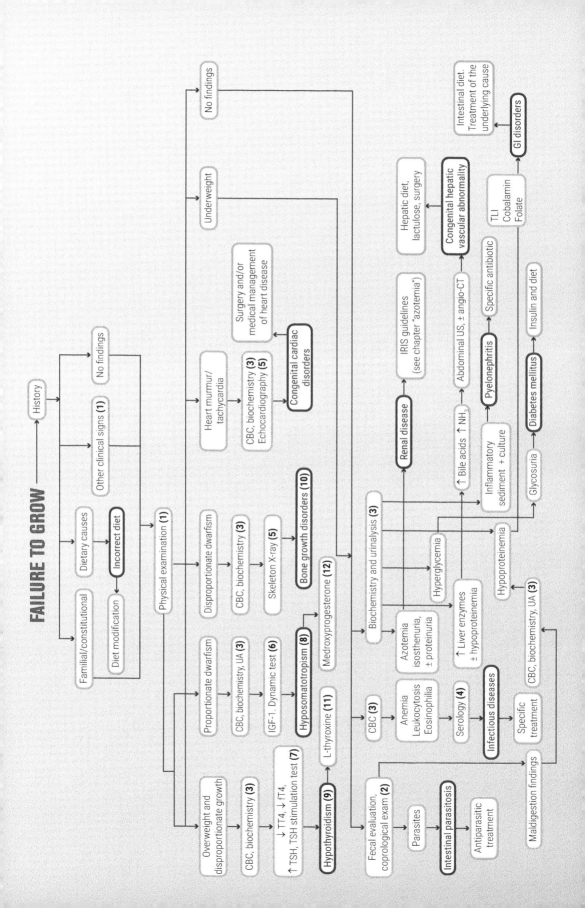

FAILURE TO GROW

- History
  - Familial/constitutional
  - Dietary causes → Incorrect diet → Diet modification
  - Other clinical signs (1)
  - No findings

- Physical examination (1)
  - Disproportionate dwarfism → CBC, biochemistry (3) → Skeleton X-ray (5) → **Bone growth disorders (10)**
  - Heart murmur/tachycardia → CBC, biochemistry (3) Echocardiography (5) → **Congenital cardiac disorders** → Surgery and/or medical management of heart disease
  - Proportionate dwarfism → CBC, biochemistry, UA (3) → IGF-1. Dynamic test (6) → **Hyposomatotropism (8)** → Medroxyprogesterone (12)
  - Overweight and disproportionate growth → CBC, biochemistry (3) → ↓ TT4, ↓ fT4, ↑ TSH, TSH stimulation test (7) → **Hypothyroidism (9)** → L-thyroxine (11)
  - Underweight
  - No findings

- Fecal evaluation, coprological exam (2)
  - Parasites → **Intestinal parasitosis** → Antiparasitic treatment

- Biochemistry and urinalysis (3)
  - Hyperglycemia
  - Azotemia isosthenuria, ± proteinuria → **Renal disease** → IRIS guidelines (see chapter "azotemia")
  - ↑ Liver enzymes ± hypoproteinemia → ↑ Bile acids → NH₃ → Abdominal US, ± angio-CT → **Congenital hepatic vascular abnormality** → Hepatic diet, lactulose, surgery
  - Inflammatory sediment + culture → **Pyelonephritis** → Specific antibiotic
  - Hypoproteinemia
  - Glycosuria → **Diabetes mellitus** → Insulin and diet
  - CBC (3) → Anemia Leukocytosis Eosinophilia → Serology (4) → **Infectious diseases** → Specific treatment
  - CBC, biochemistry, UA (3) → Maldigestion findings → TLI Cobalamin Folate → **GI disorders** → Intestinal diet. Treatment of the underlying cause

DIAGNOSTIC PROTOCOL

1. Poor appetite despite an adequate dietary protocol suggests an oropharyngeal or gastrointestinal disorder or systemic disease. Diarrhea might suggest gastrointestinal disease, polydipsia and/or polyuria might imply renal disorder, hepatic disease, or diabetes mellitus. Symmetrical truncal alopecia points to hyposomatotropism or congenital hypothyroidism; mental dullness might suggest hypothyroidism or encephalopathy. A physical examination is essential since additional findings might be present, suggesting certain disorders. Findings, such as being overweight, might suggest congenital hypothyroidism while underweight is present in malnutrition or systemic disorders. The presence of a heart murmur and/or tachycardia points to a cardiac disorder; bradycardia and bradysfigmia can be present in hypothyroidism. Disproportionate growth (relatively short limbs compared to the trunk) is common in congenital hypothyroidism or chondrodystrophy while proportionate dwarfism is seen in hyposomatotropism.

2. Intestinal parasites are an important cause, often underestimated, of failure to grow; therefore, it is important not to forget a fecal examination as the first step in the diagnostic workup.

3. Hematology, a complete biochemistry profile, and urinalyses are also needed, especially if coprological exams are unremarkable. These evaluations can identify or raise suspicion of renal or hepatic disorders, diabetes mellitus, inflammation, or infections, hypoadrenocorticism, or hypothyroidism. Anemia could be suggestive of renal disease; eosinophilia is associated with parasitism or hypoadrenocorticism. A decrease in total protein concentration could be suggestive of protein-losing enteropathy, hepatic diseases, or renal disease. Proteinuria, glycosuria, isosthenuria, or hyposthenuria can be observed in cases with renal disorders.

4. Based on clinical signs and the clinicopathological abnormalities, additional diagnostic protocols should be carried out; serology for viral diseases in kittens (FeLV-FIV, herpesvirus, calicivirus) and puppies (herpesvirus, adenovirus, coronavirus, distemper) are needed depending on clinical signs, clinical-pathological abnormalities and the vaccination protocol used. Consider additional serology for *Leptospira*, *Neospora*, and *Toxoplasma gondii*.

5. Radiological evaluation of the thorax and skeleton, and abdominal ultrasound or echocardiography are useful in congenital cardiac diseases, respiratory disorders, liver diseases, renal diseases, bone growth abnormalities, and hyposomatotropism.

6. In puppies and kittens with proportionate dwarfism and symmetrical truncal hypotrichosis or alopecia, hyposomatotropism should be evaluated by determining serum IGF-I (insulin growth factor-I) concentrations. IGF-I levels should be interpreted considering the reference range of the laboratories for growing animals. To confirm hyposomatotropism, dynamic tests with growth hormone-releasing hormone (GHRH) or ghrelin can also be carried out.

7. In kittens with failure to grow or in dogs with disproportionate dwarfism, a thyroid panel including total T_4 (TT_4), TSH, and free T_4 (fT_4) should be carried out. Secondary (pituitary) hypothyroidism can also cause congenital hypothyroidism; in these cases, the TSH is normal or low, and thus, a TSH stimulation test should be carried out.

DIAGNOSIS

8. Hyposomatotropism or pituitary dwarfism is a common endocrine cause of failure to grow in puppies. In some breeds of dogs, such as German Shepherds, Saarloos Wolfdogs, Czechoslovakian Wolfdogs, and Carelian Bears, it is an autosomal inherited disorder. Other breeds prone to the disease include Weimaraners, Spitz, Dachshunds, Corgis, and Basset Hounds. Pituitary dwarfism in dogs can also occur when the pituitary gland fails to develop normally or can also be due to pituitary cysts or tumors. A molecular genetic test to detect the mutation (deletion) in the LHX3 gene can be used for diagnosis. In these cases, there is a combined lack of GH, prolactin, and thyrotropin (TSH).

9. Congenital hypothyroidism is the most common endocrine disorder causing failure to grow in cats. Early recognition and treatment of the disease improve survival.

10. Several musculoskeletal disorders may cause failure to grow in young animals. Most of them are congenital and inherited, such as dyschondroplasia (especially in Poodles, Scottish Terriers, and Alaska Malamutes), dystrophy-like myopathies, osteochondrosis, osteochondromatosis, osteogenesis imperfecta, osteopetrosis, angular limb deformities (abnormal development of the radius and ulna), and hypertrophic osteodystrophy and glycogen storage disease. In addition, nutritional imbalances, such as nutritional secondary hyperparathyroidism, a deficiency of vitamin D and/or excessive intake of vitamin A, may cause failure to grow.

TREATMENT

11. Congenital hypothyroidism is treated with life-long supplementation of oral L-thyroxine at a dosage of 10 µg/kg PO q12h.

12. Treating canine hyposomatotropism involves administering synthetic progestins: either medroxyprogesterone acetate at a dosage of 5 mg/kg SC initially every 3 weeks and subsequently at 6-week intervals or proligestone at a dosage of 10 mg/kg SC every 3 weeks, both until 12 months of age. There are, however, some adverse effects, including recurrent periods of pruritic pyoderma and, occasionally, the development of mammary tumors. Porcine GH (pGH) is another potential option. Treatment with either progestagens or pGH should be accompanied by thyroid hormone replacement.

SUGGESTED READINGS

-   Kooistra HS. Failure to grow. In Ettinger SJ, Feldman EC, Côté E (editors). Textbook of Veterinary Internal Medicine 8th edition. St. Louis, Elsevier, 2017, pp 88-91.
-   Peterson ME. Hypothyroidism. In Feldman EC, Fracassi F, Peterson ME (editors). Feline Endocrinology. Milan, Edra, 2019, pp 281-316.

FEVER/HYPERTHERMIA

GENERAL INTERNAL MEDICINE

Johan P. Schoeman and Federico Fracassi

Fever (pyrexia) is a subset of hyperthermia, characterized by an increase in the thermoregulatory set point in the anterior hypothalamus as a consequence of the release of prostaglandin E2. This elevated thermoregulatory set point is brought about by exogenous or endogenous pyrogens, which activate physiologic responses to raise body temperature. Fever is believed to be an evolutionary adaptation to fight infection through, *inter alia*, enhanced leukocyte activity. The underlying molecular mechanisms of fever are complex and involve cytokines (IL-1, IL-6, and TNF), prostaglandins, complement factor 5a, and norepinephrine that together trigger a pyrogenic signaling cascade. Some physiological consequences of fever include increased metabolic demand (especially for fluids and calories), protein catabolism, and bone marrow suppression. If uncontrolled, fever could lead to disseminated intravascular coagulation, shock, and death.

Hyperthermia, in contrast, is not associated with a change in the thermoregulatory set point and is usually associated with exposure to increased environmental temperatures. Hence, hyperthermia in dogs and cats arises from exercise (especially in hot, humid conditions by obese or respiratory-impaired dogs), seizures, hypermetabolic disorders (hyperthyroidism and hypocalcemia), medications (such as ketamine), intoxications (such as cocaine in dogs), malignant hyperthermia and stress. As a compensatory mechanism, such hyperthermic animals make deliberate efforts to cool themselves compared to pyrexic animals at the same body temperature.

Fever of unknown origin (FUO) in dogs and cats is a chronically elevated temperature (>39.2 °C) of at least 2-weeks' duration for which an obvious cause is not immediately apparent.

FEVER/HYPERTHERMIA

Body temperature >39.2 °C (>102.5 °F)

Review history and physical examination **(1)**

History of increased environmental temperature (heat stroke), exercise, seizures, hypermetabolic disorders (hyperthyroidism and hypocalcemia), medications (e.g., ketamine), intoxications (e.g., cocaine in dogs) **(2)**

Possible FUO **(1)**

CBC, biochemistry, urinalysis

Active cooling may be required. If no underlying causes are apparent, let the patient rest for 20 minutes in a cool room with the owner present and then re-measure the temperature; if normal or only mild hyperthermia (≤39.6 °C) suggest follow-up the next day **(3)**

Normalization of the temperature?

YES → Hyperthermia

NO

Joint swelling/joint pain → Possible polyarthritis **(4)** / See dedicated algorithm/chapter

Pain → See dedicated algorithm/chapter

Mass → Aspirate → Neoplasia / Inflammation / Abscess

Leukocytosis or leukopenia with left shift → Blood and urine culture Positive? → **YES** → Sepsis

NO

Pyuria, bacteriuria → Urine culture Positive? → **YES** → Urinary tract infection

NO

Lymphadenomegaly / Thrombocytopenia / Anemia / Hyperglobulinemia → See dedicated algorithm/chapter

Bacterial infection → **YES** → 7-10 day broad-spectrum antibiotic course **(8)** Recovery?

NO → Culture blood and urine, abdominal US, thorax X-ray, echocardiography, synovial fluid collection and cytology, CSF, CT whole body, MRI (brain)

Negative clinical or laboratory findings

Evaluate for infectious diseases. Positive?

YES

dog → Rickettsial infection / Ehrlichiosis / Anaplasmosis / Babesiosis / Leishmaniasis / Fungal infection / Distemper → Specific treatment

cat → FIP / FIV / FeLV / Toxoplasmosis / Fungal infections / Hemoplasmosis → Specific treatment

NO

Thorax X-ray **(6)** / Abdominal US **(7)** / CT (if needed)

Heart murmur? → Echocardiography **(5)** / Blood and urine culture → Endocarditis → Antibiotics based on culture results **(8)**, supportive treatment

→ Pyelonephritis / Peritonitis / Pneumonia / Abscess / Cholangitis

Prednisolone **(9)** → Diagnosis obtained? → **YES** → Specific treatment

NO

1. A diagnosis of fever of unknown origin (FUO) is justified if an elevated body temperature has been documented on several occasions over a 14-day period, in the absence of confounding factors such as anxiety, elevated ambient temperatures, or a recent stressful car journey to the practice. In addition, heat stroke, over-exertion, and muscle fasciculations should be ruled out since hyperthermia induced by such incidents may require an urgent reduction of body temperature.
   As a first step, a complete physical examination in patients with FUO cannot be over-emphasized and should include rectal, fundic, dermatological, orthopedic, and neurological examinations. The clinical presentation of such animals will vary depending on the causative agent and body system involved but will invariably include non-specific clinical signs such as anorexia, lethargy, and depression. Significant pointers to a specific etiology may include pale mucous membranes (anemia/hemoparasites), generalized lymphadenopathy (infectious and neoplastic causes), neck or back pain (meningitis, meningoencephalitis, or discospondylitis), joint pain or swelling (polyarthritis), heart murmur (endocarditis), chorioretinitis (feline infectious diseases) and localized pain or swellings (tick bites or wounds and abscesses).

2. The temperature may exceed 41 °C. Physiological and behavioral signs of trying to cool down may show (panting, inactivity, peripheral vasodilation, cold seeking).

5. Echocardiography is useful for identifying vegetative cardiac valve lesions associated with bacterial endocarditis. If the echocardiogram does not suggest the diagnosis, blood cultures can diagnose bacterial causes of septicemia, especially if three samples are taken in a 24-hour period and when the patient is hyperthermic. A urine culture can also be helpful.

6. Thoracic radiographs are especially useful in cases of pneumonia, pulmonary neoplasia, and effusions. In the latter, thoracic ultrasonography may be superior in detecting smaller amounts of thoracic fluid.

7. Abdominal ultrasonography is very useful to rule out pyelonephritis, prostatitis, pancreatitis, abdominal effusions, or the identification of enlarged abdominal organs that require fine-needle aspiration.

DIAGNOSIS

4. Idiopathic polyarthritis is the most common disorder of dogs with immune-mediated polyarthritis. It occurs most commonly in pure breeds dogs between 1 and 6 years of age. The anamnesis often includes a cyclic fever associated with an intermittent, shifting leg lameness, stiffness, malaise, and anorexia. In some cases, fever is the only clinical manifestation; therefore, polyarthritis should always be a differential diagnosis, especially in dogs with FUO.

3. Acute non-specific therapy includes intravenous crystalloid fluid therapy at 1.5-2 times

maintenance rates. Mechanical cooling methods such as cool water baths or fans to increase convective heat loss should only be considered if body temperature is elevated above 41 °C. Antipyretic agents are controversial and lack a proper evidence base in dogs and cats and should be reserved for patients who are fully hydrated with fevers >40.6 °C, especially since their use can mask the effect of other therapies and they may be associated with gastrointestinal ulceration and hepatic or renal toxicities.

8. Specific treatment such as broad-spectrum antibiotics (based on the organ system involved, the most likely bacterium present, and their known antibiotic sensitivity) should be instituted once culture specimens have been obtained. Once culture results are back, antibiotic therapy should be de-escalated swiftly to an appropriate narrow-spectrum antibiotic to reduce the likelihood of gut dysbiosis. Commonly used antibiotics include amoxicillin-clavulanic acid at 10-20 mg/kg bid to tid or doxycycline at 10 mg/kg bid if tick-borne diseases are suspected.

9. The goal in all cases of FUO is to identify a specific cause and treat the patient appropriately. A therapeutic trial, especially when considering corticosteroids, should be implemented only when a specific diagnosis cannot be ascertained and after every effort has been made to rule out an infectious cause. Prednisolone should be used at 1 mg/kg bid, and a dramatic reduction in fever should be seen within 24-48 hours if it was caused by an immune-mediated condition.

SUGGESTED READINGS

- Ewart S. Thermoregulation. In Klein BG (editor). Cunningham's Textbook of Veterinary Physiology 6th edition. St. Louis, Elsevier, 2020, pp 596-607.
- Ramsey IK, Tasker S. Fever. In Ettinger SJ, Feldman EC, Côté E (editors). Textbook of Veterinary Internal Medicine 8th edition. St. Louis, Elsevier, 2017, pp. 195-203.
- Tefft KM. Fever of unknown origin. In Cohn LA, Côté E (editors). Côtè's Clinical Veterinary Advisor: Dogs and Cats 4th edition. St. Louis, Elsevier, 2020, pp 334-335.

GAIT ABNORMALITIES

Gualtiero Gandini

The majority of gait problems stem from dysfunction of the nervous or locomotor systems. The correct recognition of the system involved is crucial for planning the proper diagnostic steps.

Gait examination is of paramount importance and is a relevant part of the neurological and orthopedic examination. Evaluation of a video recording and the use of slow-motion video can be very helpful.

Gait alterations fall into three categories: lameness, paresis, and ataxia. Ataxia and paresis represent neurological deficits, while lameness is most frequently caused by disorders of the locomotor system. In a minority of cases, lameness can also result from neurological disorders. In most instances, lameness is caused by pain and, less commonly, by a mechanical impediment. In addition to lameness, the typical signs of limb pain include reluctance to move and difficulty in weight-bearing on the affected limb(s). Besides, orthopedic disorders do not usually produce neurological signs and, in most cases, only affect a single limb, less frequently two, and rarely four. The opposite happens in the case of neurologic disorders.

Ataxia defines the inability of performing normal, coordinated movements that are not caused by weakness and musculoskeletal disorders. Ataxia is classified into proprioceptive, cerebellar, and vestibular. Typically, vestibular and cerebellar ataxia affect all four limbs. Proprioceptive ataxia, depending on the site of the lesion, can involve two or all four limbs.

Paresis is the partial loss of voluntary motor function. Paralysis (or plegia) is the complete loss of this function. Paresis and paralysis are two terms defining the same type of defect, differing only quantitatively. Paresis shows different degrees of severity and can be differentiated into ambulatory paresis (when the animal can stand and walk unassisted), and non-ambulatory paresis (when the patient needs to be supported to stand and walk).

Ataxia and paresis can present simultaneously in the same patient, especially in the case of spinal cord lesions.

GAIT ABNORMALITIES

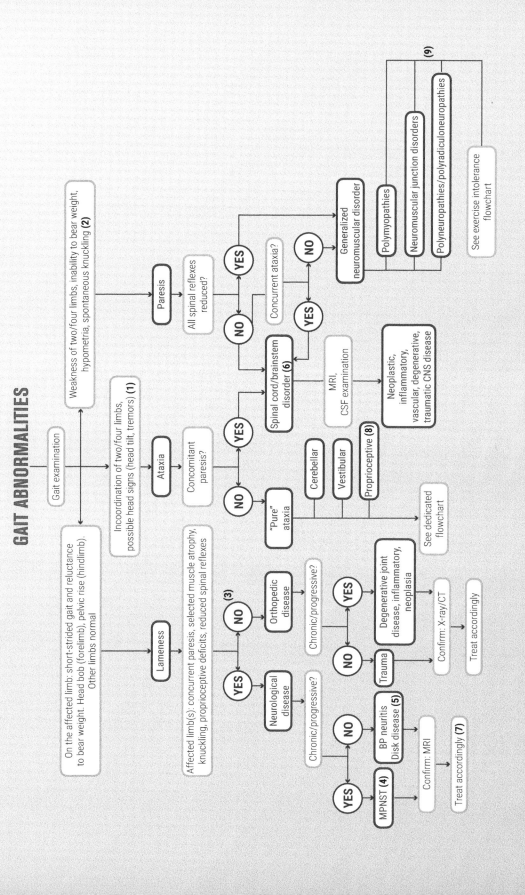

1. Proprioceptive ataxia is the only type of ataxia that only affects the hindlimbs. The presence of a head tilt is typically accompanied by vestibular ataxia. Intention tremors of the head are associated with hypermetria and spasticity, typical of cerebellar disorders.

2. The description in the algorithm refers to ambulatory paresis. More severe levels of paresis may result in the inability to ambulate without assistance.

3. Some neurological disorders may only present with lameness. This is particularly true for the early stages of malignant peripheral nerve sheath tumors (MPNSTs) and some lateralized disc herniations.

DIAGNOSIS

4. Malignant peripheral nerve sheath tumors (MPNSTs) most frequently affect the brachial plexus. The first sign is lameness, possibly followed by focal neurological signs regarding the affected limb, such as monoparesis and proprioceptive deficits.

5. Brachial plexus (BP) neuritis is a rare disease of unknown origin. It can be monolateral or bilateral. Immune-mediated pathogenesis is suspected. The typical clinical presentation is acute-onset paresis/plegia of the affected limb(s). The prognosis is guarded, and recovery, which is not guaranteed, requires a long period of time.

6. Both spinal cord and brainstem diseases can result in ataxia and paresis. Diseases affecting the brainstem should especially be noted because they can also result in impaired mental status and cranial nerve function.

8. Proprioceptive ataxia, due to the specific adjacency of the ascending proprioceptive fibers with the descending fibers of the upper motor neuron is frequently associated with a certain degree of paresis. Many superficial lesions of the spinal cord can result in proprioceptive ataxia without concomitant weakness.

9. Generalized neuromuscular disorders are characterized by weakness and the absence of primary ataxia. Based on the findings of the neurological examination, additional clinical differentiation in polymyopathies, neuromuscular junction disorders, and poly(radiculo) neuropathies is often not possible. The diagnostic workup is depicted in the flowchart of exercise intolerance.

7. Malignant peripheral nerve sheath tumors tend to have centripetal growth. In the event that they reach the spinal canal, the prognosis is poor. More distal MPNSTs can be surgically removed with amputation of the affected limb. Lateralized disc herniations can be surgically removed or conservatively treated with analgesic medications and non-steroid anti-inflammatory drugs. In the latter case healing usually takes much longer. Gabapentin can also be used.

SUGGESTED READINGS

- da Costa R. Ataxia, paresis, paralysis. In Ettinger SJ, Feldman EC, Côté E (editors). Textbook of Veterinary Internal Medicine 8th edition. St. Louis, Elsevier, 2017, pp 554-559.
- de Lahunta A, Glass E, Kent M. The neurological examination. In de Lahunta A, Glass E, Kent M (editors). De Lahunta's Veterinary Neuroanatomy and Clinical Neurology 5th edition. St Louis, Elsevier, 2020, pp 531-546.
- Dewey CW, da Costa R, Thomas WB. Performing the neurological examination. In Dewey CW, da Costa RC (editors). Practical Guide to Canine and Feline Neurology 3rd edition. Ames, Wiley Blackwell, 2015, pp 9-29.

GENERALIZED LYMPHADENOMEGALY

Laura Marconato

Generalized lymphadenomegaly is defined as the abnormal enlargement of >2 non-contiguous peripheral and/or visceral lymph nodes (LNs); it occurs more frequently in dogs, while it is rare in cats. Routinely palpable peripheral LNs in healthy dogs include mandibular, prescapular, inguinal, and popliteal LNs. LNs which may become palpable, if diseased, include facial, retropharyngeal, axillary, mesenteric, and sacral LNs.

In the case of localized lymphadenomegaly, the tissue drained by the enlarged LNs is most likely diseased. In the case of generalized lymphadenomegaly, systemic disease is usually present; the main differential diagnoses include reactive hyperplasia and cancer.

The first step of a diagnostic workup should be an accurate history, including travel to areas endemic to particular infectious diseases, exposure to possible infectious agents, recent immunization and medications, and reviewing the presence, severity, and duration of systemic signs. More often, the signs are non-specific or secondary to the compromise of adjacent organs/structures. If the flow of afferent lymph is disrupted, edema of the affected area is observed.

The severity of nodal enlargement should be noted (mild, moderate, severe), as well as whether enlarged LNs are firm, mobile, euthermic, or non-painful. In the case of lymphadenitis, LNs are typically soft and warm, and palpation is associated with discomfort.

Apart from blood and urinalysis, fine-needle aspiration of an enlarged LN is crucial. Normal LNs contain a heterogeneous lymphoid population, with the predominant cell type represented by small mature lymphocytes, making up 90-95% of the entire population. Fewer than 5% of the remaining cells are large lymphoid cells. Plasma and inflammatory cells are rare.

Only positive findings are useful for diagnostic purposes since the absence of cellular anomalies leads to an uncertain diagnosis. In case of doubt, it is necessary to biopsy the LN. Lymphadenectomy, instead of biopsy, is the preferred technique.

If an infectious disease is suspected, then specific etiologies must be confirmed by culture, serology, or PCR testing. Imaging (thoracic radiographs, abdominal ultrasound, and/or tetrahedron beam CT) is useful for refining a differential diagnosis list.

GENERALIZED LYMPHADENOMEGALY

Enlargement of >2 non-contiguous lymph nodes

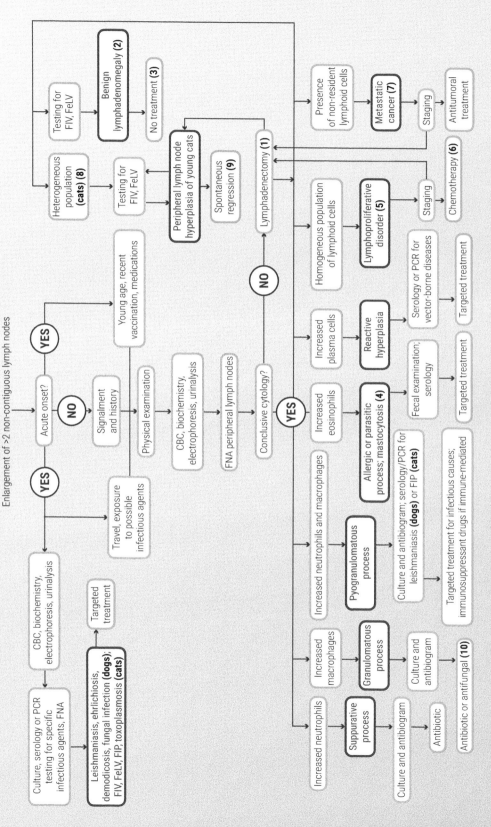

DIAGNOSTIC PROTOCOL

1. Lymphadenectomy provides a conclusive diagnosis in most cases. The entire lymph node should be removed instead of a biopsy. It allows for the examination of the overall structure of the organ and for highlighting areas affected by infiltrations of abnormal cells or the disappearance of normal structural elements. This is especially true in the case of lymphoma since lymphadenectomy allows obtaining the correct histotype and has prognostic and therapeutic relevance. Lymphadenectomy also provides a sufficient amount of tissue to be used for culture and to undergo special staining or clonal testing, if indicated. In addition to its diagnostic role, therapeutic and prognostic relevance has been documented for lymphadenectomy of the sentinel lymph node in dogs with mast cell tumors.

8. Atypical follicular lymphoid hyperplasia has been described in young cats, for which a retroviral cause has been hypothesized. A pleomorphic infiltrate of lymphocytes, plasma cells, and immunoblasts marks the lymph node. In the majority of cases, lymphadenomegaly is transient, requiring no treatment. However, progression to lymphoma has occasionally been reported.

DIAGNOSIS

2. In these cases, however, another possible differential diagnosis should be hypothesized. Small lymphocytic lymphoma is characterized by a homogeneous population of small lymphocytes, thus representing a diagnostic challenge. Flow cytometry and/or histopathology with immunohistochemistry and/or molecular testing should be carried out in doubtful cases.

4. In dogs with mast cell tumors, the occurrence of disseminated nodal metastasis has not been reported. Conversely, in cats with diffuse cutaneous mastocytosis, mast cells may be increased in the peripheral lymph nodes.

5. Lymphoproliferative disorders include lymphomas and leukemias. A complete staging workup should include a complete blood count with a differential, serum biochemistry profile, thoracic radiographs, abdominal ultrasound, cytologic evaluation of the liver and spleen regardless of the ultrasonographic appearance, and immunophenotype determined by flow cytometry on a lymph node aspirate, peripheral blood, and a bone marrow aspirate. Lymphadenectomy of a peripheral enlarged lymph node allows obtaining the lymphoma histotype.

7. Numerous solid cancers spread to the lymph nodes. Lymphadenectomy confirms the diagnosis and allows defining whether isolated neoplastic cells, micrometastasis, or macrometastasis are present. Staging and treatment depend on the type of cancer that has metastasized.

TREATMENT

3. If a small lymphocytic lymphoma is diagnosed, treatment should then be considered.

6. Chemotherapy is the gold standard for lymphomas and leukemias. Immunotherapy may be an option for some dogs, and consultation with an oncologist is necessary for evaluating all treatment options.

9. Some cats may need symptomatic treatment or immunosuppressive drugs.

10. Dermatopathic lymphadenopathy is a granulomatous lymphadenitis that occurs with skin disorders. Treatment depends on the cause.

SUGGESTED READINGS

- Brooks M, Harr K, Seelig D, Wardrop KJ, Weiss DJ (editors). Schalm's Veterinary Hematology 7th edition. Wiley Blackwell, 2022.
- Day MJ, Whitbread TJ. Pathological diagnoses in dogs with lymph node enlargement. *Vet Rec* 136:72-73, 1995.

HEART MURMUR

Serena Crosara

A heart murmur is a sound made by turbulent blood in or near the heart. This condition can be due to a reduction in blood viscosity, an increase in blood volume, or the presence of a shunt. A murmur can be caused by extracardiac causes, such as anemia, fever, hyperthyroidism, and others. A murmur is defined as "innocent" when it is not associated with cardiac disease; this category is typical of puppies and is systolic, left basal, low-intensity (I-II/VI) and usually disappears with growth. In cats, the presence of a cardiac murmur without a structural cardiac anomaly is frequent at any age; for this reason, the specificity and sensitivity of a cardiac murmur are very low and an echocardiogram is always required every time there is a cardiac murmur in a cat. Cardiac murmurs are defined based on the point of maximum intensity (PMI), duration and intensity. The PMI can be left basal (aortic and pulmonic valves, patent ductus arteriosus [PDA]), left apical (mitral valve), or right (tricuspid valve). In cats, most murmurs are audible along the sternum. Murmurs can be systolic (between the first and the second tone), diastolic (after the second tone or before the first tone), or continuous (during systole and diastole). Systolic murmurs are due to atrioventricular valve insufficiency, semilunar valve stenosis, or a left-to-right shunt ventricular septal defect (VSD). Diastolic murmurs are rare in pets and are due to semilunar valve insufficiency or atrioventricular valve stenosis. Continuous murmurs are due to left-to-right shunt PDA or a combination of systolic and diastolic murmurs (defined to-and-fro murmur). Intensity is based on the Levine scale. Murmurs can be very soft and difficult to hear (I/VI), soft but easily audible (II/VI), clearly audible and possibly irradiated (III/VI), loud (IV/VI); associated with a precordial thrill (V/VI) or audible without the stethoscope (VI/VI). The intensity of the murmur is not always correlated with the severity of the disease.

HEART MURMUR

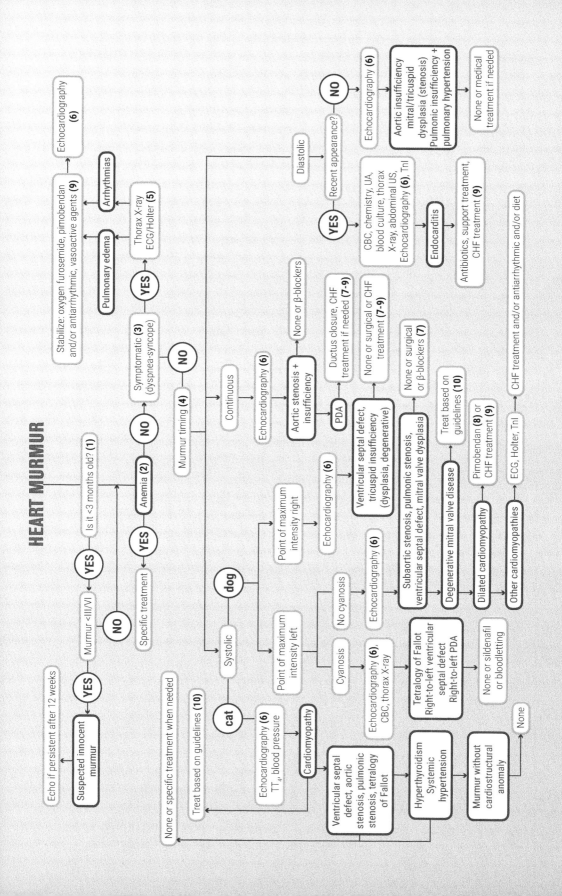

1. The approach to a heart murmur is different depending on the animal's age. It might be an innocent murmur if it is less than 3 months old. However, if the murmur is loud (≥III/VI) or associated with symptoms, or persists over time, congenital heart disease is likely.

3. If the heart murmur is associated with other symptoms, diagnostics should be addressed to define the origin and the severity of the condition. If dyspnea or cough are the main complaints, thoracic radiographs should be performed to rule out pulmonary edema. If syncope or weakness is present, an ECG and thoracic radiographs are recommended. Before the stabilization of the patient, a complete echocardiographic examination is not indicated.

4. The correct definition of a heart murmur in terms of localization, duration, and intensity is mandatory. A left basal continuous murmur is caused by a left-to-right PDA. A to-and-fro murmur (e.g., aortic stenosis and aortic insufficiency) could be mistaken for a continuous murmur. Diastolic murmurs are rare in small animals. When it is of recent appearance, bacterial endocarditis is the prime suspect. For the most part, it affects aortic and mitral valves; the trigger is the presence of any bacterial infection, and dogs with valvular disease are predisposed. Complete bloodwork, urinalysis, blood culture, abdominal ultrasound, and TnI are suggested. Systolic murmurs with the point of maximum intensity on the right chest could be due to tricuspid insufficiency or a ventricular septal defect. Left side systolic murmurs are mostly related to aortic, pulmonic, and mitral valves. Congenital disease is more likely in puppies; if cyanosis is present, tetralogy of Fallot, right-to-left shunt PDA, or a ventricular septal defect are the prime causes. If the animal is not cyanotic, the main differentials are aortic/subaortic stenosis, pulmonic stenosis (PS), mitral valve dysplasia, and a left-to-right ventricular septal defect. In adult dogs, a left systolic murmur is generally associated with mitral insufficiency. In large breed dogs, mitral insufficiency could be secondary to cardiomyopathy, while, in small-medium breed dogs, the most likely diagnosis is a chronic degenerative mitral valve disease (MMVD).

5. Thoracic radiographs are mandatory in the case of respiratory symptoms to rule out pulmonary edema or pulmonary congestion. A dilated cardiac silhouette could suggest cardiac disease underlying the respiratory symptoms. Holter or ECG monitoring is needed in the case of suspected arrhythmia.

6. Echocardiogram is the gold standard for diagnosing most cardiovascular diseases. Advanced diagnostics (e.g., transesophageal echocardiography, contrast study, angiography) may be needed to diagnose specific conditions.

DIAGNOSIS

2. Any systemic conditions which could cause a murmur should always be ruled out before a specialistic cardiologic consult. Anemia is a common cause of a cardiac murmur. In cats, frequent differentials are hyperthyroidism and systemic hypertension.

TREATMENT

7. Several congenital conditions (e.g., PDA, pulmonic stenosis, ventricular/atrial septal defects, tricuspid dysplasia) can be treated with minimally invasive/hybrid/thoracic surgery. The treatment can be curative or palliative, according to the case.

8. Pimobendan is indicated for treating asymptomatic dogs with chronic degenerative mitral valve disease stage ACVIM B2 and dogs with preclinical dilated cardiomyopathy. Both these conditions should be diagnosed by echocardiography before starting treatment.

9. Patients with symptoms of congestive heart failure should be treated with oxygen, loop diuretics, and pimobendan. Antiarrhythmic and vasoactive agents are used when needed.

10. Specific guidelines for managing chronic degenerative mitral valve disease and feline cardiomyopathies at different stages have been published.

SUGGESTED READINGS

- Keene BW, Atkins CE, Bonagura JD, et al. ACVIM consensus guidelines for the diagnosis and treatment of myxomatous mitral valve disease in dogs. *J Vet Intern Med* 33:1127-1140, 2019.
- Luis Fuentes V, Abbott J, Chetboul V, et al. ACVIM consensus statement guidelines for the classification, diagnosis, and management of cardiomyopathies in cats. *J Vet Intern Med* 34:1062-1077, 2020.
- Macdonald K. Infective endocarditis in dogs: diagnosis and therapy. *Vet Clin North Am Small Anim Pract* 40:665-684, 2010.
- Oliveira P, Domenech O, Silva J, et al. Retrospective review of congenital heart disease in 976 dogs. *J Vet Intern Med* 25:477-483, 2011.
- Summerfield NJ, Boswood A, O'Grady MR, et al. Efficacy of pimobendan in the prevention of congestive heart failure or sudden death in Doberman Pinschers with preclinical dilated cardiomyopathy (the PROTECT study). *J Vet Intern Med* 26:1337-1349, 2012.

HEMATEMESIS

Harry Swales

Hematemesis is defined as the process of vomiting blood from the gastrointestinal (GI) tract. "Pseudohematemesis" is an important differential diagnosis for hematemesis and commonly refers to vomiting blood that originated from outside of the GI tract, such as epistaxis or hemoptysis. Finally, repetitive bouts of vomiting can result in GI bleeding leading to "flecks" of blood admixed with vomit/saliva; this is not typically considered hematemesis in the strictest sense of the word.

Aspects of the history may help narrow differential diagnoses, such as recent administration of non-steroidal anti-inflammatory drugs (NSAIDs) and/or glucocorticoids or ingestion of a caustic substance. Sled dogs, as well as search and rescue dogs, can develop gastric ulceration and erosion (GUE) following strenuous exercise. Animals with hepatic disease also have an increased risk of GUE, although whether uremia is a risk factor for GUE remains controversial. The extent of the investigations into hematemesis depends on both the severity and duration of hematemesis.

As with all hemorrhages, it is important to differentiate between hemorrhage from a local lesion (e.g., gastric ulcer) and hemorrhage because of a coagulopathy (e.g., immune-mediated thrombocytopenia). Ruling out pseudohematemesis is essential and often overlooked. An important point of note is that causative lesions are often inconspicuous on endoscopy, especially in the presence of digested blood. No lesion should be overlooked, regardless of how insignificant it may appear.

Owing to a paucity of veterinary research into hematemesis, a number of protocols from human medicine are suggested in this chapter, which may have a theoretical benefit in animals, but have no evidence to support their use or safety in animals; these are denoted by (H). Furthermore, the causes of GI hemorrhage in human patients differ from those in animals, and consequently, the clinician should make a risk-benefit analysis.

Omitted from the recommendations is tranexamic acid (TXA), whose use is discouraged in human medicine, and limited evidence in animals does not suggest a benefit. TXA may also cause vomiting.

HEMATEMESIS (1)

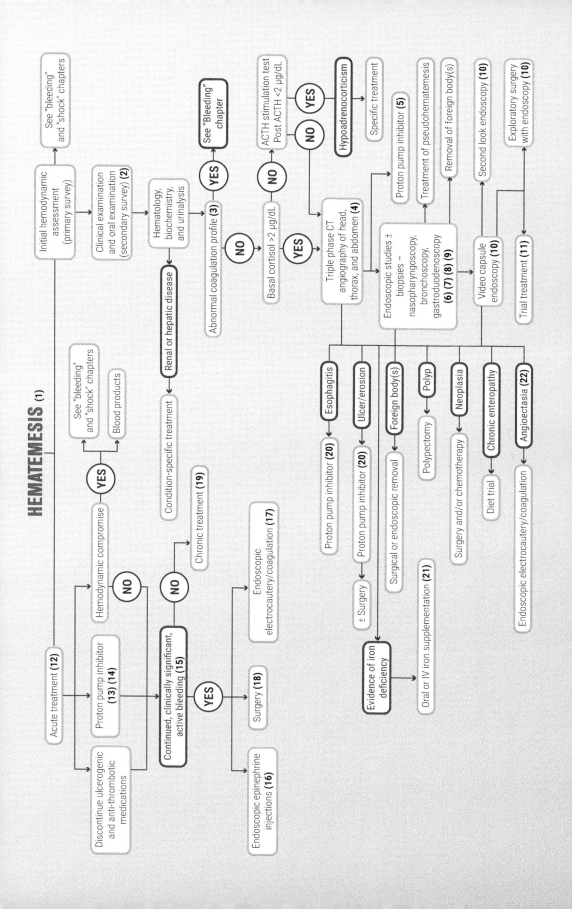

Initial hemodynamic assessment (primary survey) → See "bleeding" and "shock" chapters

Clinical examination and oral examination (secondary survey) (2)

Hematology, biochemistry, and urinalysis

Abnormal coagulation profile (3) — YES → See "Bleeding" chapter
— NO → Basal cortisol >2 μg/dL
— NO → ACTH stimulation test Post ACTH <2 μg/dL
— YES → **Hypoadrenocorticism** → Specific treatment
— NO → Proton pump inhibitor (5)
— YES → Triple phase CT angiography of head, thorax, and abdomen (4)
→ Treatment of pseudohematemesis
→ Removal of foreign body(s)

Endoscopic studies ± biopsies – nasopharyngoscopy, bronchoscopy, gastroduodenoscopy (6) (7) (8) (9)

Video capsule endoscopy (10) → Second look endoscopy (10)
→ Exploratory surgery with endoscopy (10)

Trial treatment (11)

Renal or hepatic disease → Condition-specific treatment → Chronic treatment (19)

Hemodynamic compromise — YES → See "bleeding" and "shock" chapters / Blood products
— NO →

Acute treatment (12)
Proton pump inhibitor (13) (14)
Discontinue ulcerogenic and anti-thrombotic medications

Continued, clinically significant, active bleeding (15)
— NO → Chronic treatment (19)
— YES → Surgery (18)
→ Endoscopic epinephrine injections (16)
→ Endoscopic electrocautery/coagulation (17)

Esophagitis → Proton pump inhibitor (20)

Ulcer/erosion → Proton pump inhibitor (20) → ± Surgery

Foreign body(s) → Surgical or endoscopic removal

Polyp → Polypectomy

Neoplasia → Surgery and/or chemotherapy

Chronic enteropathy → Diet trial

Angioectasia (22) → Endoscopic electrocautery/coagulation

Evidence of iron deficiency → Oral or IV iron supplementation (21)

1. Investigations and treatment are split into two pathways. The decision as to whether to follow these in a stepwise manner or simultaneously depends on the clinical presentation.

2. Clinical examination should assess for signs suggestive epistaxis or hemoptysis, which may suggest pseudohematemesis as well as signs of systemic coagulopathy. An in-depth oral examination should be repeated under a general anesthetic.

3. A basic coagulation profile should consist of platelet count, buccal mucosal bleeding time, APTT, PT, and fibrinogen (see "bleeding" chapter).

4. There is growing evidence regarding the benefit of CT angiography to investigate the GI tract. CT of the head and thorax will also help assess for signs of pseudohematemesis and abdominal CT of the stomach, duodenum, and liver. Recent evidence suggests that CT may be superior to ultrasound in the detection of perforated gastric ulcers and gastric neoplasia. If CT is not available, orthogonal head, thoracic, and abdominal radiographs may detect some abnormalities but have poor sensitivity for gastric ulceration.

6. (H) Administration of erythromycin (0.5-1 mg/kg IV) 30-120 minutes prior to endoscopy for GI hemorrhage improves lesion detection (H). Although this author has not used erythromycin in this setting, he has extensive experience with its use as a prokinetic agent.

7. If there is a high suspicion of gastric ulceration and erosion, or evidence is present on imaging, endoscopy should be performed cautiously with gentle insufflation and sampling to avoid inadvertent perforation.

8. The GI tract should be examined meticulously for evidence of hemorrhage. It is important to rotate the animal through each lateral recumbency in case lesions are hidden under gastric contents. Do not underestimate the clinical significance of a lesion.

9. As well as assessing the GI tract for evidence of hemorrhage, the respiratory tract (including nasopharynx) should be assessed for evidence of epistaxis or hemoptysis as causes of pseudohematemesis.

10. Video capsule endoscopy may provide better magnification of vascular lesions in the proximal small intestine. Allowing time for digested blood to clear may allow identification of lesions on a "second look" endoscopy. If the severity of hematemesis is enough to cause anemia, then exploratory celiotomy could be considered. However, the likelihood of finding a causative lesion is low. Intraoperative endoscopy may be of benefit.

DIAGNOSIS

15. That is not the result of a coagulopathy and is significant enough to warrant intervention.

22. Poorly described in animals.

TREATMENT

5. (H) Administration of a proton pump inhibitor (PPI) prior to endoscopy improves outcome in cases of GI bleeding (H).

11. Given the low yield of exploratory surgery, trial treatment could be considered.

12. Acute treatment may be indicated in animals with acute onset hematemesis and/or those with hemodynamic compromise.

13. IV PPI administration may not be necessary for non-acute or mild presentations.

14. (H) 1 mg/kg omeprazole or esomeprazole IV q12h for at least 72 hours (H).

16. (H) Endoscopic injection of 0.01 mg/kg of diluted (1:10,000-1:20,000) epinephrine in 0.5-2.0 mL aliquots around the base of an actively bleeding lesion has both vasoconstrictive and tamponade effects. It is not recommended as a sole treatment and is considered a temporary stopgap. Its efficacy has been demonstrated in animal models (H).

17. (H) If available (H).

18. If hemorrhage is severe enough to be life-threatening, non-abetting, and able to be addressed surgically, then surgical intervention may be warranted following hemodynamic stabilization.

19. If the presentation does not warrant acute treatment pathway or is a chronic presentation (see specific diagnoses).

20. 1 mg/kg omeprazole PO q12h for 4-6 weeks, tapering prior to discontinuation.

21. Oral iron absorption may be reduced in the presence of PPIs – consider packed red blood cell transfusion or (H) intravenous iron formulations (H).

SUGGESTED READINGS

-   Fitzgerald E, Barfield D, Lee KCL, et al. Clinical findings and results of diagnostic imaging in 82 dogs with gastrointestinal ulceration. *J Small Anim Pract* 58:211-218, 2017.
-   Marks SL, Kook PH, Papich MG, et al. ACVIM consensus statement: support for rational administration of gastrointestinal protectants in dogs and cats. *J Vet Intern Med* 32:1823-1840, 2018.
-   Stiller J, Defarges AM, Brisson BA, et al. Feasibility, complications, and quality of visualization using video capsule endoscopy in 40 dogs with overt or questionable gastrointestinal bleeding. *J Vet Intern Med* 35:1743-1753, 2021.
-   Willard, MD. Hemorrhage (Gastrointestinal). In Washabu RJ, Day MJ (editors). Canine and Feline Gastroenterology. St. Louis, Elsevier, 2013, pp 129-134.

HEMATURIA

Sofia Segatore

Hematuria means that excessive red blood cells (RBCs) are present in the urine. A low number of RBCs are usually found in the urine of dogs and cats; it is considered normal for up to 5 RBCs/HPF (high power field) on a free urine catch. However, the numbers may be increased when urine is collected by catheterization or cystocentesis (<20 RBC/HPF). Hematuria can be classified into microscopic (detectable only on a dipstick or microscopic examination) or macroscopic (grossly visible). An erythrocyte/hemoglobin dipstick is also positive in the presence of hemoglobinuria, methemoglobinuria, and myoglobinuria. Due to intravascular hemolysis, hemoglobinuria is expected to result in pink-tinged plasma, whereas plasma would be clear with myoglobinuria or hematuria. Hematuria is most often secondary to urinary or genital tract problems; however, it can be caused by systemic diseases (primary or secondary hemostatic diseases) or trauma. Several causes of hematuria have been reported; therefore, it is essential to investigate the patient's history, evaluate the signalment and carry out a thorough direct physical examination before starting a diagnostic protocol. It is important to investigate possible trauma, pharmacological treatment (e.g., cyclophosphamide), other sites of bleeding (melena, hematemesis, hemoptysis), or the presence of other urological clinical signs (such as pollakiuria, stranguria, and dysuria). Identifying at which stage of urination the hematuria occurs can help the clinician identify the problem site. In fact, initial hematuria suggests a problem affecting the prostate, urethra, penis, uterus, or vagina; terminal hematuria is more typical of prostatic or bladder problems, and constant hematuria suggests kidney or ureter disease (but sometimes bladder or prostate disorders). The only possible therapy for hematuria is identifying and resolving the underlying cause.

HEMATURIA

Hematuria → Microscopical examination of urine sediment: erythrocytes?

YES → Erythrocyte lysis → Unconcentrated urine (USG <1.015) o alkaline pH? **(2)**

NO → Positive dipstick heme reaction?

- **NO** → Is hemoglobinemia present? **(1)**
  - **NO** → Hemoglobinuria ± methemoglobinuria / Myoglobinuria
  - **YES** → **Intravascular hemolysis** → CBC, biochemistry, PT and aPTT, urinalysis

- Hemoglobinuria ± methemoglobinuria → **False-positive reaction (3)**
- Myoglobinuria → History, elevated creatine kinase and/or aspartate aminotransferase activity
  - **Excessive exertion**
  - **Muscular trauma**
  - → Fluid therapy and supportive treatments
- **Intravascular hemolysis** → Identify and treat the underlying cause, supportive care

Signalment and history →
- Estrus
- Trauma
- **Previous cyclophosphamide treatment (4)**

Physical examination →
- Enlarged prostate or kidney or urethral mass
- Vaginal or penile mass → Staging and, if possible, surgical treatment
- Prolapsed urethra (males)
- Other bleeding sites → Suspected coagulopathy

CBC, biochemistry, PT and aPTT, urinalysis →
- Bacteriuria ± active urine sediment
- Possibly normal
- Suspected coagulopathy → Thrombocytopenia or abnormal PT or aPTT? → **Primary or secondary hemostatic disorders** → Identify and treat the underlying cause

Imaging (X-ray ± contrast medium, abdominal US) →
- Normal → CT, video endoscopy → Normal → **Idiopathic renal hematuria (5)** → Sclerotherapy/ureteroscopy + endoscopic electrocautery
- **Urinary tract infection/pyelonephritis or prostatitis** → Quantitative urine culture or urine specimen testing pre- and postprostatic massage → Antibiotic treatment; if possible, choose antibiotic therapy according to an antibiogram
- **Urolithiasis (kidneys, ureters, bladder or urethra) (6)** → Quantitative urine culture → Medical and/or surgical approach depending on the presumed nature of the stones. If urinary tract infection is present, carry out antibiotic treatment based on an antibiogram
- **Feline idiopathic cystitis (cat) (7)** → Dietary therapy (wet diet), increase water intake and behavioral therapy
- **Benign prostatic hyperplasia** → Surgical or medical castration
- **Kidney, bladder, urethral or vaginal neoplasia** → CT, FNA + cytology or endoscopy + histology → Surgical treatment and/or chemotherapy
- **Prostatic neoplasia (8)** → CT, FNA + cytology or biopsy + histology → Chemotherapy and/or palliative therapy

1. Intravascular hemolysis occurs because of the direct lysis of red blood cells due to complement-activated antibodies, infectious agents, drugs or toxins, metabolic imbalances, or an increase in red blood cell fragmentation. In diagnosing hemoglobinemia, it is necessary to detect signs of hemolysis, such as suggestive changes in the blood smear, alterations of the iron profile, and a discrepancy between mean cellular hemoglobin concentration (MCHC) and the cellular hemoglobin concentration mean (CHCM) and/or the presence of hemoglobinuria. The features that allow differentiating the presence of hemoglobinuria from hematuria are a) hematocrit value (decreased versus normal); b) plasma color (pink to red versus normal); and c) red blood cells in the urine sediment (absent in hemoglobinuria versus present in hematuria).

2. Several laboratory studies in humans have investigated the best urine collection and storage methods. As a result of these studies, it was noted that the presence of red blood cells in hypo- or isosthenuric urine (urine specific gravity [USG] <1.015) or those having an alkaline pH decreasing over time during storage due to their lysis. Therefore, it is important to analyze the urine soon after its collection in patients with suspected hematuria or hemoglobinuria.

DIAGNOSIS

3. Falsely increased reactions may occur due to the presence of peroxidase-producing microorganisms and leukocytes within the urine tested or contamination of the sample with oxidizing compounds, such as hypochlorite (bleach).

4. Sterile hemorrhagic cystitis is a complication of cyclophosphamide administration due to the effect of direct urothelial irritation caused by acrolein (an inactive metabolite). The risk in dogs may depend on the protocol of cyclophosphamide administration and cumulative doses. Cats may be at a lower risk of developing sterile hemorrhagic cystitis; however, caution should be used when predisposing factors (e.g., feline idiopathic cystitis) are present. First and foremost, it is imperative to discontinue administering the causative agent indefinitely and confirm sterile hemorrhagic cystitis by ruling out other differentials.

5. Idiopathic renal hematuria is a rare condition seen in young large breed dogs; however, it has also been reported in older dogs and cats of various ages. This condition results in persistent red urine, and may be progressive, become bilateral, result in ureteral or urethral obstructions due to blood clots or result in progressive anemia. The lesion is usually of benign origin and can be an angioma, hemangioma, or an ulcerative lesion of the renal pelvis. Traditionally, ureteronephrectomy has been performed to treat this condition; however, >30% of affected animals develop bilateral disease over time.

6. A diagnosis of urolithiasis without predicting the composition of the uroliths is insufficient for optimally selecting an effective treatment. For predicting the urolith composition, survey radiography (first step), detection of stone prevalence, and identifying the breed and gender of the animal should be considered. In addition, a serum biochemistry profile should be carried out in patients with urolithiasis, especially for those with liver disease or urethral obstruction.

7. Feline idiopathic cystitis is commonly observed in younger and middle-aged cats. More than half of the cats with lower urinary tract signs have feline idiopathic cystitis. Risk factors include being overweight, young (<10 years), neutered/spayed, experiencing stress (such as a new house or another cat in the house, an increased number of cats in the household), a lower activity level, less water intake, using a single litter box and having less access to the exterior environment. The precise etiology and pathogenesis are unknown but are hypothesized to involve multiple factors, including increased bladder wall permeability, neurological abnormalities, stress, and environmental and genetic factors. Periuria, pollakiuria, stranguria, and gross hematuria are the most common clinical pathologies observed in cats with nonobstructive idiopathic cystitis and may precede the obstructive form of the disease. The diagnosis of feline idiopathic cystitis is reached by excluding the other causes which determine lower urinary tract signs. Up to 90% of cats with acute non-obstructive idiopathic cystitis resolve their clinical signs in a few days without treatment; therefore, diagnostics may not be needed for young cats presented for the first episode of lower urinary tract signs. However, relapses of clinical signs are frequent within one to two years after the initial episode, and additional evaluation is indicated for cats with recurrent signs.

8. Stranguria, dysuria, tenesmus, lumbar pain, and gait abnormalities are common clinical signs. Tumors are often detected after metastatic spread since clinical signs occur late. Postrenal azotemia can occur if the mass is obstructive, causing hydroureter and hydronephrosis. Ultrasonography and US-guided fine-needle aspiration or biopsy are helpful in reaching a diagnosis; however, histology is usually required to differentiate tumor type.

SUGGESTED READINGS

-   Ettinger SJ, Feldman EC, Côté E (editors). Textbook of Veterinary Internal Medicine 8th edition. St. Louis, Elsevier, 2017.
-   Kruger JM, Osborne CA, Lulich JP. Changing paradigms of feline idiopathic cystitis. *Vet Clin North Am Small Anim Pract* 39:15-40, 2009.
-   Nelson RW, Couto CG (editors). Small Animal Internal Medicine 6th edition. St. Louis, Elsevier, 2019.
-   Scott MA, Stockham SL (editors). Fundamentals of Veterinary Clinical Pathology 2nd edition. John Wiley & Sons, 2013.
-   Weiss DJ, Wardrop KJ (editors). Schalm's Veterinary Hematology 6th edition. John Wiley & Sons, 2011.

HYPERCALCEMIA

Carolina Arenas

Calcium is required for a number of intra- and extracellular functions, such as nerve conduction, neuromuscular transmission, muscle contraction, transport of substances across membranes, cell membrane excitability, blood clotting, cell growth, and division as well as skeletal support. The major part of the calcium in the body (>99%) is in the bone, which acts as a reservoir of calcium. Calcium is found in three forms in the circulation: ionized calcium (iCa), which is the biologically active form (approximately 55%), protein-bound calcium (35%, mainly albumin), and calcium complexed with anions (10%).

The regulation of serum calcium is complex and involves the parathyroid glands, kidneys, intestine, and bone. The main hormones involved in calcium regulation are the parathyroid hormone (PTH) and 1,25-dihydroxyvitamin D_3 (calcitriol). PTH secretion increases calcium concentrations by enhancing renal tubular reabsorption of calcium, resulting in less calcium loss in the urine, mobilizing calcium from skeletal reserves into the extracellular fluid, and increasing the production of 1,25-dihydroxyvitamin D_3, thus increasing the intestinal absorption of calcium. PTH also causes phosphaturia, which decreases serum phosphorus. Calcitriol enhances the intestinal absorption of calcium and phosphate and stimulates bone resorption, causing an additional increase in circulating calcium concentrations. Dogs and cats are dependent on vitamin D in their diet. Once in the circulation, it is metabolized to calcidiol (25-hydroxyvitamin D (25[OH]D), the major circulating form of vitamin D) before undergoing additional hydroxylation to calcitriol.

Clinical signs might result from the hypercalcemia itself, be due to the underlying disease-causing hypercalcemia, or a combination. Clinical signs vary upon the magnitude of the hypercalcemia, its duration, and the rate of onset. Electrolyte, acid-base, and renal dysfunction, which may arise due to hypercalcemia, could also contribute to the clinical signs. Clinical signs can be vague and non-specific and can include anorexia, lethargy, polyuria/polydipsia (most commonly), vomiting and constipation, muscular weakness and/or twitching/shivering, cardiac arrhythmias, hypertension, and seizures. Cats do not exhibit polyuria/polydipsia as often as dogs. Some animals (especially cats) may not show any clinical signs.

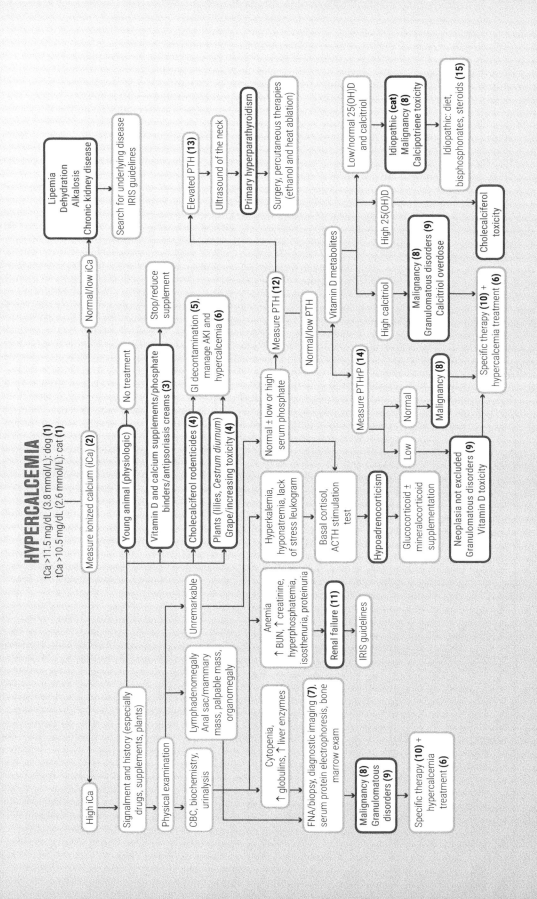

HYPERCALCEMIA

tCa >11.5 mg/dL (3.8 mmol/L): dog (1)
tCa >10.5 mg/dL (2.6 mmol/L): cat (1)

Measure Ionized calcium (iCa) (2)

High iCa

Normal/low iCa

Lipemia
Dehydration
Alkalosis
Chronic kidney disease

Search for underlying disease
IRIS guidelines

Signalment and history (especially drugs, supplements, plants)

Physical examination

Young animal (physiologic) → No treatment

Vitamin D and calcium supplements/phosphate binders/antipsoriasis creams (3) → Stop/reduce supplement

Cholecalciferol rodenticides (4) → GI decontamination (5), manage AKI and hypercalcemia (6)

Plants (lilies, *Cestrum diurnum*) Grape/increasing toxicity (4)

Lymphadenomegaly Anal sac/mammary mass, palpable mass, organomegaly

CBC, biochemistry, urinalysis

Unremarkable

Cytopenia, ↑ globulins, ↑ liver enzymes

FNA/biopsy, diagnostic imaging (7), serum protein electrophoresis, bone marrow exam

Malignancy (8) Granulomatous disorders (9)

Specific therapy (10) + hypercalcemia treatment (6)

Anemia ↑ BUN, ↑ creatinine, hyperphosphatemia, isosthenuria, proteinuria

Renal failure (11)

IRIS guidelines

Hyperkalemia, hyponatremia, lack of stress leukogram

Basal cortisol, ACTH stimulation test

Hypoadrenocorticism

Glucocorticoid ± mineralocorticoid supplementation

Neoplasia not excluded Granulomatous disorders (9) Vitamin D toxicity

Normal ± low or high serum phosphate

Measure PTH (12)

Elevated PTH (13)

Ultrasound of the neck

Primary hyperparathyroidism

Surgery, percutaneous therapies (ethanol and heat ablation)

Normal/low PTH

Measure PTHrP (14)

Low

Normal → Malignancy (8)

Vitamin D metabolites

Specific therapy (10) + hypercalcemia treatment (6)

High calcitriol → Malignancy (8) Granulomatous disorders (9) Calcitriol overdose

High 25(OH)D → Cholecalciferol toxicity

Low/normal 25(OH)D and calcitriol

Idiopathic (cat) (8) Malignancy (8) Calcipotriene toxicity

Idiopathic: diet, bisphosphonates, steroids (15)

DIAGNOSTIC PROTOCOL

1. When the product of total serum calcium (tCa) × phosphorus (mg/dL) exceeds 70, mineralization and nephrotoxicity are likely. Do not use adjustment formulas to correct the tCa.

2. The serum iCa concentration is approximately 4.5-5.5 mg/dL (1.1-1.4 mmol/L). The serum is typically used for iCa measurement; however, heparinized plasma or whole blood (lower values than serum) can be used. Do not use EDTA plasma since it chelates calcium.

7. Abdominal ultrasound, thoracic and/or bone radiographs should be evaluated for cranial mediastinal masses, thoracic metastasis, lytic lesions in the vertebrae or long bones, osteoporosis, and organomegaly. These could indicate malignancy-associated hypercalcemia and/or granulomatous disease.

12. PTH should be evaluated relative to the serum calcium concentration.

13. A PTH level above the reference range or in the upper half of the reference range in the presence of hypercalcemia is consistent with primary hyperparathyroidism.

14. Parathyroid hormone-related protein (PTHrP) is secreted by some types of cancer cells. It has the same physiological effects as PTH.

DIAGNOSIS

3. Vitamin D toxicosis can be chronic (as it may develop with the ingestion of supplements or antipsoriasis-containing calcipotriol and calcipotriene creams) and may require weeks until clinical signs develop.

4. Acute vitamin D toxicity seems to be the most common form of toxicosis in dogs and cats. It can cause hypercalcemia, acute kidney injury (AKI), and soft tissue mineralization.

8. The most frequent neoplasias causing hypercalcemia are lymphoma and adenocarcinoma of the apocrine glands of the anal sac (in dogs). Other neoplasias reported are multiple myeloma, mammary carcinoma, squamous cell carcinoma, lung carcinoma, thymoma, and malignant melanoma. Causes of hypercalcemia include PTHrP secretion, bone resorption by hematologic tumors present in the bone, and metastasis to the bone.

9. Some granulomatous diseases associated with hypercalcemia are: blastomycosis, aspergillosis, schistosomiasis, hepatozoonosis, histoplasmosis, *Angiostrongylus* spp., nocardiosis, and panniculitis.

11. The presence of concurrent azotemia, hyperphosphatemia, and hypercalcemia might represent a diagnostic dilemma, as hypercalcemia could be the cause or the consequence of renal disease. Other tests might be necessary to support a diagnosis of renal disease (UP/C, abdominal ultrasound to evaluate renal size, echotexture, and architecture) (see the chapter on "azotemia").

TREATMENT

5. Decontamination by emesis or gastric lavage if <2-3 hours of exposure. In case of cholecalciferol rodenticide ingestion, activated charcoal should be used q4-6h during the first 24 hours since it enters the enterohepatic circulation.

6. Management of acute or severe hypercalcemia:
   6.1. Fluid therapy: it is the first-line treatment for all patients with hypercalcemia. Fluid therapy enhances renal calcium excretion. Sodium chloride 0.9% is the fluid of choice.
   6.2. Furosemide (following rehydration): it promotes additional calciuresis. Dose: 2-4 mg/kg IV, IM, SC, PO q8-12h.
   6.3. Sodium bicarbonate. It is useful in patients who remain acidotic despite adequate rehydration.
   6.4. Glucocorticoids: they increase calciuresis and decrease bone resorption. They cause rapid tumor lysis and reduce the secretion of PTHrP. They should be avoided when a diagnosis has not been reached. Dosage: prednisolone 1-2 mg/kg IV, PO q12h or dexamethasone 0.1-0.2 mg/kg IV, SC q12h.
   6.4. Salmon calcitonin: it inhibits osteoclasts activity. Typically given when a diagnosis has not been reached instead of glucocorticoids. It has a rapid effect. Resistance to it may develop in a few days. Dosage: 4 U/kg IV followed by 4-6 U/kg SC q12-24h.
   6.6. Bisphosphonates: they inhibit bone resorption. Pamidronate: 1-2 mg/kg IV over 2 h. Onset action: 1-4 days. Zoledronate: 0.25 mg/kg IV over 15 minutes. Alendronate: 2-4 mg/kg PO once weekly.

10. Treatment of the underlying disease may indirectly decrease serum calcium concentrations.

15. High fiber diets, renal diets, and diets formulated for the management of calcium oxalate might be useful. Wet diets can be used to increase water consumption and dilute the urine, promoting calciuresis. If diet fails to normalize the calcium, bisphosphonates (e.g., alendronate) can be used. If hypercalcemia does not resolve with bisphosphonates, glucocorticoids can be used.

SUGGESTED READINGS

- Feldman EC, Nelson RW, Reusch CE, Scott-Moncrieff JCR, Behrend E (editors). Canine and Feline Endocrinology 4th edition. St. Louis, Elsevier, 2015.
- Galvao JB, Schenck P, Chew D. A quick reference on hypercalcemia. *Vet Clin North Am Small Anim Pract* 47:241-248, 2017.
- Graves TK. Hypercalcemia. In Feldman EC, Fracassi F, Peterson ME (editors). Feline Endocrinology. Milan, Edra, 2019, pp. 579-591.
- Skelly B. Primary hyperparathyroidism. In Ettinger SJ, Feldman EC, Côté E (editors). Textbook of Veterinary Internal Medicine 8th edition. St. Louis, Elsevier, 2017, pp 1715-1727.

HYPERGLOBULINEMIA

Eugenio Faroni

Hyperglobulinemia can be due to several conditions, such as inflammatory, infectious, or neoplastic diseases, and it is the main cause of increased total protein concentration.

Serum globulin concentration is not measured but is calculated by subtracting serum albumin concentration from total serum protein concentration, both of which are obtained using standard biochemical assays. Any laboratory error causing erroneous total protein and/or albumin measurement will interfere with globulin concentration estimates and should prompt careful evaluation.

When hyperproteinemia is recorded, evaluation of the albumin to globulin (A:G) ratio is mandatory for differentiating panhyperproteinemia (normal A:G ratio), which derives from hemoconcentration due to dehydration, from selective hyperproteinemia (shifted A:G ratio). A decreased A:G ratio is usually due to an increase in globulin concentration.

Globulins include immunoglobulins (IgG, IgM, IgA, and IgE), which represent the main component, and several other proteins with a role in oncotic support, blood buffering, hormone and drug transport, and coagulation. Increased globulin concentration is generally due to increased production, which may be a consequence of antigenic stimulation (from infectious or inflammatory diseases) or may be caused by production of clones of an immunoglobulin (or part of it) by B-cell lymphoma/leukemia or plasma cell neoplasm.

Serum protein electrophoresis helps to accurately separate globulin fractions by allowing the classification of a patient's hyperglobulinemia in one of the diagnostic categories used in veterinary medicine: acute-phase protein response, polyclonal gammopathy, restricted polyclonal/oligoclonal gammopathy, and monoclonal gammopathy. However, it is known that different diseases can produce very similar electrophoretic patterns. Medical history, physical examination, blood and urine tests, diagnostic imaging, or more specific tests based on clinical suspicion should all be considered and correlated with the electrophoretic pattern to define the cause of hyperglobulinemia.

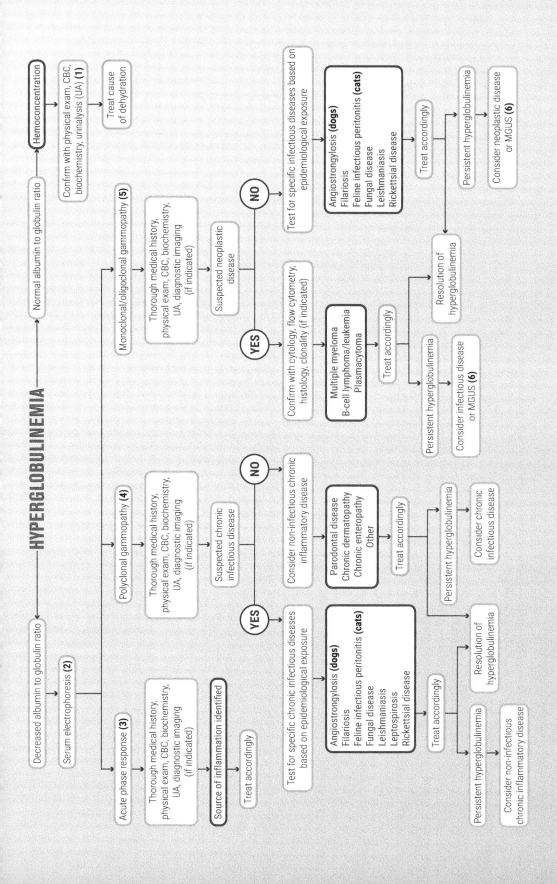

HYPERGLOBULINEMIA

Decreased albumin to globulin ratio

Normal albumin to globulin ratio

Hemoconcentration

Confirm with physical exam, CBC, biochemistry, urinalysis (UA) **(1)**

Treat cause of dehydration

Serum electrophoresis **(2)**

Acute phase response **(3)**

Thorough medical history, physical exam, CBC, biochemistry, UA, diagnostic imaging (if indicated)

Source of inflammation identified

Treat accordingly

Polyclonal gammopathy **(4)**

Thorough medical history, physical exam, CBC, biochemistry, UA, diagnostic imaging (if indicated)

Suspected chronic infectious disease

YES

Test for specific chronic infectious diseases based on epidemiological exposure

Angiostrongylosis **(dogs)**
Filariosis
Feline infectious peritonitis **(cats)**
Fungal disease
Leishmaniasis
Leptospirosis
Rickettsial disease

Treat accordingly

Resolution of hyperglobulinemia

Persistent hyperglobulinemia

Consider non-infectious chronic inflammatory disease

NO

Consider non-infectious chronic inflammatory disease

Parodontal disease
Chronic dermatopathy
Chronic enteropathy
Other

Treat accordingly

Persistent hyperglobulinemia

Consider chronic infectious disease

Monoclonal/oligoclonal gammopathy **(5)**

Thorough medical history, physical exam, CBC, biochemistry, UA, diagnostic imaging (if indicated)

Suspected neoplastic disease

YES

Confirm with cytology, flow cytometry, histology, clonality (if indicated)

Multiple myeloma
B-cell lymphoma/leukemia
Plasmacytoma

Treat accordingly

Resolution of hyperglobulinemia

Persistent hyperglobulinemia

Consider infectious disease or MGUS **(6)**

NO

Test for specific infectious diseases based on epidemiological exposure

Angiostrongylosis **(dogs)**
Filariosis
Feline infectious peritonitis **(cats)**
Fungal disease
Leishmaniasis
Rickettsial disease

Treat accordingly

Persistent hyperglobulinemia

Consider neoplastic disease or MGUS **(6)**

DIAGNOSTIC PROTOCOL

1. Hemoconcentration due to dehydration is one of the main causes of hyperproteinemia. In order to confirm suspected hemoconcentration, panhyperproteinemia should be correlated with clinical findings (e.g., loss of skin elasticity, dry mucous membranes, sunken eyes) and/or blood and urine test abnormalities, such as increased hematocrit, azotemia with high urinary specific gravity, or increased sodium concentration. The focus should be placed on determining and treating the cause of dehydration.

2. There are different methods for obtaining electrophoretic separation of proteins into fractions based on size and charge, and the most common are agarose gel electrophoresis, cellulose acetate electrophoresis, and capillary zone electrophoresis. The capillary zone method is considered to be more accurate; however, for the most part, the results are mostly similar in all methods. It is important to note that every method needs specific reference intervals. In dogs and cats, the typical electrophoretic pattern allows the distinction of albumin, and α1, α2, β1, β2 and γ globulins. Hemolysis-hemoglobin and lipemia may interfere with the electrophoretic pattern in the β-globulin and α-globulin regions, respectively. Fibrinogen and other clotting proteins may cause a peak in the β-globulin region when protein electrophoresis is performed on plasma and not on serum samples.

3. Although rare, increased production of acute-phase proteins (APPs), such as haptoglobin, ceruloplasmin, C-reactive protein, serum amyloid A, α1-lipoprotein, or α2-macroglobulin, may cause hyperglobulinemia. Most APPs migrate in the α-globulin fraction of the electrophoretic pattern, thereby causing a typical acute-phase response pattern characterized by an α-globulin peak. Inflammation also usually down-regulates the production of negative-phase proteins, such as albumin and transferrin, possibly causing a decrease in the albumin peak. This electrophoretic pattern is not pathognomic for any cause of inflammation and should be correlated with other findings.

4. Chronic antigenic stimulation is responsible for the increased production of immunoglobulins of different sizes and charges by multiple plasma cell lineages. A typical electrophoretic pattern is represented by a broad-based peak ranging from β-globulin to γ-globulin fractions. Although chronic hepatopathies have also been reported, chronic infectious and chronic non-infectious inflammatory diseases are the main causes of polyclonal gammopathies.

5. Single peaks as high as or higher than, and as narrow as or narrower than the albumin peak, or peaks with a height:width ratio of 4:1 should be considered a monoclonal gammopathy pattern. A less typical pattern is biclonal gammopathy, in which two restricted bands are found on the electrophoretic tract; however, its distinction from a true monoclonal pattern is usually not clinically relevant. Monoclonal gammopathies typically derive from the increased neoplastic production of a single immunoglobulin by clonal expansion of a single B-lymphocyte or plasma cell. Interestingly, primary hyperparathyroidism has been reported to be a cause of monoclonal gammopathy. It is important to note that the antibodies produced during infectious diseases may sometimes be so similar in size and charge that they migrate in the same fraction, causing a narrow band spike on a broad polyclonal base, a pattern called oligoclonal (or restricted polyclonal) gammopathy, which is very similar to the monoclonal track. Protein electrophoresis is rarely capable of reliably differentiating monoclonal from oligoclonal gammopathies, requiring a comprehensive view of the case by the clinician.

6. The term monoclonal gammopathy of unknown significance (MGUS) is used in human medicine to identify a single and distinct monoclonal peak on the electrophoretic tract after the exclusion of a neoplastic disease. MGUS has rarely been reported in veterinary medicine, and its diagnosis relies on a confirmed monoclonal pattern at protein electrophoresis without any clinical or clinicopathological evidence of a neoplastic or infectious disease. In human medicine, MGUS is considered to be a pre-malignant state and requires life-long monitoring since some patients may develop multiple myeloma.

SUGGESTED READINGS

-   Burton S. Hypoproteinemia, hyperproteinemia. In Ettinger SJ, Feldman EC, Côté E (editors). Textbook of Veterinary Internal Medicine 8th edition. St. Louis, Elsevier, 2017, pp. 243-245.
-   McGrotty Y, Bell R, McLauchlan G. Disorders of plasma proteins. In Villiers E, Ristic J (editors). BSAVA Manual of Canine and Feline Clinical Pathology 3rd edition. Gloucester, British Small Animal Veterinary Association, 2016, pp. 123-141.
-   Moore AR, Avery PR. Protein characterization using electrophoresis and immunofixation; a case-based review of dogs and cats. *Vet Clin Pathol* 48 Suppl 1:29-44, 2019.
-   Stockham SL, Scott MA. Fundamentals of Veterinary Clinical Pathology 2nd edition. Ames, Blackwell publishing, 2008.

HYPERGLYCEMIA

Lucy Davison

Hyperglycemia is defined by a blood glucose value above the reference range, typically >117 mg/dL (6.5 mmol/L) in dogs and >130 mg/dL in cats (7.2 mmol/L). Mild or transient hyperglycemia is most commonly encountered in stressed animals and is rarely associated with any clinical signs. In contrast, persistent hyperglycemia in dogs and cats is most commonly associated with diabetes mellitus, which can progress to life-threatening diabetic ketoacidosis (DKA) or hyperglycemic hyperosmolar syndrome (HHS) if not treated.

Blood glucose homeostasis depends on a range of hormones, as well as the interaction between food absorption, storage of glycogen in the liver and skeletal muscles, and production of glucose from amino acids in the liver by gluconeogenesis. Insulin is released from the beta cells of the pancreas during periods of hyperglycemia. Activation of the insulin receptor results in the co-transport of glucose with potassium from the bloodstream into cells. Insulin is antagonized by several hormones, including glucagon, cortisol, growth hormone, progestogens, and catecholamines, all of which are able to elevate blood glucose via their effects on glucose metabolism and insulin sensitivity. Dogs and cats with conditions associated with high levels of insulin-antagonistic hormones (e.g., hyperadrenocorticism, hypersomatotropism, diestrus) are likely to be hyperglycemic. Obesity, particularly in cats, can also be associated with insulin resistance and hyperglycemia. Transient stress hyperglycemia, which is particularly common in cats, arises from the combined activity of cortisol and adrenaline.

The most common cause of persistent hyperglycemia in dogs and cats is diabetes mellitus. Diabetes is a heterogeneous group of diseases with multiple etiologies, characterized by hyperglycemia resulting from inadequate insulin secretion, inadequate insulin action, or both. Recently agreed criteria for diagnosis of diabetes in dogs (European Society for Veterinary Endocrinology (ESVE) Project ALIVE https://www.esve.org/alive/search.aspx) include documentation of a random (fasted or unfasted) BG ≥200 mg/dL (11.1 mmol/L) in the presence of classic clinical signs of hyperglycemia (with no other plausible cause) or hyperglycemic crisis. Where BG is >126 mg/dL (7 mmol/L) ≤200 mg/dL (11.1 mmol/L), diabetes is differentiated from stress hyperglycemia in dogs by documentation of persistent fasting hyperglycemia for more than 24 hours or increased glycated proteins.

In cats, the criteria for diabetes mellitus diagnosis are more stringent due to the higher prevalence of stress hyperglycemia in this species, which may result in a blood glucose value above 360 mg/dL (20 mmol/L). Feline diabetes mellitus is suspected where a random (fasted or unfasted) BG is ≥270 mg/dL (15 mmol/L) accompanied by classic clinical signs of hyperglycemia (with no other plausible cause) or hyperglycemic crisis. However, to confirm a diagnosis, and address the possibility of stress hyperglycemia masquerading as diabetes, documentation of increased glycated proteins or repeated glycosuria on a naturally voided sample acquired in a home environment must be undertaken. Where BG is >126 mg/dL (7 mmol/L) ≤270 mg/dL (15 mmol/L), both an elevation in glycated proteins and glycosuria must be documented for diabetes to be diagnosed.

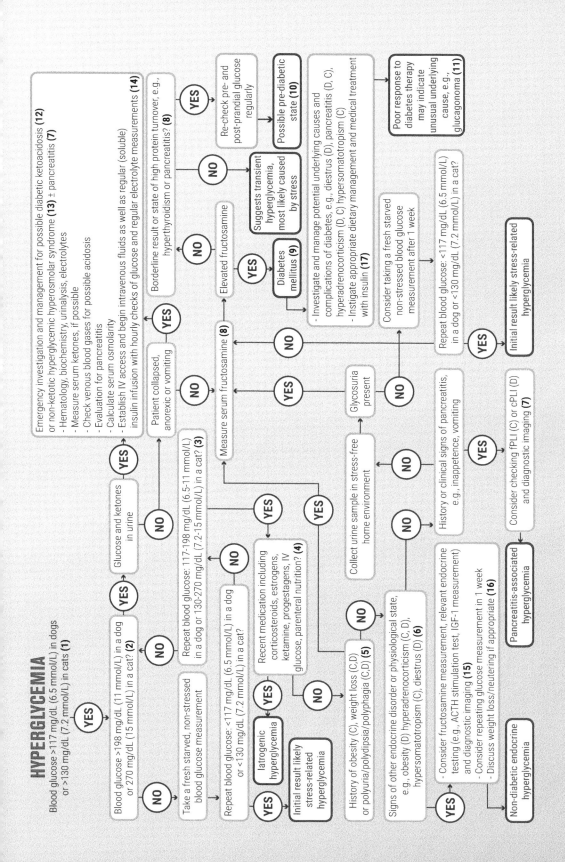

HYPERGLYCEMIA

Blood glucose >117 mg/dL (6.5 mmol/L) in dogs or >130 mg/dL (7.2 mmol/L) in cats **(1)**

Blood glucose >198 mg/dL (11 mmol/L) in a dog or 270 mg/dL (15 mmol/L) in a cat? **(2)**

YES → Glucose and ketones in urine

YES → Glucose and ketones in urine

YES → Emergency investigation and management for possible diabetic ketoacidosis **(12)** or non-ketotic hyperglycemic hyperosmolar syndrome **(13)** ± pancreatitis **(7)**
- Hematology, biochemistry, urinalysis, electrolytes
- Measure serum ketones, if possible
- Check venous blood gases for possible acidosis
- Evaluation for pancreatitis
- Calculate serum osmolarity
- Establish IV access and begin intravenous fluids as well as regular (soluble) insulin infusion with hourly checks of glucose and regular electrolyte measurements **(14)**

NO → Borderline result or state of high protein turnover, e.g., hyperthyroidism or pancreatitis? **(8)**

YES → Re-check pre- and post-prandial glucose regularly → Possible pre-diabetic state **(10)**

NO → Suggests transient hyperglycemia, most likely caused by stress

Measure serum fructosamine **(8)**

Elevated fructosamine

YES → Diabetes mellitus **(9)** → Investigate and manage potential underlying causes and complications of diabetes, e.g., diestrus (D), pancreatitis (D, C), hyperadrenocorticism (D, C) hypersomatotropism (C)
- Instigate appropriate dietary management and medical treatment with insulin **(17)**

Poor response to diabetes therapy may indicate unusual underlying cause, e.g., glucagonoma **(11)**

NO → Patient collapsed, anorexic or vomiting

YES →

NO →

Consider taking a fresh starved non-stressed blood glucose measurement after 1 week

Repeat blood glucose: <117 mg/dL (6.5 mmol/L) in a dog or <130 mg/dL (7.2 mmol/L) in a cat?

YES → Initial result likely stress-related hyperglycemia

NO → Take a fresh starved, non-stressed blood glucose measurement

Repeat blood glucose: 117-198 mg/dL (6.5-11 mmol/L) in a dog or 130-270 mg/dL (7.2-15 mmol/L) in a cat? **(3)**

NO → Repeat blood glucose: <117 mg/dL (6.5 mmol/L) in a dog or < 130 mg/dL (7.2 mmol/L) in a cat?

YES → Iatrogenic hyperglycemia

NO → Initial result likely stress-related hyperglycemia

YES → Recent medication including corticosteroids, estrogens, ketamine, progestagens, IV glucose, parenteral nutrition? **(4)**

YES → Iatrogenic hyperglycemia

NO → History of obesity (C), weight loss (C,D) or polyuria/polydipsia/polyphagia (C,D) **(5)**

YES → Signs of other endocrine disorder or physiological state, e.g., obesity (D) hyperadrenocorticism (C, D), hypersomatotropism (C), diestrus (D) **(6)**

YES → - Consider fructosamine measurement, relevant endocrine testing (e.g. ACTH stimulation test, IGF-1 measurement) and diagnostic imaging **(15)**
- Consider repeating glucose measurement in 1 week
- Discuss weight loss/neutering if appropriate **(16)**

→ Non-diabetic endocrine hyperglycemia

NO → Glycosuria present

YES →

NO → Collect urine sample in stress-free home environment

NO → History or clinical signs of pancreatitis, e.g., inappetence, vomiting

YES → Consider checking fPLI (C) or cPLI (D) and diagnostic imaging **(7)**

→ Pancreatitis-associated hyperglycemia

DIAGNOSTIC PROTOCOL

1. This algorithm applies to canine and feline patients who have not previously been diagnosed with diabetes mellitus. Every attempt should be made to minimize stress to the animal undergoing blood sampling (especially cats) because of the risk of cortisol and adrenaline release leading to stress hyperglycemia. If a sample from a hyperglycemic patient is stored before analysis, the result may be artefactually low since the erythrocytes continue to consume glucose unless the sample is preserved in a fluoride oxalate tube. Point-of-care glucometers for evaluating blood glucose must also be used with care, ensuring the correct volume of blood is used and a meter calibrated for veterinary species.

2. Setting a threshold minimizes the risk of stress hyperglycemia being diagnosed as diabetes mellitus, but as cats are more susceptible to this phenomenon, thresholds are different for dogs and cats.

3. This glucose threshold is set by the European Society for Veterinary Endocrinology ALIVE criteria for diagnosis of diabetes. In this blood glucose range, diabetes may be suspected but must be confirmed by further robust diagnostic criteria.

4. A range of different pharmacological agents and the use of total parenteral nutrition can all cause hyperglycemia, which usually resolves when the agent is withdrawn. Corticosteroid treatment should not be withdrawn suddenly.

5. Clinical signs associated with diabetes mellitus are part of the ESVE/ALIVE diagnostic criteria, but it should be noted that the signs listed are not unique to diabetes.

6. Clinical signs of hyperadrenocorticism may include thin skin (skin tearing in cats), bilaterally symmetrical alopecia, and a pot-bellied appearance. Signs of hypersomatotropism may include a large tongue, altered facial appearance, renomegaly, and widened inter-dental spaces.

7. Diagnostic tests for pancreatitis have relatively poor sensitivity and specificity. Pancreatitis may appear clinically silent in some cases.

8. Fructosamine is glycosylated albumin and reflects the average blood glucose concentration during the preceding 1-2 weeks. Persistent hyperglycemia leads to high fructosamine concentration. Increased protein turnover may artefactually reduce fructosamine concentration.

DIAGNOSIS

9. See ESVE/ALIVE diagnostic criteria and definitions for a diagnosis of diabetes to be confirmed in a dog or cat.

10. According to the ESVE/ALIVE criteria, pre-diabetes in human medicine is defined as hyperglycemia below the cut-off for diabetes mellitus and/or impaired glucose tolerance. This definition may also be applicable for dogs and cats with hyperglycemia and diagnostic criteria below the cut-off for diabetes. In these cases, further future monitoring and avoidance of potential environmental triggers of fulminant diabetes may be appropriate, e.g., neutering entire female dogs or encouraging weight loss in overweight cats.

11. Glucagonoma is a very rare glucagon-secreting neuroendocrine tumor of the alpha cells of the pancreas. Glucagonoma patients may also present with crusting erythematous exudative skin lesions (superficial necrolytic dermatitis).

TREATMENT

12. Diabetic ketoacidosis (DKA) is characterized by the presence of profound hyperglycemia and elevation of serum beta-hydroxybutyrate and/or acetoacetate, as well as metabolic acidosis on venous blood gas analysis. Concurrent disorders, e.g., urinary tract infection, pyometra, pancreatitis, and hyperadrenocorticism, are common in DKA patients. DKA is a life-threatening complication of diabetes mellitus, more common in dogs than cats, and requires early recognition and intensive in-patient therapy.

13. Hyperglycemic hyperosmolar syndrome (HHS) is characterized by severe hyperglycemia (>600 mg/dL or >33.3 mmol/L) and serum osmolality >350 mOsm/kg. Osmolality is calculated by [Osm = (Na + K) 2 + Glu/18] with the glucose concentration in mg/dL. HHS is a life-threatening complication of diabetes mellitus, more common in dogs than cats. Similar to DKA, HHS requires early recognition and intensive in-patient therapy.

14. Glucose and potassium are co-transported into cells in the presence of insulin, so it is important to monitor for potential hypokalemia in hyperglycemic animals receiving an insulin infusion. Care must also be taken to avoid rapid changes in osmolality, which may result in neurological signs due to myelinolysis.

15. Therapy for hypersomatotropism (acromegaly) may include radiation, hypophysectomy, or injectable somatostatin agonists, as well as insulin if the cat is diabetic. Therapy for hyperadrenocorticism may include medical management with trilostane or surgical adrenalectomy or hypophysectomy. Whilst not all cats with hypersomatotropism or hyperadrenocorticism have concurrent diabetes, the majority of cats will. Serum IGF-1 will usually be elevated in cats with hypersomatotropism but may not reach maximum concentration in diabetic cats until 6-8 weeks after beginning insulin therapy, so borderline results may require re-testing. Diagnostic imaging may include evaluation of adrenals, pancreas, or pituitary gland, dependent on which disorder is suspected.

16. Weight loss in cats and neutering in entire female dogs reduces the potential for further insulin resistance and diabetes mellitus to develop in the future.

17. Treatment with insulin, reduced carbohydrate diet, and weight loss in cats can lead to diabetes remission. Diabetes is likely to be permanent in dogs, even if an underlying cause can be identified and addressed. Regular blood glucose and fructosamine monitoring are required lifelong. Continuous interstitial glucose monitoring with a subcutaneous sensor can provide an excellent alternative to repeated venipuncture during diabetes management.

SUGGESTED READINGS

- Behrend E, Holford A, Lathan P, et al. 2018 AAHA Diabetes Management Guidelines for Dogs and Cats. *J Am Anim Hosp Assoc* 54:1-21, 2018.
- Frezoulis PS, Oikonomidis IL, Saridomichelakis MN, Kasabalis D, et al. Prevalence, association with systemic inflammatory response syndrome and outcome of stress hyperglycaemia in sick cats. *J Small Anim Pract* 63:197-202, 2022.
- Gilor C, Niessen SJ, Furrow E, DiBartola SP. What's in a name? Classification of diabetes mellitus in veterinary medicine and why it matters. *J Vet Intern Med* 30:927-940, 2016.
- Hagley SP, Hopper K, Epstein SE. Etiology and prognosis for dogs with abnormal blood glucose concentrations evaluated in an emergency room. *J Vet Emerg Crit Care (San Antonio)* 30:567-573, 2020.
- Thomovsky E. Fluid and electrolyte therapy in diabetic ketoacidosis. *Vet Clin North Am Small Anim Pract* 47:491-503, 2017.

HYPERKALEMIA

Federica Alessandrini

Hyperkalemia is defined as a serum potassium concentration that exceeds 5.5 mEq/L, becoming a life-threatening disorder when the serum potassium exceeds 7.5 mEq/L. Clinical signs depend on the severity of the potassium concentration, and usually, the greater the potassium concentration, the more severe the symptoms. The main effect of hyperkalemia occurs at the neuromuscular cell membrane due to depolarization with weakness, paresthesias, and paralysis. Cardiac toxicity usually appears when the serum potassium concentration exceeds 7.5 mEq/L and seems more severe when associated with hyponatremia, as seen in Addison's disease. An electrocardiogram (ECG) can be excellent support for the suspicion and monitoring of hyperkalemia. A prolonged PR interval, the disappearance of the P wave, prolonged QRS complex, a complete heart block, bradycardia, ectopic beats, sine wave complexes, and ventricular fibrillation reaching a ventricular block can be a consequence of hyperkalemia. The main causes of hyperkalemia are increased potassium intake (less common when the renal excretion is normal), decreased renal potassium excretion (e.g., oliguric/anuric state, renal failure, ruptured bladder/uroperitoneum, urethral obstruction, Addison's disease, pleural effusion), and transcellular maldistribution as in metabolic acidosis (e.g., diabetes mellitus/diabetic ketoacidosis, reperfusion injury, massive trauma). The first group refers to excessive potassium supplementation or the administration of medications known to predispose to hyperkalemia with concurrent potassium supplementation (e.g., ACE inhibitors, non-specific beta-blockers). Hyperkalemia observed in pleural effusion (e.g., chylous ascites, neoplastic effusion, feline infectious peritonitis) is assumed to arise as decreased renal excretion due to a state of hypovolemia. In metabolic acidosis, the potassium shifts from the intracellular space into the extracellular space secondary to the tendency of the excess hydrogen ions to remain in the extracellular fluid space, thus maintaining electroneutrality. In addition, in metabolic acidosis, the increase in hydrogen ions produces a decreased excretion of potassium ions by the renal tubular cells.

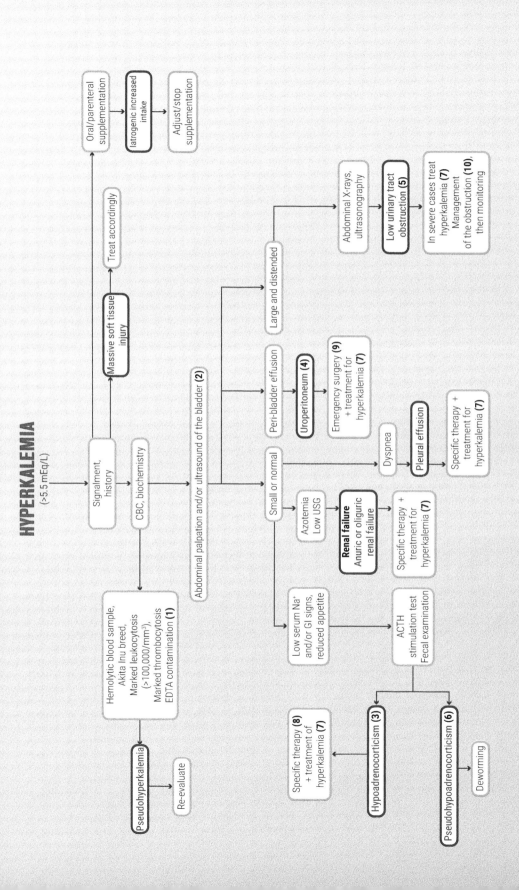

HYPERKALEMIA
(>5.5 mEq/L)

Signalment, history

CBC, biochemistry

Massive soft tissue injury

Treat accordingly

Oral/parenteral supplementation

Iatrogenic increased intake

Adjust/stop supplementation

Hemolytic blood sample, Akita Inu breed, Marked leukocytosis (>100,000/mm³), Marked thrombocytosis EDTA contamination **(1)**

Pseudohyperkalemia

Re-evaluate

Abdominal palpation and/or ultrasound of the bladder **(2)**

Large and distended

Abdominal X-rays, ultrasonography

Low urinary tract obstruction **(5)**

In severe cases treat hyperkalemia **(7)** Management of the obstruction **(10)**, then monitoring

Peri-bladder effusion

Uroperitoneum **(4)**

Emergency surgery **(9)** + treatment for hyperkalemia **(7)**

Small or normal

Dyspnea

Pleural effusion

Specific therapy + treatment for hyperkalemia **(7)**

Azotemia Low USG

Renal failure
Anuric or oliguric renal failure

Specific therapy + treatment for hyperkalemia **(7)**

Low serum Na⁺ and/or GI signs, reduced appetite

ACTH stimulation test
Fecal examination

Hypoadrenocorticism **(3)**

Specific therapy **(8)** + treatment of hyperkalemia **(7)**

Pseudohypoadrenocorticism **(6)**

Deworming

1. Artifactual/pseudohyperkalemia, resulting from contamination of the sample with EDTA (in these cases, hyperkalemia is usually associated with artifactual hypocalcemia), thrombocytosis, extreme leukocytosis, physiologic increased intracellular K^+ (e.g., the Akita breed is predisposed to a higher concentration of potassium within the red blood cells which, as a result of hemolysis, causes an increase in serum potassium), should be ruled out.

2. Once iatrogenic and artificial causes are excluded, if the palpation of the bladder does not clearly define the degree of distension, an ultrasound evaluation allows for determining the bladder size and any peribladder deposits.

DIAGNOSIS

3. Hypoadrenocorticism (Addison's disease) is an endocrine condition usually characterized by both mineralocorticoid and glucocorticoid deficiency, resulting in hyponatremia and/or hyperkalemia and signs of cortisol deficiency. Much less commonly, dogs have signs of cortisol deficiency but no electrolyte changes.

4. Uroperitoneum should be suspected in patients presenting with a history of trauma, acute abdomen, or bradycardia. If suspected, a suitable diagnostic protocol should include abdominal radiographs, abdominal ultrasound/FAST to identify free fluid in the abdomen or retroperitoneal space, and abdominal fluid analysis. The aim of the fluid analysis is to compare the concentration of potassium and creatinine in the abdominal fluid with the potassium and creatinine in a blood sample; it can be defined as uroperitoneum in dogs when the potassium ratio of the abdominal fluid is 1.6 times the concentration of the blood potassium, and, in cats, when it is 1.9 times the concentration of the blood potassium, and when the creatinine ratio is twice the concentration of creatinine in both. It is essential to identify the location of the disruption to the urinary tract with a contrast retrograde/anterograde urethrocystogram and then treat the patient surgically.

5. Lower urinary tract obstruction can be due to calculi, tumors, foreign bodies, plugs, or feline idiopathic cystitis. To identify the primary disease, a complete diagnostic protocol should include medical history, physical examination, CBC, biochemistry, urinalysis, abdominal ultrasound, abdominal radiographs, and/or a contrast retrograde urethrocystogram.

6. Pseudohypoadrenocorticism is caused not by aldosterone deficiency but occurs with trichuriasis. It is characterized by electrolyte abnormalities similar to hypoadrenocorticism and is associated with GI signs.

7. Managing the ECG abnormalities requires a slow intravenous bolus of 10% calcium gluconate (0.5-1.5 mL/kg) to counteract the direct cardiotoxic effects of hyperkalemia by causing decreased membrane potential and decreased cardiac membrane excitability. The purpose of administering calcium gluconate is cardiac stabilization of the patient.

Unfortunately, calcium gluconate does not reduce the blood potassium concentration. To reduce hyperkalemia, dextrose and insulin can be used. Insulin produces the simultaneous shift of glucose and potassium into the cells. Recommended dosages are 0.5 U/kg IM or IV of regular crystalline insulin and 2 g of dextrose (50% dextrose solution) IV for every calculated unit of insulin administered intravenously. Another effective treatment is intravenous sodium bicarbonate infusion (1-2 mEq/kg). The resulting alkalosis, due to the bicarbonate supplementation, determines an alteration of the acid-base equilibrium between the intracellular fluid (ICF) and the extracellular fluid (ECF). Plasma alkalosis attracts hydrogen ions (H^+) from the ICF to the ECF, determining the transition of potassium from the ECF to the ICF, leading to a reduction in serum potassium.

8. Treatment of dogs with an acute presentation of hypoadrenocorticism prioritizes correcting the hypovolemia, hyperkalemia, acidosis, and, if present, hypoglycemia. Fluid therapy addresses the majority of these issues, but other specific treatments are usually required, especially in the most severe cases (e.g., calcium gluconate, dextrose, glucocorticoids, supportive treatment). For long-term management, all patients with Addison's disease require replacement of glucocorticoids (e.g., prednisone 0.1 to 0.22 mg/kg/day PO), and most patients require replacement of the mineralocorticoids with either desoxycorticosterone pivalate (1.5 mg/kg SC every 25-30 days;) or fludrocortisone acetate (0.02 mg/kg once daily or divided q12h PO).

9. Following patient stabilization, it is important to correct the electrolyte blood acid-base balance abnormalities before surgery. Temporarily, a peritoneal drainage catheter and a urinary catheter to allow drainage of any urine in the bladder can be placed. After identifying the location of the disrupture, surgical treatment should be carried out.

10. Lower urinary tract obstruction can represent a life-threatening emergency. Therefore, it is important to first stabilize the patient by treating the acidosis, hyperkalemia, and uremia, and subsequently urgently manage the obstruction, for example, with catheterization (where possible).

SUGGESTED READINGS

-   DiBartola SP (editor). Fluid, Electrolyte, and Acid-Base Disorders in Small Animal Practice 4th edition. St. Louis, Elsevier, 2012.
-   Feldman EC, Nelson RW, Reusch CE, Scott-Moncrieff JCR, Behrend E (editors). Canine and Feline Endocrinology 4th edition. St. Louis, Elsevier, 2015.
-   Stockham SL, Scott MA (editors). Fundamentals of Veterinary Clinical Pathology 2nd edition. Iowa, Wiley Blackwell, 2008.

HYPERLIPIDEMIA

Panagiotis G. Xenoulis

Hyperlipidemia is a common condition in dogs but less common in cats. In the last decade, several studies in both humans and dogs have associated specific forms of hyperlipidemia with a much wider range of diseases than previously thought. Postprandial hyperlipidemia is physiologic and typically resolves within 7-12 hours after a meal. Therefore, the determination of serum lipid concentrations should always follow a fast of at least 12 hours. Persistent fasting hyperlipidemia can be either primary (typically due to an inborn inherited error in lipid metabolism) or secondary to other diseases or drug administration. Secondary hyperlipidemia is the most common form of hyperlipidemia in dogs and cats. Most commonly, secondary hyperlipidemia (hypertriglyceridemia and/or hypercholesterolemia) is the result of an endocrine disorder such as hypothyroidism, diabetes mellitus, or hyperadrenocorticism. Hyperlipidemia (hypertriglyceridemia and/or hypercholesterolemia) has also been associated with naturally occurring pancreatitis in dogs. Another important cause of secondary hyperlipidemia in dogs and cats is obesity. Other possible causes of hyperlipidemia in dogs and/or cats include protein-losing nephropathy (nephrotic syndrome), cholestasis, high-fat diets (dogs), hepatic lipidosis (cats), and possibly other conditions (e.g., infections, inflammation, neoplasia, congestive heart failure). Administration of certain drugs, mainly glucocorticoids and estrogens (such as megestrol acetate), can induce marked hyperlipidemia. Other drugs reported to cause hyperlipidemia in dogs (such as phenobarbital, potassium bromide, and progestagens) may also cause hyperlipidemia in cats. In dogs, primary lipid abnormalities are usually, but not always, associated with certain breeds. Primary hyperlipidemia is very common in Miniature Schnauzers. Other breeds, such as Shetland Sheepdogs, Beagles, Briards, Doberman Pinschers, and Rottweilers, may also have different forms of primary hyperlipidemias. Primary lipid abnormalities are uncommon in cats. Hyperlipidemia per se does not appear to lead to any clinical signs. However, many animals with hyperlipidemia develop diseases because of hyperlipidemia, and clinical signs develop as a result of those diseases. Such diseases include pancreatitis, hepatobiliary disease (vacuolar hepatopathy and gallbladder mucocele), atherosclerosis, ocular disease, xanthomatosis (benign granulomatous lesions in the skin or internal organs), proteinuria and glomerular lipidosis, and neurologic disease (e.g., seizures, ischemic strokes).

HYPERLIPIDEMIA

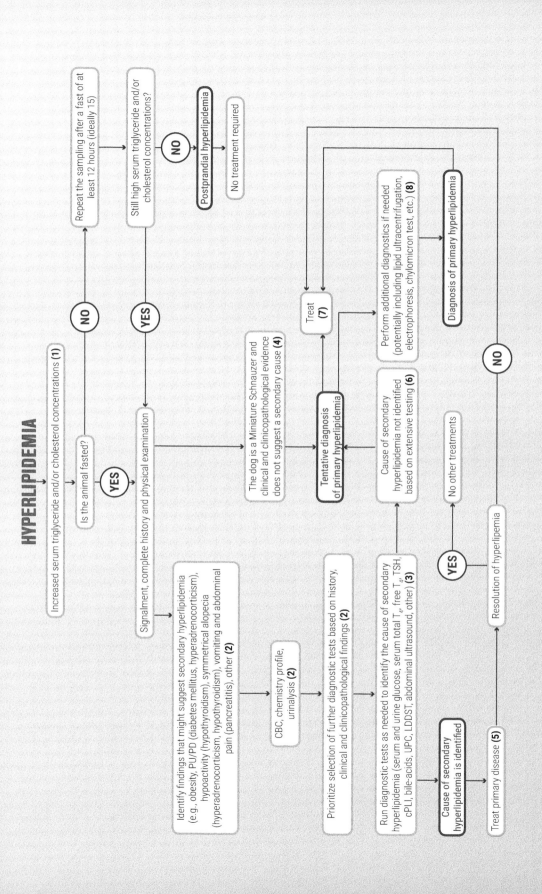

Increased serum triglyceride and/or cholesterol concentrations **(1)**

Is the animal fasted?

YES → Signalment, complete history and physical examination

NO → Repeat the sampling after a fast of at least 12 hours (ideally 15)

Still high serum triglyceride and/or cholesterol concentrations?

NO → Postprandial hyperlipidemia → No treatment required

YES ↓

Identify findings that might suggest secondary hyperlipidemia (e.g., obesity, PU/PD (diabetes mellitus, hyperadrenocorticism), hypoactivity (hypothyroidism), symmetrical alopecia (hyperadrenocorticism, hypothyroidism), vomiting and abdominal pain (pancreatitis), other **(2)**

CBC, chemistry profile, urinalysis **(2)**

Prioritize selection of further diagnostic tests based on history, clinical and clinicopathological findings **(2)**

Run diagnostic tests as needed to identify the cause of secondary hyperlipidemia (serum and urine glucose, serum total T_4, free T_4, TSH, cPLI, bile-acids, UPC, LDDST, abdominal ultrasound, other) **(3)**

The dog is a Miniature Schnauzer and clinical and clinicopathological evidence does not suggest a secondary cause **(4)**

Tentative diagnosis of primary hyperlipidemia

Cause of secondary hyperlipidemia is identified

YES → Treat primary disease **(5)** → Resolution of hyperlipemia

NO → Cause of secondary hyperlipidemia not identified based on extensive testing **(6)**

Treat **(7)**

YES → Resolution of hyperlipemia

NO → No other treatments

Perform additional diagnostics if needed (potentially including lipid ultracentrifugation, electrophoresis, chylomicron test, etc.) **(8)**

Diagnosis of primary hyperlipidemia

DIAGNOSTIC PROTOCOL

1. Hyperlipidemia is typically diagnosed by measuring fasting serum triglyceride and cholesterol concentrations. In some cases, especially in cats, fasting serum triglyceride concentrations may be normal, while abnormal hypertriglyceridemia might be evident postprandially.

2. After hyperlipidemia has been diagnosed, the next step is to determine whether the patient has a primary or a secondary lipid disorder, based initially on clinical presentation and results from routine testing. This is crucial because animals with secondary hyperlipidemia typically show clinical signs of the primary disease (e.g., obesity, polyuria, and polydipsia in cats with diabetes mellitus) and/or laboratory abnormalities (e.g., hyperglycemia and glucosuria in diabetes mellitus), which can help prioritize the selection of diagnostic tests and lead the way towards an appropriate diagnostic plan. Dogs and cats with primary hyperlipidemia commonly do not have clinical signs unless hyperlipidemia has led to a secondary disease (such as pancreatitis or biliary mucocele).

3. Specific diagnostic investigations should be performed to diagnose or rule out specific diseases that can cause secondary hyperlipidemia. The selection of tests to be performed is based on information from the history and physical examination and is tailored to each individual case. A more general and wide selection of tests might be necessary for patients with vague or no clinical signs.

4. One possible exception is the Miniature Schnauzer, in which primary hyperlipidemia is common. A detailed diagnostic investigation of hyperlipidemia might not be necessary for this breed in the absence of clinical signs and routine clinicopathologic testing not suggesting an underlying cause, because primary hyperlipidemia is very common and well-characterized in this breed. The main clinicopathological finding in these dogs is hypertriglyceridemia. Hypercholesterolemia might also be present but isolated hypercholesterolemia is not a feature of primary hyperlipidemia in this breed.

6. If secondary hyperlipidemia is excluded, a tentative diagnosis of a primary lipid disorder can be made.

8. In some cases, additional specialized testing might be implemented to determine the nature of hyperlipidemia (e.g., ultracentrifugation to determine the lipoprotein fractions responsible for the hyperlipidemia). For example, hypertriglyceridemia resulting from increased chylomicrons is more likely to respond to dietary treatment as opposed to increased VLDLs.

TREATMENT

5. If hyperlipidemia is secondary, the condition causing hyperlipidemia should be treated. This typically resolves or at least improves hyperlipidemia. If severe hyperlipidemia persists after treatment of the primary disease, treatment for hyperlipidemia should be implemented (see treatment).

7. Treatment of primary or persistent secondary hypertriglyceridemia is clinically important. Management of hypercholesterolemia seems to be of less clinical importance. In most

cases, treatment should initially be pursued with dietary management, while drug therapy can be initiated later if deemed necessary. The most commonly used and likely most effective dietary option for hyperlipidemia in dogs and cats is feeding an appropriate low-fat diet (<25 g of total fat per 1,000 Kcal (metabolizable energy). Omega-3 fatty acids, niacin, chitosan, and 5-aminolevulinic acid might also help, although they are not routinely used. Medical management includes fibrates (which is the most commonly used drug class in dogs) such as bezafibrate (4-10 mg/kg q24h) and fenofibrate (10 mg/kg, q24h) and was found to be highly effective. Statins are mainly cholesterol-lowering drugs, and this makes them less than ideal for cases with hypertriglyceridemia as the main lipid abnormality.

SUGGESTED READINGS

- Xenoulis PG. Disorders of lipid metabolism. In Feldman EC, Fracassi F, Peterson ME (editors). Feline endocrinology. Edra, Milan, 2019, pp 609-620.
- Xenoulis PG, Steiner JM. Canine hyperlipidaemia. *J Small Anim Pract* 56:595-605, 2015.

HYPERNATREMIA

Francesco Lunetta

Hypernatremia is an electrolyte alteration caused by an increased sodium concentration ($[Na^+]$) in the water content of the extracellular fluid (ECF). The solute concentration (osmolarity) in the plasma of dogs and cats is directly proportional to the Na^+, blood urea nitrogen (BUN), and glucose concentrations. Since BUN can move freely between cells and glucose is balanced by insulin (in non-diabetic patients), plasma osmolarity is mainly influenced by $[Na^+]$. In healthy patients, an increase in $[Na^+]$ is quickly corrected by raising the component of free water in the ECF by means of an increased thirst stimulus and an increased release of antidiuretic hormone (ADH). This hormone is produced by the hypothalamus, and its action is carried out by reabsorbing free water in the renal tubules. The causes of hypernatremia can be a pure water deficit, a hypotonic fluid loss, or an impermeant solute $[Na^+]$ gain. Assessing the volemic status and the hydration state of the patient, and the presence of polyuria and polydipsia can be useful in defining the cause of hypernatremia. Clinical signs of hypernatremia are primarily neurological (lethargy, weakness, tremors, seizure, coma, and death). These signs are related to the dehydration of cerebral cells caused by the elevated osmolarity in the ECF. In severe cases, the rapid decrease in brain volume may result in rupture of the cerebral vessels and cerebral hemorrhage. The severity of the clinical signs is usually related to the rapidity of the onset of hypernatremia. A slow increase (>48h) in $[Na^+]$ allows the cerebral cells to adapt to the high osmolarity of ECF (production of intracellular osmolytes, uptake of Na^+ and potassium). Therefore, patients affected by chronic hypernatremia can be relatively asymptomatic. The main goal in treating hypernatremic patients is to restore normal $[Na^+]$, usually by administering intravenous (IV) hypotonic fluids (e.g., 5% dextrose or 0.45% NaCl solutions). Secondary, it is mandatory to diagnose and treat the underlying disorder.

HYPERNATREMIA

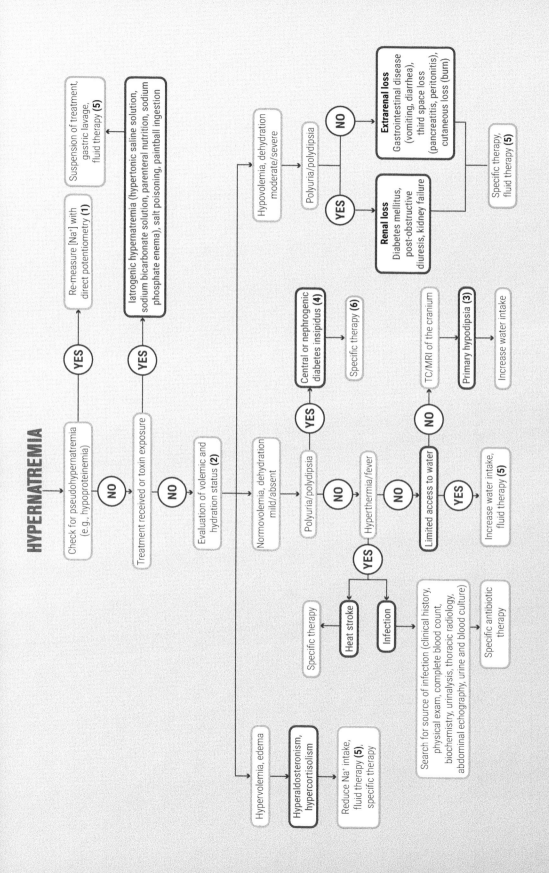

Check for pseudohypernatremia (e.g., hypoproteinemia)

YES → Re-measure [Na⁺] with direct potentiometry **(1)** → Suspension of treatment, gastric lavage, fluid therapy **(5)**

NO →

Treatment received or toxin exposure

YES → **Iatrogenic hypernatremia (hypertonic saline solution, sodium bicarbonate solution, parenteral nutrition, sodium phosphate enema), salt poisoning, paintball ingestion**

NO →

Evaluation of volemic and hydration status (2)

Hypervolemia, edema
→ **Hyperaldosteronism, hypercortisolism** → Reduce Na⁺ intake, fluid therapy **(5)**, specific therapy

Normovolemia, dehydration mild/absent

Polyuria/polydipsia

YES → **Central or nephrogenic diabetes insipidus (4)** → Specific therapy **(6)**

NO → **Hyperthermia/fever**

  YES →
    Heat stroke → Specific therapy
    Infection → Search for source of infection (clinical history, physical exam, complete blood count, biochemistry, urinalysis, thoracic radiology, abdominal echography, urine and blood culture) → Specific antibiotic therapy

  NO → **Limited access to water**
    YES → Increase water intake, fluid therapy **(5)**
    NO → TC/MRI of the cranium → **Primary hypodipsia (3)** → Increase water intake

Hypovolemia, dehydration moderate/severe

Polyuria/polydipsia

YES → **Renal loss** Diabetes mellitus, post-obstructive diuresis, kidney failure

NO → **Extrarenal loss** Gastrointestinal disease (vomiting, diarrhea), third space loss (pancreatitis, peritonitis), cutaneous loss (burn)

→ Specific therapy, fluid therapy **(5)**

1. Direct potentiometry methodology is not affected by hypoproteinemia when measuring [Na$^+$]. Instead, if indirect potentiometry is used, the sample is diluted before measurement. In this case, hypoproteinemic samples can falsely detect increased [Na$^+$].

2. Assessing the patient's volume status and hydration is helpful in determining the cause of hypernatremia. Cutaneous edema, jugular vein distention, or pulmonary edema suggest hypervolemia caused by an excessive Na$^+$ intake. Instead, normovolemic patients without dehydration signs suggest a pure water deficit. However, these patients can become dehydrated if their access to water is limited. The clinical signs of hypovolemia (e.g., tachycardia, hypotension, tachypnea) and severe dehydration (dry mucous membranes and skin) are suggestive of a hypotonic fluid loss.

DIAGNOSIS

3. Patients developing chronic hypernatremia with free access to water can be affected by an abnormal release of ADH. A congenital hypothalamic malformation can cause defective osmoregulation of ADH and an abnormal thirst mechanism, resulting in hypodipsia.

4. Central (neurogenic) diabetes insipidus is due to ADH deficiency. It can be congenital or acquired. In the second case, the cause may be a brain tumor, a head injury, granulomatous disease, or an immune-mediated process. Nephrogenic diabetes insipidus can be: 1) congenital, due to agenesis of ADH receptors or aquaporins, or 2) acquired, for example, as a result of toxic or infectious tubular damage (e.g., the outcome of pyelonephritis).

5. The administration of IV hypotonic fluid solutions is the therapy indicated for correcting hypernatremia. Estimating the water deficit (WT) in these patients is necessary for the correct use of these fluids, using the formula

    WT (L)= 0.6 × weight (kg) × [([Na$^+$] patient/[Na$^+$] desired) − 1]

    where 0.6 is the assumed water percentage (60%) of body weight. If the rise in [Na$^+$] is acute (onset <48h), a rapid correction of [Na$^+$] is indicated using IV hypotonic fluids (e.g., 5% dextrose solution) at a rate of 5-10 mL/kg/h and a correction rate of 2 mEq/L/h until the signs of hypernatremia are resolved. In chronic hypernatremia (onset >48h), the correction should be lowered to 10 mEq/L/day due to potential cerebral edema caused by a rapid correction of [Na$^+$]. In patients affected by hypovolemia, fluid resuscitation can be achieved using a crystalloid having a [Na$^+$] similar to that of the patient, for example, adding hypertonic saline fluid to a crystalloid fluid. After the correction of the volemic state, hypotonic fluids can be administered. Moreover, hypernatremic patients with a hypervolemic state due to excessive sodium intake can be treated by reducing the intake of sodium and the slow administration of IV hypotonic fluid solution, leading to natriuresis and diuresis. Careful monitoring of fluid overload is necessary for hypervolemic patients suffering from cardiac or renal diseases in which IV fluid therapy can lead to pulmonary edema. Promoting natriuresis and diuresis with a loop diuretic (e.g., furosemide) may be necessary.

6.   DDAVP is a synthetic analog of ADH. Initial therapy includes doses of 0.05 mg PO q12h for dogs <5 kg and cats, 0.1 mg PO q12h for dogs between 5 to 20 kg, 0.2 mg PO q12h for dogs >20 kg, up to a maximum of 0.4 mg q8h. If these doses are not enough to control the polyuria and polydipsia, it is possible to try the administration q8h. If necessary, the conjunctival or subcutaneous route can also be used.

SUGGESTED READINGS

-   DiBartola SP. Disorders of sodium and water: hypernatremia and hyponatremia. In DiBartola SP (editor). Fluid, Electrolyte, and Acid-base Disorders in Small Animal Practice. St. Louis, Elsevier, 2012, pp 45-79.
-   Rosenberg D. Sodium, chloride. In Ettinger SJ, Feldman EC, Côté E (editors). Textbook of Veterinary Internal Medicine 8th edition. St. Louis, Elsevier, 2017, pp 805-821.
-   Stockam SL, Scott MA. Monovalent electrolytes and osmolality. In Stockam SL, Scott MA (editors). Fundamentals of Veterinary Clinical Pathology. Blackwell Publishing, 2008, pp 495-557.
-   Ueda Y, Hopper K. Sodium and water balance. In Drobatz KJ, Hopper K, Rozanski E, Silverstein DC (editors). Textbook of Small Animal Emergency Medicine. Wiley Blackwell, 2019, pp 690-699.

HYPERTENSION

Rosanne E. Jepson

Systemic hypertension (SH) is defined as a persistent increase in systolic blood pressure (SBP) >160 mmHg that can cause target organ damage (TOD) to the eyes, cardiovascular system, kidney, and central nervous system. Normal SBP in cats and dogs ranges from 120-160 mmHg, which increases with age. Breed differences in dogs (not cats) are recognized: e.g., Sighthounds have SBP 10-20 mmHg higher than crossbred dogs, and brachycephalic breeds have higher SBP. Measuring SBP should be "routine" in older dogs and cats as a component of any wellness examination as well as those with signs of hypertensive TOD or a condition associated with SH. Systemic hypertension can be categorized as idiopathic (no underlying cause or associated disease condition identified), secondary (an underlying disease process or drug associated with hypertension), or situational (short-term increase in SBP associated with stress or anxiety).

Dog and cat SBPs are usually assessed with a Doppler or high definition oscillometric (HDO) SBP machine, measured from the forelimb, the hindlimb or the tail. The location used should be consistent with each pet. SBP can be dramatically affected by the environment, the pet's temperament and/or position, the measurement method, and the operator's experience. Using standardized methods in accordance with the American College of Veterinary Medicine (ACVIM) hypertension guidelines provides the best opportunity for accurate and reliable results.

Key principles:
- Ensure a quiet, stress-free environment.
- Allow a period of acclimatization for 5-10 minutes.
- Allow the pet to choose a comfortable position (ideally the same for each recheck).
- Ensure the cuff is 30-40% of limb circumference.
- Discard first reading and then take 5-7 readings.
- Average the readings to give a mean SBP.

Staging systems (see table below) can guide the diagnosis and treatment of systemic hypertension (ACVIM) with the goal of preventing TOD.

Systolic blood pressure category	Systolic blood pressure (mmHg)	Target organ risk category
Normotensive	<140	Minimal
Prehypertensive	140-159	Low
Hypertensive	160-179	Moderate
Severe hypertension	≥180	High

SYSTEMIC HYPERTENSION

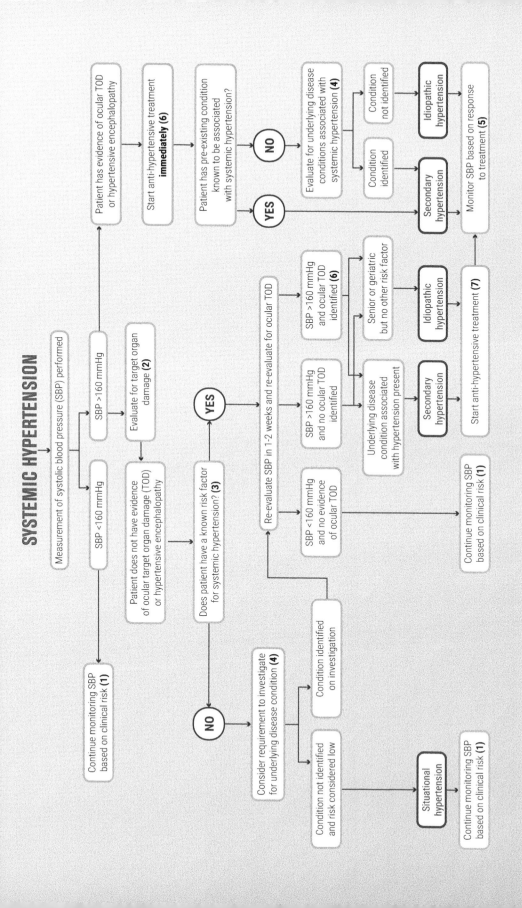

Measurement of systolic blood pressure (SBP) performed

SBP <160 mmHg
- Continue monitoring SBP based on clinical risk **(1)**

SBP >160 mmHg
- Evaluate for target organ damage **(2)**

Patient has evidence of ocular TOD or hypertensive encephalopathy
- Start anti-hypertensive treatment **immediately (6)**
- Patient has pre-existing condition known to be associated with systemic hypertension?

YES → Secondary hypertension

NO → Evaluate for underlying disease conditions associated with systemic hypertension **(4)**
- Condition identified → Secondary hypertension
- Condition not identified → Idiopathic hypertension

Monitor SBP based on response to treatment **(5)**

Patient does not have evidence of ocular target organ damage (TOD) or hypertensive encephalopathy
- Does patient have a known risk factor for systemic hypertension? **(3)**

YES → Re-evaluate SBP in 1-2 weeks and re-evaluate for ocular TOD
- SBP <160 mmHg and no evidence of ocular TOD → Continue monitoring SBP based on clinical risk **(1)**
- SBP >160 mmHg and no ocular TOD identified → Underlying disease condition associated with hypertension present → Secondary hypertension
- SBP >160 mmHg and ocular TOD identified **(6)** → Senior or geriatric but no other risk factor → Idiopathic hypertension

Start anti-hypertensive treatment **(7)**

NO → Consider requirement to investigate for underlying disease condition **(4)**
- Condition identified on investigation
- Condition not identified and risk considered low → Situational hypertension → Continue monitoring SBP based on clinical risk **(1)**

DIAGNOSTIC PROTOCOL

1. Monitor SBP based on the risk of developing SH. Screening SBP recommended q6-12 months for cats >8-9 years and senior dogs. Measurement at least q3-6 months is indicated for pets with conditions associated with SH (see point 3) or those given drugs modulating SBP. Assess all pets with signs of hypertensive TOD (see point 2).

2. Ocular target organ damages (TODs) (retinal detachment, focal bullous retinal detachment, retinal hemorrhage, iris aneurysm, hyphema) are recognized via recognized via fundic/ocular examination. Pets with hypertensive encephalopathy exhibit behavioral and mentation changes and/or seizures. Cardiac TOD identified with echocardiography includes left ventricular wall thickening but must be differentiated from primary cardiac disease. Hypertensive kidney injury is difficult to differentiate from a primary process. Assess renal function (creatinine, urea, symmetric dimethylarginine and urine specific gravity), and check proteinuria (urine protein to creatinine ratio) in all patients with SH.

3. Known SH risk factors and disease conditions:
   a. Age: SBP increases with age; SH is more likely in senior dogs and cats older than 8-9 years.
   b. Clinical conditions associated with hypertension in cats (prevalence of hypertension):
   - i. Chronic kidney disease (19-65%).
   - ii. Hyperthyroidism (5-10% pre-treatment, 22-25% post-treatment).
   - iii. Hyperaldosteronism (Conn's syndrome 50-100%; rare condition).
   - iv. Acute kidney injury (20-80%).
   - v. Hyperadrenocorticism (rare condition).
   c. Clinical conditions associated with hypertension in dogs:
   - i. Chronic kidney disease (14-93%).
   - ii. Acute kidney injury (15-81%).
   - iii. Hyperadrenocorticism (20-73%).
   - iv. Diabetes mellitus (24-67%).
   - v. Hyperaldosteronism (rare condition).
   - vi. Pheochromocytoma (43-86%, rare condition).
   d. Drugs that may increase SBP (treat by stopping or lowering dose):
   - i. Glucocorticoids.
   - ii. Mineralocorticoids.
   - iii. Erythrocyte-stimulating drugs.
   - iv. Phenylpropanolamine (rare at therapeutic dose).
   - v. Phenylephrine/ephedrine.
   - vi. Toceranib.

4. High SBP without a known pre-existing risk factor for SH (see point 3): investigate for an underlying disease contributing to SH. Other investigations should be tailored to the individual.

5. After anti-hypertensive treatment has started, monitor to ensure SBP <160 mmHg (prehypertensive) or ideally <140 mmHg (normotensive), whilst avoiding hypotension (SBP <120 mmHg). Initial review after 3-14 days is appropriate for most. Consider hospitalization for hypertensive emergency. Gradually dose-adjust anti-hypertensive medication to reach target with repeat monitoring q3-14 days. Thereafter, SBP monitor q3-4 months or sooner with clinical concern.

TREATMENT

6. Hypertensive emergency: start anti-hypertensive treatment immediately. If the patient can tolerate oral drugs, amlodipine besylate (0.2-0.5 mg/kg PO q24h) or hydralazine (0.5-2 mg/kg PO q12h) can be used. When oral medications are not appropriate, e.g., altered mentation, consider parenteral drugs (e.g., fenoldepam, labetolol, hydralazine, nitroprusside). Intensive monitoring is required. Consider direct arterial BP monitoring for critical patients. Oral anti-hypertensive therapy is usually appropriate for patients with acute onset ocular TOD without neurological signs (see below). Hospitalization can be considered or early review after 24-72 hours on an outpatient basis. Rarely ocular TOD is recognized with SPB <160 mmHg. Where convincingly due to SH, start anti-hypertensive treatment. Monitor carefully for hypotension.

7. The choice of an anti-hypertensive agent depends on the individual patient, licensing regulation and underlying disease conditions.

    Cats: first-line treatment includes amlodipine besylate (0.125-0.25 mg/kg PO q24h) or telmisartan (2 mg/kg PO q24h). Monotherapy is often successful. Angiotensin-converting enzyme inhibitors (ACEi), e.g., benazepril, are not effective anti-hypertensive agents and are not recommended first-line.

    Dogs: due to the high prevalence of proteinuric CKD-associated hypertension, RAS inhibitors are first-line agents, e.g., ACEi enalapril 0.5 mg/kg PO q12h, benazepril 0.5 mg/kg PO q12h or the angiotensin receptor blocker telmisartan 1-2 mg/kg PO q24h. Multimodal anti-hypertensive treatment is often required including the addition of amlodipine besylate 0.2-0.5 mg/kg PO q24h.

    In cats and dogs, the use of RAS inhibition is contraindicated to treat hypertension in severe acute kidney injury due to a potential decline in GFR.
    Specific anti-hypertensive agents are required for certain conditions, e.g., aldosterone receptor blocker for patients with hyperaldosteronism- and, alpha-blocker for patients with pheochromocytoma.

SUGGESTED READINGS

- Acierno MJ, Brown S, Coleman AE, et al. ACVIM consensus statement: guidelines for the identification, evaluation, and management of systemic hypertension in Dogs and Cats. *J Vet Intern Med* 32:1803-1822, 2018.
- Elliot J, Syme HM, Jepson RE (editors). Hypertension in the Dog and Cat. Switzerland, Springer Nature Publications, 2020.
- Taylor SS, Sparkes AH, Briscoe K, et al. ISFM Consensus Guidelines on the Diagnosis and Management of Hypertension in Cats. *J Feline Med Surg* 19: 288-303, 2017.

HYPOALBUMINEMIA

Andrea N. Johnston

Hypoproteinemia is a reduction of the plasma protein pool below 50 g/L (5 g/dL). Albumin is the most abundant plasma protein, accounting for at least half of the total protein content and the primary intravascular osmotic colloid. Hypoalbuminemia is defined as plasma albumin less than 30 g/L (3.0 g/dL). Albumin homeostasis is influenced by the rate of production, distribution, loss, and degradation. Hepatocytes synthesize most plasma proteins (albumin, antithrombin, α2 macroglobulin, α1 antitrypsin, and protein C), excluding immunoglobulins, factor VIII, and von Willebrand factor. Albumin is used as a marker of synthetic liver function; however, the sensitivity of hypoalbuminemia for liver disease is poor because serum albumin is influenced by many other physiologic variables. More than 80% of functional hepatic parenchyma must be lost before a reduction in serum albumin is detectable.

Decreased albumin production is also caused by reduced delivery of metabolites and pro-synthetic signals from the portal circulation to the liver due to chronic anorexia or hypoperfusion; the negative acute-phase inflammatory response, wherein transcription is downregulated by proinflammatory cytokine release; or increased oncotic pressure caused by severe hyperglobulinemia (e.g., multiple myeloma). Expansion of the plasma volume leads to a relative reduction in plasma levels. Causes include free water excess due to iatrogenic or pathophysiologic overhydration, compensatory ADH response to reduced effective circulatory volume, and third space sequestration of albumin. Albumin loss occurs with proteinuria, protein-losing enteropathy, exudative skin lesions, or extracorporeal hemorrhage. Albumin catabolism due to a negative nitrogen balance can occur in cachexic, protein malnourished patients, or associated with neoplasia. Albumin degradation is enhanced by structural modifications or post-translational oxidation and glycosylation. While a shortened albumin half-life is difficult to identify in a clinical setting, it should be considered in pets with diabetes mellitus, chronic inflammation, and oxidant injury.

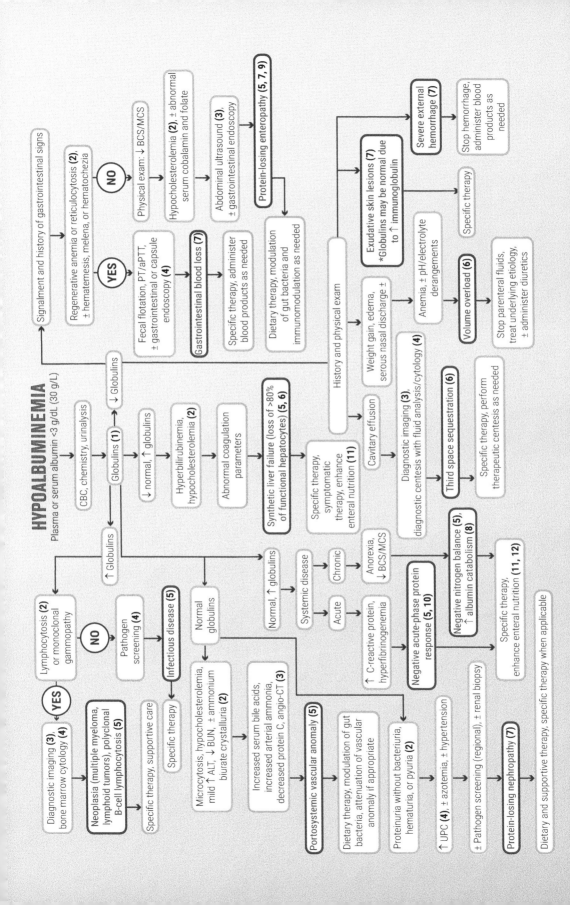

HYPOALBUMINEMIA

Plasma or serum albumin <3 g/dL (30 g/L)

CBC, chemistry, urinalysis

↓ Globulins

↑ Globulins

Globulins **(1)**

→ normal, ↑ globulins

Hyperbilirubinemia, hypocholesterolemia **(2)**

Abnormal coagulation parameters

Synthetic liver failure (loss of >80% of functional hepatocytes) **(5, 6)**

Specific therapy, symptomatic therapy, enhance enteral nutrition **(11)**

Lymphocytosis **(2)** or monoclonal gammopathy

YES

Diagnostic imaging **(3)**, bone marrow cytology **(4)**

Neoplasia (multiple myeloma, lymphoid tumors), polyclonal B-cell lymphocytosis **(5)**

Specific therapy, supportive care

NO

Pathogen screening **(4)**

Infectious disease **(5)**

Specific therapy

Normal globulins

Microcytosis, hypocholesterolemia, mild ↑ ALT, ↓ BUN, ± ammonium biurate crystalluria **(2)**

Increased serum bile acids, increased arterial ammonia, decreased protein C, angio-CT **(3)**

Portosystemic vascular anomaly **(5)**

Dietary therapy, modulation of gut bacteria, attenuation of vascular anomaly if appropriate

Systemic disease

Chronic

Acute

Anorexia, ↓ BCS/MCS

↑ C-reactive protein, hyperfibrinogenemia

Negative nitrogen balance **(5)**, ↑ albumin catabolism **(8)**

Negative acute-phase protein response **(5, 10)**

Specific therapy, enhance enteral nutrition **(11, 12)**

Normal, ↑ globulins

Proteinuria without bacteriuria, hematuria, or pyuria **(2)**

↑ UPC **(4)**, ± azotemia, ± hypertension

± Pathogen screening (regional), ± renal biopsy

Protein-losing nephropathy **(7)**

Dietary and supportive therapy, specific therapy when applicable

Signalment and history of gastrointestinal signs

Regenerative anemia or reticulocytosis **(2)**, ± hematemesis, melena, or hematochezia

YES

NO

Physical exam: ↓ BCS/MCS

Fecal flotation, PT/aPTT, ± gastrointestinal or capsule endoscopy **(4)**

Gastrointestinal blood loss **(7)**

Specific therapy, administer blood products as needed

Hypocholesterolemia **(2)**, ± abnormal serum cobalamin and folate

Abdominal ultrasound **(3)**, ± gastrointestinal endoscopy

Protein-losing enteropathy **(5, 7, 9)**

Dietary therapy, modulation of gut bacteria and immunomodulation as needed

History and physical exam

Weight gain, edema, serous nasal discharge

Diagnostic imaging **(3)**, diagnostic centesis with fluid analysis/cytology **(4)**

Cavitary effusion

Third space sequestration **(6)**

Specific therapy, perform therapeutic centesis as needed

Exudative skin lesions **(7)**
*Globulins may be normal due to ↑ immunoglobulin

Severe external hemorrhage **(7)**

Stop hemorrhage, administer blood products as needed

Anemia, ± pH/electrolyte derangements

Specific therapy

Volume overload **(6)**

Stop parenteral fluids, treat underlying etiology, ± administer diuretics

DIAGNOSTIC PROTOCOL

1. The signalment, history, clinical signs, and findings from the minimum database dictate the appropriate diagnostic protocol for hypoalbuminemic patients. Of the biochemical parameters, globulin is the first decision node by which the causes of hypoalbuminemia can be differentiated.

2. Ancillary results from the CBC, chemistry, and urinalysis further hone the diagnostic plan.

3. In some cases, diagnostic imaging provides supportive evidence (radiographs – osteolysis associated with multiple myeloma) or a definitive diagnosis (angio-CT – portosystemic vascular anomaly).

4. Targeted testing is needed for definitive diagnosis in many cases.

DIAGNOSIS

5. Reductions in albumin production are caused by numerous physiologic stimuli, including nutrient depletion (chronic anorexia, protein starvation, cachexia, reduced delivery of trophic factors to the liver), increased presinusoidal colloid osmotic pressure (hyperglobulinemia, dextran administration), severe inflammation (negative acute-phase response), and synthetic liver failure. The normal half-life of albumin is 8-10 days in the dog and 5-6 days in the cat, so changes in plasma albumin are not immediately apparent with synthetic downregulation.

6. Albumin is normally distributed between the intravascular and the extravascular space. Expansion of the total distribution area due to volume excess will reduce plasma albumin. In pathologic effusions, plasma albumin may reduce due to compensatory sodium and water retention or vascular and lymphatic leakage, resulting in sequestration of albumin in a "third space".

7. Albumin can be lost with globulins through severe external and internal hemorrhage, exudative cutaneous lesions, and protein-losing enteropathies. In instances where bleeding is mild, or there is a concurrent immunoglobin response, globulins can be normal. Albumin loss unaccompanied by globulin depletion occurs with protein-losing nephropathies.

8. The rate of albumin catabolism increases with protein starvation or negative energy balance to replenish the depleted amino acid pool. Enhanced degradation of albumin also occurs with changes to the physical or chemical structure of albumin and possibly with patient age, although this is less well characterized in dogs and cats.

9. Basenjis with small intestinal lymphoproliferative disease have normal globulin levels.

10. Aside from the negative acute phase response, in some cases of critical illness such as sepsis, hypoalbuminemia may occur secondary to vascular leakage and increased rates of catabolism.

TREATMENT

11. Appropriate enteral nutrition is critical in hypoalbuminemic patients. Feeding tube placement is indicated if voluntary food intake is inadequate. Consultation with a nutritionist for diet formulation is recommended to meet specific nutritional requirements.

12. Clinical manifestations of hypoalbuminemia, including edema or anasarca, do not usually occur until serum albumin levels are less than 20 g/L (2.0 g/dL). Although administration of canine-specific albumin will increase albumin and colloid osmotic pressure in dogs, the high risk of immediate and delayed-type hypersensitivity reactions precludes its routine use. There is an ongoing debate whether the benefits of albumin infusions outweigh the risks in hypoalbuminemic humans with sepsis and severe burns; whether survival outcomes improve with albumin infusion in this subset of veterinary patients is unknown. Increasing canine serum albumin by 0.5 g/dL requires 450 mg/kg of canine albumin. Canine and feline plasma products are approximately 50% albumin.

SUGGESTED READINGS

- Busher JT. Serum albumin and globulin. In Walker HK, Hall WD, Hurst JW (editors). Clinical Methods: The History, Physical, and Laboratory Examinations 3rd edition. Boston, Butterworths, 1990. Available from: https://www.ncbi.nlm.nih.gov/books/NBK204/
- eClinPath.com, Cornell University. Available from: https://eclinpath.com/chemistry/proteins/albumin/
- Mazzaferro EM, Edwards T. Update on albumin therapy in critical illness. *Vet Clin North Am Small Anim Pract* 50:1289-1305, 2020.
- McPherson RA. Specific proteins. In McPherson RA, Pincus MR (editors). Henry's Clinical Diagnosis and Management 23rd edition. St. Louis, Elsevier, 2017, pp 253-256.
- Scott MA, Stockham SL. Proteins. In Scott MA, Stockham SL (editors). Fundamentals of Veterinary Clinical Pathology 2nd edition. Ames, Blackwell Publishing, 2008, pp 385-392.

HYPOCALCEMIA

Antonio Maria Tardo

Hypocalcemia is an electrolyte abnormality commonly encountered in veterinary medicine and, if unrecognized, can result in potentially life-threatening consequences. Calcium is essential for many physiological processes, including muscle contraction, neurotransmission, hormone secretion, blood clotting, enzymatic reactions, bone metabolism, and others. Calcium homeostasis is complex and strictly regulated through the concerted actions of the parathyroid hormone (PTH), 1,25-dihydroxyvitamin D_3 (calcitriol), and calcitonin. Hypocalcemia occurs when there is a derangement in calcium-regulating hormones and in cases of calcium precipitation or chelation.

Serum total calcium (tCa) exists in 3 forms: protein-bound (predominantly albumin), ionized calcium (iCa), and complexed calcium. Ionized calcium is the biologically active form and accounts for approximately 50% of the serum tCa concentration. Total calcium is the most used indicator of calcium status in veterinary patients, even though it does not always correlate well with iCa, and changes in serum proteins may alter its concentration. Correction formulas have been developed to adjust the tCa measurement relative to serum total protein or albumin; however, they are no longer used due to their poor performance and the increased availability of benchtop analyzers suitable for iCa measurement. Ionized calcium should always be measured to assess calcium status accurately. When this is not possible, total calcium should be interpreted with caution and in the context of serum albumin concentration.

Clinical signs of hypocalcemia can affect nearly all body systems. The severity of clinical signs depends on the magnitude of hypocalcemia; most animals show no symptoms until serum tCa is less than 7 mg/dL (1.75 mmol/L) and iCa is less than approximately 0.8 mmol/L (3.2 mg/dL). Early signs of hypocalcemia are nonspecific and include anorexia, lethargy, facial rubbing, growling, nervousness, and a stiff gait. Subsequently, the signs can progress to muscle tremor or cramping, hyperventilation, and generalized tetany, which may culminate in seizures. Once hypocalcemia is recognized, clinicians are encouraged to determine the cause to establish an adequate therapeutic protocol and formulate a correct prognosis.

HYPOCALCEMIA

Severely symptomatic at the time of detection? (e.g., tetany and/or seizures)

YES → Calcium salts slow intravenous infusion **(1)**

NO → **Confirm result (2)**

- Normal calcium → EDTA sample contamination / Laboratory error
- → Signalment, history and physical examination
  - Improper diet / Pathologic fractures → Nutritional secondary hyperparathyroidism / Nutritional vitamin D deficiency (rare) → Dietary modification
  - Acute trauma (rare)
  - Known malignancies → Consider tumor lysis syndrome (rare)
- → CBC, biochemistry, blood gas analysis, urinalysis
  - Hyperphosphatemia
  - Hypomagnesemia (see dedicated chapter)
  - Normal

Supportive and specific treatment

- Toxin ingestion (e.g., ethylene glycol)
- Recent neck surgery → Surgically-induced hypoparathyroidism **(3)** → Oral calcium supplementation **(5)**
- Lactating bitch or queen → Eclampsia → Phosphate-containing enema / Phosphate or sodium bicarbonate infusion / Blood transfusion using citrated anticoagulant
- Iatrogenic causes
- Palpable thyroid nodule → Consider hyperthyroidism (in cats)(rare)
- Vomiting, anorexia and/or abdominal pain → Consider pancreatitis
  - Elevated DGGR lipase → Abdominal US, cPLI/fPLI → Pancreatitis → Supportive and symptomatic treatments
  - Elevated/reduced WBC, left shift, increased bilirubin and C-reactive protein → Imaging (US, CT), blood culture, infectious disease testing, echocardiogram → Sepsis → Fluid therapy, antibiotics, supportive treatments

Oral vitamin D **(4)** and calcium supplementation **(5)**

Normal renal function?

- **YES** → PTH concentration **(7)**
  - High **(9)**
  - Low/normal → Hypoparathyroidism: - Naturally-occurring **(8)** - Surgically induced → Oral vitamin D **(4)** and calcium supplementation **(5)**
  - Consider hereditary rickets (rare) → Imaging (X-rays, CT) → 1,25,dihydroxy-vitamin D (calcitriol) concentration
    - Low → Vitamin D-dependent rickets type I → Oral vitamin D **(4)** and calcium supplementation **(5)**
    - High → Vitamin D-dependent rickets type II

- **NO** → Imaging (US, X-rays), UPC, urinary culture → Chronic kidney disease / Acute kidney injury / Urinary tract obstruction / Ethylene glycol toxicity → Supportive and symptomatic treatments

Hypoalbuminemia (6)

- iCa, abdominal US, UPC, serum bile acids, intestinal biopsy → Protein-losing enteropathy (in dogs) → Dietary therapy, immunosuppressive drugs, supportive treatments
- Hyperglycemia / Glycosuria / Ketonuria → Diabetes mellitus / Ketoacidosis → Insulin, fluid therapy, supportive treatments

2. It is important to confirm hypocalcemia since several factors can lead to inaccurate measurement. When tCa concentration is decreased, clinicians should measure iCa to determine whether the dog or cat has ionized hypocalcemia. Serum can be used to measure iCa concentrations but should ideally be collected anaerobically. Exposure to air leads to loss of CO_2 from the sample, increased pH, and falsely lowered iCa. Many benchtop analyzers carry out iCa measurements on heparinized plasma or whole blood. iCa is less stable in whole or heparinized blood compared with serum and must therefore be analyzed immediately. In addition, liquid heparin can dilute the sample and falsely decrease iCa concentration. Hence, commercially available syringes containing a premeasured quantity of dry heparin should be used. Ethylenediaminetetraacetic acid (EDTA) contamination should be avoided because EDTA chelates calcium, resulting in very low iCa concentration.

7. Clinicians should follow their laboratory protocols regarding sample collection and processing. Handling of the sample is crucial for an appropriate diagnosis because parathyroid hormone (PTH) may degrade if subjected to warm temperatures.

9. Every cause of hypocalcemia, except for hypoparathyroidism, can lead to an increased serum PTH concentration. At this point in the algorithm, it has been assumed that clinicians have ruled out most differential diagnoses, and the patient is eating a nutritionally balanced diet.

DIAGNOSIS

3. A risk of thyroid, parathyroid, or other neck surgeries, is hypoparathyroidism. Due to the high incidence of hyperthyroidism in cats and because canine thyroid tumors are often malignant, thyroid surgery is common in both species. The incidence of surgically-induced hypoparathyroidism is now decreased because surgical techniques have improved, and surgeons are more aware of this complication. Hypocalcemia may occur following surgical removal or ablation of a parathyroid adenoma; however, it is generally transient, as normal atrophied parathyroid cells return to function.

6. Hypoalbuminemia is a common explanation for apparent hypocalcemia because it causes a decrease in the protein-bound form of circulating calcium. This hypocalcemia is not usually clinically relevant unless iCa concentrations are decreased, which can occur in dogs with protein-losing enteropathy.

8. Naturally-occurring hypoparathyroidism can be primary or secondary to non-parathyroid disease in the neck. Primary hypoparathyroidism is uncommon in dogs and is even less often encountered in cats. The etiology of primary hypoparathyroidism is thought to be immune-mediated. Spontaneous infarction of a parathyroid gland adenoma, resulting in acute hypoparathyroidism, has been described in two dogs.

1. A solution of 10% calcium gluconate is recommended and should be slowly administered IV (0.5-1.5 mL/kg), over 20-30 minutes, or until it takes effect. Thereafter, a continuous rate

infusion can be given at 2.5-3.75 mg/kg/h elemental calcium (6.5-9.75 mL/kg/day of 10% calcium gluconate). It is useful to dilute the dose required into a larger volume of 0.9% saline. An ECG is advisable to monitor cardiac effects. It is worth mentioning that all calcium salts are highly irritating when extravasated or administered for a prolonged period IV.

4. Calcitriol is the preferred active vitamin D metabolite, given its quick onset of action (1-4 days), short plasma half-life, and relatively short biologic half-life. Calcitriol is administered at a loading dose of 20-30 ng/kg/day OS for 2-4 days, then decreased to a maintenance dose of 5-15 ng/kg/day OS, divided q12h. The reformulation of calcitriol is sometimes necessary by specialty pharmacies, especially for small dogs and cats. The goal of therapy is to achieve iCa or tCa concentrations just below or within the low-normal range.

5. Calcium carbonate is the most commonly used calcium supplement at a dosage of 25-50 mg/kg/day of elemental calcium OS, divided q12h. In treated hypoparathyroid animals, once calcitriol reaches a steady level, oral calcium can usually be tapered off or stopped as dietary calcium should be sufficient to supply the need of the pet.

SUGGESTED READINGS

-   Feldman EC. Hypocalcemia and primary hypoparathyroidism. In Feldman EC, Nelson RW, Reusch CE, Scott-Moncrieff JCR, Behrend EN (editors). Canine and Feline Endocrinology 4th edition. St Louis, Elsevier, 2015, pp 625-648.
-   Holowaychuk MK. Hypocalcemia of critical illness in dogs and cats. *Vet Clin North Am Small Anim Pract* 43:1299-1317, 2013.
-   Schenck PA, Chew DJ. Calcium: total or ionized? *Vet Clin North Am Small Anim Pract* 38:497-502, 2008.
-   Skelly BJ. Feline primary hypoparathyroidism and hypocalcemia. In Feldman EC, Fracassi F, Peterson ME (editors). Feline Endocrinology. Milan, Edra, 2019, pp 335-354.

HYPOGLYCEMIA

ENDOCRINOLOGY

Federico Fracassi and Lucy Davison

Hypoglycemia is defined as a blood glucose concentration below 60 mg/dL (3.5 mmol/L). In healthy dogs and cats, the blood glucose concentrations are kept within the normal range thanks to complex neuroendocrine and cellular mechanisms linked together. Carbohydrate homeostasis is maintained by the interaction between food absorption, liver deposits and their release, and the effects of the main hormones that control blood glucose (insulin and glucagon). The liver acts as a storage organ for glucose, which is stored as glycogen and can be released following glycogenolysis or through the mobilization of fatty acids or amino acids (gluconeogenesis). Other hormones, in addition to insulin and glucagon, are also involved in glycemic control, increasing the release of glucose by the liver or by influencing the cellular response to insulin; these include glucocorticoids, thyroid hormones, catecholamines, and progesterone. Glucose is the primary energy source for the body; in particular, the central nervous system cannot synthesize or store glucose and is totally dependent on plasma glucose concentrations. Therefore, a condition of neuroglycopenia produces neurological clinical signs of a central origin, typically characterized by lethargy, trembling, depression, ataxia, or, in severe cases, seizures and coma. However, the clinical manifestations depend on the duration and intensity of the hypoglycemic episode; clinical signs are usually evident when blood glucose concentration is below 45 mg/dL (2.5 mmol/L). Dogs may remain asymptomatic at blood glucose as low as 45 mg/dL (2.5 mmol/L), but the more rapid the fall in glucose concentration, the more likely clinical signs are to be present. Clinical signs of hypoglycemia range from mild trembling, behavioral changes and lethargy to ataxia, collapse, seizures, and death. Clinical signs can be acute or progress over time. The hypoglycemic condition can be the result of several mechanisms, such as the excessive consumption of glucose by healthy or neoplastic cells (insulinoma and insulin growth factor 2 [IGF-2]-secreting neoplasms), abnormalities of hepatic gluconeogenesis and/or glycogenolysis, a deficiency of counterregulatory hormones (e.g., hypoadrenocorticism), an insufficient dietary intake of glucose (especially in young animals, or a combination of one or more of these mechanisms). Furthermore, it can derive from the administration or ingestion of drugs or toxins such as insulin, sulphonylurea, and xylitol. The best therapy for hypoglycemia is always that aimed at resolving the determining cause.

173

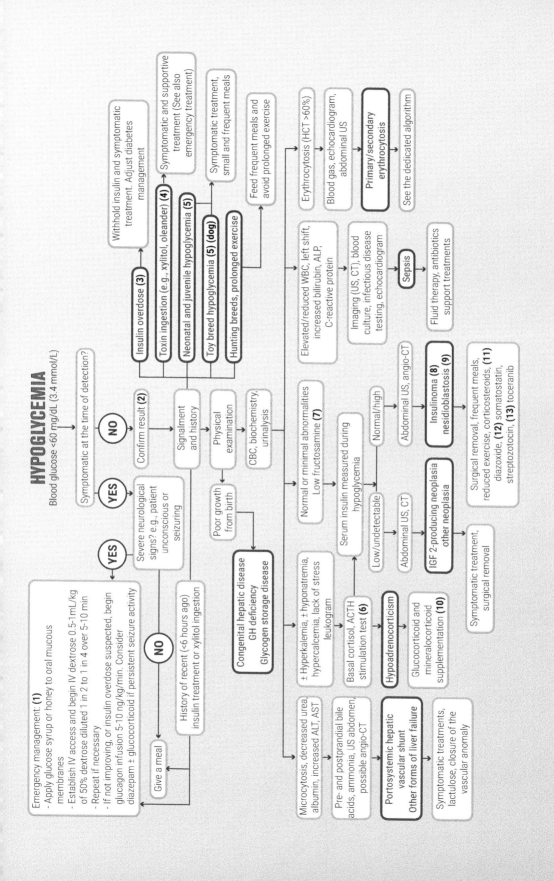

HYPOGLYCEMIA

Blood glucose <60 mg/dL (3.4 mmol/L)

Emergency management: (1)
- Apply glucose syrup or honey to oral mucous membranes
- Establish IV access and begin IV dextrose 0.5-1mL/kg of 50% dextrose diluted 1 in 2 to 1 in 4 over 5-10 min
- Repeat if necessary
- If not improving, or insulin overdose suspected, begin glucagon infusion 5-10 ng/kg/min. Consider diazepam ± glucocorticoid if persistent seizure activity

Symptomatic at the time of detection?

NO → Confirm result **(2)**

YES → Severe neurological signs? e.g., patient unconscious or seizuring

YES → (Emergency management)

NO → History of recent (<6 hours ago) insulin treatment or xylitol ingestion → Give a meal

Confirm result **(2)** → Signalment and history → Physical examination → CBC, biochemistry, urinalysis

Insulin overdose (3) → Withhold insulin and symptomatic treatment. Adjust diabetes management

Toxin ingestion (e.g., xylitol, oleander) (4) → Symptomatic and supportive treatment (See also emergency treatment)

Neonatal and juvenile hypoglycemia (5) → Symptomatic treatment, small and frequent meals

Toy breed hypoglycemia (5) (dog)

Hunting breeds, prolonged exercise → Feed frequent meals and avoid prolonged exercise

Erythrocytosis (HCT >60%) → Blood gas, echocardiogram, abdominal US → **Primary/secondary erythrocytosis** → See the dedicated algorithm

Elevated/reduced WBC, left shift, increased bilirubin, ALP, C-reactive protein → Imaging (US, CT), blood culture, infectious disease testing, echocardiogram → **Sepsis** → Fluid therapy, antibiotics support treatments

Poor growth from birth

Normal or minimal abnormalities
Low fructosamine **(7)**

Serum insulin measured during hypoglycemia

Normal/high → Abdominal US, angio-CT → **Insulinoma (8) nesidioblastosis (9)** → Surgical removal, frequent meals, reduced exercise, corticosteroids, **(11)** diazoxide, **(12)** somatostatin, streptozotocin, **(13)** toceranib

Low/undetectable → Abdominal US, CT → **IGF 2-producing neoplasia other neoplasia** → Symptomatic treatment, surgical removal

Congenital hepatic disease
GH deficiency
Glycogen storage disease

± Hyperkalemia, ± hyponatremia, hypercalcemia, lack of stress leukogram → Basal cortisol, ACTH stimulation test **(6)** → **Hypoadrenocorticism** → Glucocorticoid and mineralocorticoid supplementation **(10)**

Microcytosis, decreased urea, albumin, increased ALT, AST
Pre- and postprandial bile acids, ammonia, US abdomen, possible angio-CT → **Portosystemic hepatic vascular shunt Other forms of liver failure** → Symptomatic treatments, lactulose, closure of the vascular anomaly

DIAGNOSTIC PROTOCOL

2. The finding of low blood glucose concentrations can also be an artifact, that is the result of too long an interval of time before the separation of serum or plasma from a blood sample; the erythrocytes are, in fact, able to consume glucose and the decrease in blood sugar is about 7-10 mg/dL/h (0.4-0.5 mmol/L/h). Many human portable glucose meters tend to underestimate the real blood glucose concentration of dogs and cats.

6. If no causes of hypoglycemia are found, it may be useful to carry out an ACTH stimulation test also in normokalemic and normonatremic dogs. Serum basal cortisol assessment can also be useful. A basal serum cortisol >2 µg/dL excludes hypoadrenocorticism. If basal cortisol <2 µg/dL is found, the ACTH stimulation test should always be performed to confirm or exclude the disease.

7. Fructosamine is glycosylated albumin and reflects the average blood glucose during the preceding 1-2 weeks. Persistent hypoglycemia leads to low fructosamine concentration.

DIAGNOSIS

3. A diabetic patient receiving insulin injections is at risk of hypoglycemia in three scenarios. Firstly, an accidental insulin overdose; secondly, the provision of insulin when a patient has not consumed sufficient calories (e.g., inappetence, vomiting); and thirdly, when endogenous insulin concentration or sensitivity begins to recover (diabetes remission or resolution of insulin resistance), and exogenous insulin is no longer required. Diabetes remission is much more likely in cats. In case of massive overdose, hypoglycemia can last several days and requires intensive care treatment with constant rate infusion of glucose, with careful electrolyte management.

4. Oral hypoglycemic drugs such as metformin, sulfonylureas, and glipizide, as used to treat human type 2 diabetes and some cases of feline diabetes, will cause hypoglycemia if ingested. The artificial sweetener xylitol, commonly found in "sugar-free" products such as chewing gum, may also cause signs of hypoglycemia by stimulating the release of insulin from beta cells.

5. Limited hepatic glycogen stores, small muscle mass, lack of adipose tissue, and decreased use of free fatty acids as an alternative source place the neonate/young animal at risk of developing hypoglycemia within hours of fasting. A similar condition can be observed in toy breed dogs.

8. Functional tumors arising from the beta cells of the pancreatic islets are usually malignant tumors that secrete insulin. The detection of metastasis at the time of diagnosis is common. The most common sites of tumor spread are the regional lymphatics and lymph nodes (duodenal, mesenteric, hepatic, splenic), the liver, and the peripancreatic omentum. Pulmonary metastases are uncommon.

9. Nesidioblastosis (non-insulinoma pancreatic hypoglycemia syndrome) is an increasingly recognized syndrome in people that can be congenital or acquired. It is secondary to focal or diffuse, non-neoplastic beta-cell hypertrophy and/or hyperplasia within the pancreas. This

condition has also been described in dogs and cats, and the diagnosis is reached based on the histopathology of the pancreas. Partial pancreatectomy is the treatment of choice.

TREATMENT

1. In emergency management of hypoglycemia in insulinoma (or suspected insulinoma) patients, it is preferable to avoid infusion with intravenous dextrose since this can induce further insulin release from the tumor and result in worse rebound hypoglycemia. Glucose and potassium are co-transported into cells in the presence of insulin, so it is important to monitor for potential hypokalemia in hypoglycemic animals receiving dextrose and carefully supplement potassium where necessary.

10. In the case of normokalemic and normonatremic hypoadrenocorticism, it is possible to administer only glucocorticoids without the addition of mineralocorticoids. Physiological replacement of glucocorticoids can be provided with prednisolone at 0.1 to 0.5 mg/kg daily.

11. Prompt surgical removal is the mainstay of treatment. If the surgical approach is declined and medical management is chosen, small frequent meals, reduced exercise, and the administration of prednisolone at 0.5 mg/kg PO q24h are recommended.

12. Diazoxide is a benzothiadiazine derivative, the main action of which is to inhibit insulin secretion. It also increases glycogenolysis and gluconeogenesis, inhibiting the tissue uptake of glucose. Approximately 70% of dogs exhibit a response to diazoxide doses of 10 to 40 mg/kg/day PO divided q12h or q8h. Begin with the lowest dosage and gradually increase as needed

13. The multi-receptor tyrosine kinase inhibitor (toceranib) was reacently evaluated in 30 dogs with insulinoma. The median progression-free interval and overall survival time were 561 days (95% confidence interval (CI): [246, 727 days]) and 656 days (95% CI: [310, 1045 days]), respectively.

SUGGESTED READINGS

- Feldman EC, Nelson RW, Reusch CE, Scott-Moncrieff JCR, Behrend E (editors). Canine and Feline Endocrinology 4th edition. St. Louis, Elsevier, 2015.
- Schoeman JP. Hypoglycemia. In Feldman EC, Fracassi F, Peterson ME (editors). Feline Endocrinology. Milan, Edra, 2019, pp 579-591.
- Sheppard-Olivares S, Bello NM, Johannes CM, et. al. Toceranib phosphate in the management of canine insulinoma: A retrospective multicentre study of 30 cases (2009-2019). *Vet Rec Open*. 20; e27, 2022

HYPOKALEMIA

Federica Alessandrini

Potassium (K⁺), the body's primary intracellular cation, is essential for several physiologic processes, including enzymatic action, cardiac and neuromuscular contraction, and routine cell function.

The ratio of K⁺ between intracellular and extracellular fluid is one of the major components of resting cell membrane potentials; 95% of K⁺ is in the intracellular fluid (ICF) and only 5% in the extracellular fluid (ECF). The homeostasis of K⁺ depends on dietary intake and absorption from the gastrointestinal tract, aldosterone concentration, and renal excretion. Aldosterone, the main mineralocorticoid steroid hormone produced by the zona glomerulosa of the adrenal cortex, plays a critical role in determining the amount of K⁺ excreted from the distal renal tubule and is thus a primary regulator of the K⁺ balance.

Other factors that influence the blood K⁺ concentrations are insulin, catecholamines, and pH. Insulin and epinephrine are known to increase K⁺ uptake by the muscle and liver cells; changes in pH result in an alteration of the potassium concentration to compensate for the acid-base balance between the ICF and the ECF. Hypokalemia is commonly defined as a serum/plasma potassium concentration lower than 3.5 mEq/L (normal range: 3.5-5.5 mEq/L). However, internal reference intervals for serum/plasma K⁺ concentrations should be determined by each laboratory.

Hypokalemia is often asymptomatic; however, it could produce different clinical signs according to the severity and duration of the condition. Significant hypokalemia (e.g., ≤2.5-3.0 mEq/L for most laboratories) usually results in mild to profound muscle weakness, decreased urinary concentrating ability (resulting in polyuria and secondary polydipsia), and cardiac conduction abnormalities (such as sinus bradycardia, primary heart block, paroxysmal atrial tachycardia, and atrioventricular dissociation) as a result of a hyperpolarization block at the neuromuscular junction.

Severe or chronic deficiencies (≤2.0 mEq/L) have been associated with rhabdomyolysis, respiratory muscle paralysis, paresthesia, anorexia, vomiting, and decreased bowel motility.

The main causes of hypokalemia are classified into four major groups:
    a) Decreased intake.
    b) Transcellular maldistribution between the ECF and the ICF.
    c) Loss of potassium by way of the gastrointestinal tract.
    d) Loss of potassium through the renal tract (urine).

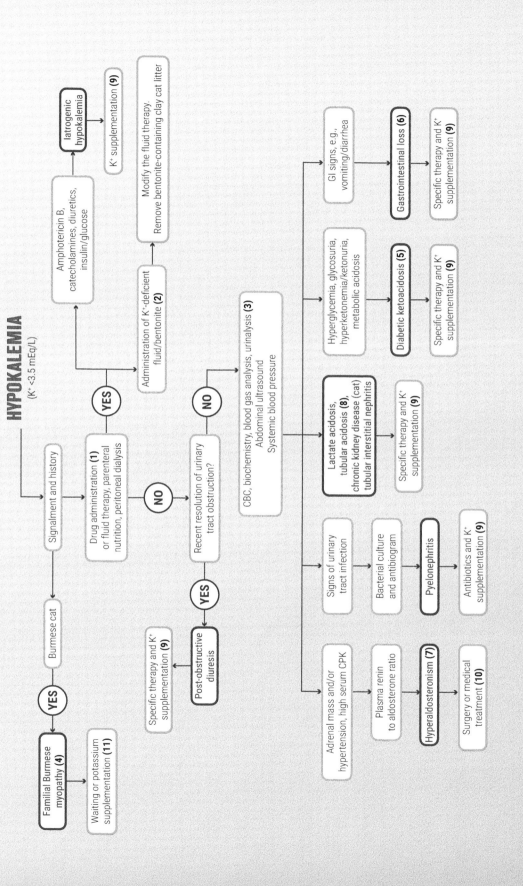

HYPOKALEMIA

(K⁺ <3.5 mEq/L)

Signalment and history

Burmese cat

YES → Familial Burmese myopathy **(4)** → Waiting or potassium supplementation **(11)**

Drug administration **(1)** or fluid therapy, parenteral nutrition, peritoneal dialysis

YES → Amphotericin B, catecholamines, diuretics, insulin/glucose → Iatrogenic hypokalemia → K⁺ supplementation **(9)**

Administration of K⁺-deficient fluid/bentonite **(2)** → Modify the fluid therapy. Remove bentonite-containing clay cat litter

NO → Recent resolution of urinary tract obstruction?

YES → Post-obstructive diuresis → Specific therapy and K⁺ supplementation **(9)**

NO → CBC, biochemistry, blood gas analysis, urinalysis **(3)**
Abdominal ultrasound
Systemic blood pressure

GI signs, e.g., vomiting/diarrhea → Gastrointestinal loss **(6)** → Specific therapy and K⁺ supplementation **(9)**

Hyperglycemia, glycosuria, hyperketonemia/ketonuria, metabolic acidosis → Diabetic ketoacidosis **(5)** → Specific therapy and K⁺ supplementation **(9)**

Lactate acidosis, tubular acidosis **(8)**, chronic kidney disease (cat) tubular interstitial nephritis → Specific therapy and K⁺ supplementation **(9)**

Signs of urinary tract infection → Bacterial culture and antibiogram → Pyelonephritis → Antibiotics and K⁺ supplementation **(9)**

Adrenal mass and/or hypertension, high serum CPK → Plasma renin to aldosterone ratio → Hyperaldosteronism **(7)** → Surgery or medical treatment **(10)**

DIAGNOSTIC PROTOCOL

1. It is important to identify any treatment carried out. In fact, the administration of specific drugs, such as amphotericin B, catecholamines, diuretics (furosemide, thiazides, hydrochlorothiazide), or insulin, could cause hypokalemia. Insulin promotes the K^+ cellular uptake by means of the activation of the Na^+-K^+-ATPase pump. The administration of exogenous insulin in an animal with diabetic ketoacidosis or a release of endogenous insulin after IV glucose administration may cause hypokalemia.

2. The ingestion of bentonite-containing clay cat litter can bind K^+ within the gastrointestinal tract.

3. A minimum database needs to be built to investigate the causes of hypokalemia, in particular linked to renal losses. Glucosuria and Na^+-losing nephropathies determine a polyuric state which promotes hypokalemia. On the other hand, ketonuria, lactaturia, and bicarbonaturia cause a consequent increased renal excretion of anions (such as K^+) to maintain an electrical balance.

DIAGNOSIS

4. Familial Burmese myopathy is a congenital disease typical of Burmese kittens. The pathogenesis is unknown, but it may be due to a sudden shift of K^+ from the ECF to the ICF. Burmese kittens show hypokalemia, muscle weakness, and high serum creatine kinase.

5. With diabetic ketoacidosis (DKA), dogs/cats could develop hypokalemia due to anorexia, vomiting, diarrhea, and polyuria. The intensive insulin treatment for DKA also produces a shift in potassium from the ECF to the ICF. Therefore, appropriate K^+ supplementation (usually potassium chloride [KCl]) and frequent monitoring of blood K^+ during the treatment of DKA are mandatory to avoid severe hypokalemia.

6. Vomiting and/or diarrhea are common causes of K^+ gastrointestinal losses. Vomiting may cause a loss of K^+.

7. Hyperaldosteronism:

   7.1 Cats:
   The disease is most commonly due to an adrenal tumor (aldosteronoma) of one or both adrenal glands; however, it can also be related to adrenal hyperplasia. The majority of the clinical signs and laboratory findings are related to hypokalemia (weakness, cervical ventroflexion, ataxia, severely increased serum creatine phosphokinase [CPK] or systemic hypertension (blindness, retinal detachment). Most cats with hyperaldosteronism have had moderate to severe hypokalemia caused by an increased renal loss.

   7.2 Dogs:
   This is a rare condition in dogs (with fewer than five cases described), usually due to an adrenal tumor. The clinical signs include lethargy, anorexia, and weakness caused by hypokalemia. In dogs, hypertension is also a common finding.

8. Renal tubular acidosis (RTA) is characterized by hypercloridremic metabolic acidosis. Various types of RTA have been described based on the area of the renal tubules affected. With proximal RTA, the urinary pH is <6.0, and the fractional excretion of $HCOP_3^-$ is <15%; with distal RTA, the urinary pH is >6.0, and the fractional excretion of $HCOP_3^-$ is >15%.

TREATMENT

9. Chronic mild hypokalemia (3.0-3.5 mEq/L) can be treated with dietary measures, including commercial oral potassium supplement tablets and elixirs. The dosage of these oral preparations is 0.5 to 1.0 mEq/kg mixed in the food once or twice daily. The treatment of severe (K^+ <2.5 mEq/L) or acute hypokalemia with or without metabolic alkalosis requires the intravenous administration of potassium chloride. The supplementation rate should not exceed 0.5 mEq/kg/h or, if increased to 1.5 mEq/kg/h, the dog/cat should be monitored with electrocardiogram monitoring.

Serum K^+ concentration (mEq/L)	KCl (mEq) added to 250 mL fluid	KCl (mEq) added to 1000 mL fluid	Maximal fluid infusion rate (mL/kg/h)
<2	20	80	6
2.1-2.5	15	60	8
2.6-3	10	40	12
3.1-3.5	7	28	18
3.6-5	5	20	25

10. Adrenalectomy is the treatment of choice. For the stabilization of the patient before surgery or when adrenalectomy is not an option, medical treatment includes oral K^+ supplementation, mineralocorticoid receptor blockers (spironolactone, 1-2 mg/kg PO twice daily), and anti-hypertensive drugs (amlodipine, dog 0.2 mg/kg PO once daily; cat 0.625-1.25 mg/cat PO once daily).

11. Clinical signs in Burmese kittens are reversible. In some cases, they are resolved without additional treatment; however, potassium supplementation is sometimes required. Subsequent continued treatment includes potassium chloride (4 mmol/cat *per os* once to twice daily).

SUGGESTED READINGS

- Feldman EC, Nelson RW, Reusch CE, Scott-Moncrieff JCR, Behrend E (editors). Canine and Feline Endocrinology 4th edition. St. Louis, Elsevier, 2015.
- Stockham SL, Scott MA (editors). Fundamentals of Veterinary Clinical Pathology 2nd edition. Iowa, Blackwell Publishing, 2008.

HYPONATREMIA

Francesco Lunetta

Hyponatremia is an electrolyte alteration caused by a decreased sodium concentration ($[Na^+]$) in plasma, usually associated with hypoosmolarity. This alteration can be a consequence of water retention in the extracellular fluid (ECF), commonly as a consequence of the increased activity of the antidiuretic hormone (ADH). If the patient shows hyponatremia with a normal or increased plasma osmolality, it is usually artifactual hyponatremia due to hyperproteinemia, hyperlipidemia, or hyperglycemia. Assessing the volemic state can be helpful in defining the cause of hyponatremia (see algorithm). The clinical signs of hyponatremia are related to its severity and the rapidity of onset. Neurological dysfunction (nausea, weakness, obtundation, seizures, and coma) because of cerebral edema is associated with an acute onset (<48h) of hyponatremia; a severe increase in intracranial pressure could also lead to brain herniation and sudden death. In comparison, a slow decrease (>48h) in $[Na^+]$ can lead to adaptive responses from brain cells to the change in ECF osmolarity and, consequently, patients with chronic hyponatremia are usually asymptomatic. The focus of the treatment is to restore normal $[Na^+]$, identifying and resolving the underlying disease. In patients with neurological signs, increasing $[Na^+]$ is necessary by means of an intravenous infusion of hypertonic saline solution (e.g., 3% NaCl). Once the neurological signs are resolved, or if the patient has asymptomatic chronic hyponatremia, a rapid increase in $[Na^+]$ should be avoided due to the risk of central pontine and extrapontine myelinolysis.

HYPONATREMIA

Check for pseudohyponatremia (e.g., hyperproteinemia, lipemia) **(1)**

YES → Re-measure [Na⁺] with direct potentiometry

NO → Hyperglycemia **(2)**

Hyperglycemia **(2)**

YES → Diagnostic workup for hyperglycemia → Specific treatment for hyperglycemia (no specific treatment for hyponatremia is warranted)

NO → Toxin exposure

Toxin exposure

YES
- Ethylene glycol → Specific treatment. Fluid therapy **(8)**
- **Therapy (hypotonic fluids, diuretics, antidiuretic drugs)** → Suspension of treatment. Fluid therapy **(8)**
- **Steroid synthesis inhibitors** → Stop the treatment. Glucocorticoid and mineralocorticoid Supplementation. Fluid therapy **(8)**

NO → Evaluation of volemic status **(3)**

Evaluation of volemic status **(3)**
- Hypervolemia
- Normovolemia
- Hypovolemia

Additional diagnostic investigation (complete blood count, biochemistry analysis, urinalysis, diagnostic imaging [e.g., ultrasound, echocardiography])

Normovolemia

Polyuria/polydipsia

YES → Primary (psychogenic) polydipsia → Behavioral therapy

NO → U[Na⁺] >30 mEq/L **(4)**

U[Na⁺] >30 mEq/L **(4)**
- **YES** → **SIADH (7)** → Specific therapy. Water restriction. Fluid therapy **(8)**
- **NO** → **Excessive exercise (e.g., endurance)** → Suspension of exercise. Increase Na⁺ intake

U[Na⁺] ≤30 mEq/L **(4)**
- **NO** → T₄ and cTSH measurement → **Possible hypothyroid myxedema coma** → Thyroid hormone supplementation

Hypervolemia

Congestive heart failure. End-stage kidney disease. Severe liver disease. Nephrotic syndrome → Specific treatment. Fluid therapy **(8)**

Hypovolemia

U[Na⁺] >30 mEq/L **(4)** → **Renal loss**

Renal loss
- ACTH stimulation test → **Hypoadrenocorticism (6)** → Glucocorticoid and mineralocorticoid supplementation
- Blood gas analysis → **Proximal renal tubular acidosis (5)** → Sodium bicarbonate or potassium citrate supplementation

U[Na⁺] ≤30 mEq/L **(4)**

Extrarenal loss
Gastrointestinal disease (vomiting, diarrhea). Third space loss (pancreatitis, peritonitis). Cutaneous loss (burn). Chronic hemorrhage
→ Specific treatment. Fluid therapy **(8)**

1. Direct potentiometry methodology is not affected by lipemia or hyperproteinemia when measuring [Na$^+$]. Instead, if indirect potentiometry is used, the sample is diluted before measurement. In this case, lipemic or hyperproteinemic samples can falsely detect decreased [Na$^+$] (pseudohyponatremia). The plasma osmolality is expected to be normal in this case, since "real" hyponatremia is usually associated with plasma hypoosmolarity.

2. The high plasma concentration of an impermeant solute (e.g., glucose) leads to water translocation in ECF. Consequently, the plasma Na$^+$ is diluted (hyponatremia) while plasma osmolality remains high (hyperosmolality) due to the high glucose concentration.

3. Physical examination can be useful to assess the patient's blood volume status. Heart rate, pulse quality, capillary refill time, blood pressure, jugular distension, and the presence of peripheral/pulmonary edema, and/or intracavitary fluids should be considered. A history of fluid loss (e.g., polyuria, vomiting/diarrhea) could support the suspicion of hypovolemia. Performing an ultrasonography/echocardiography can also be helpful.

4. Assessing the urinary [Na$^+$] can be helpful; however, it is not commonly carried out in clinical practice. If not available, clinical assessment alone can be useful in proceeding with the following diagnostic steps.

DIAGNOSIS

5. A defect in the Na$^+$ and bicarbonate cotransporter in the proximal renal tubules causes reduced plasma bicarbonate concentration and hyperchloremic metabolic acidosis. This defect can could also occur as part of an inherited tubular defect (Fanconi's syndrome), associated with glucosuria and osmotic diuresis.

6. Both mineralocorticoid and glucocorticoid deficiency in hypoadrenocorticism can contribute to the development of hyponatremia. Although aldosterone deficiency is the main cause of Na$^+$ loss, hyponatremia could also occur due to the absence of negative feedback from cortisol in the release of the ADH, leading to water retention in the ECF and dilutional hyponatremia. Furthermore, vomiting and diarrhea are non-specific clinical signs associated with hypoadrenocorticism, which contribute to the development of acute hyponatremia in these patients, if a severe hypotonic fluid loss is present.

7. The syndrome of inappropriate antidiuretic hormone secretion (SIADH) occurs in patients with increased release of the ADH in the absence of appropriate stimuli. In dogs, it has been associated with severe liver disease, antidiuretic drugs (e.g., narcotics, barbiturates, vinblastine), dirofilariasis, pulmonary carcinoma, hypothalamic neoplasia, amebic meningoencephalitis, and hydrocephalus. Some cases, classified as idiopathic SIADH, have demonstrated a pattern called "reset osmostat" in which ADH release is triggered at a lower plasma osmolarity threshold than normal; consequently, plasma osmolarity fails to increase appropriately in these patients.

TREATMENT

8. The main goal of fluid therapy is to raise serum [Na+] at a safe rate. If the patient has neurological signs, usually for the acute onset of hyponatremia (<48h), a rapid increase in [Na+] is recommended, using intravenous (IV) hypertonic fluids (e.g., 3% NaCl) at a rate of 1-2 mL/kg given over 10-20 minutes; the goal is to increase [Na+] by 4-6 mEq/L or until the neurological signs are resolved. In asymptomatic patients with hypovolemic hyponatremia, restoring a status of euvolemia using IV fluids with low [Na+] (e.g., crystalloids), is sufficient to remove the ADH stimulus release and, consequently, to correct hyponatremia. In asymptomatic chronic hyponatremia (onset >48h), the Na+ correction rate should be lowered to 10 mEq/L/day due to potential myelinolysis caused by the rapid correction of [Na+]. Estimating the Na+deficit in these patients is necessary for the correct use of these fluids, using the formula:

Na+ deficit (mEq/L) = 0.6 × weight (kg) × ([Na+] desired − [Na+] patient),

where 0.6 is the assumed water percentage (60%) of the body weight. The calculated Na+ deficit can be restored by means of the IV administration of isotonic fluids (e.g., 0.9% NaCl, crystalloids) or by adding isotonic fluids with a hypertonic solution. Monitoring the patient for potassium depletion and avoiding a rapid rise in [Na+] is recommended using frequent electrolyte monitoring (every 4-6h). Concurrent correction of hypokalemia might be necessary.

SUGGESTED READINGS

- DiBartola SP. Disorders of sodium and water: hypernatremia and hyponatremia. In DiBartola SP (editor). Fluid, Electrolyte, and Acid-base Disorders in Small Animal Practice. St. Louis, Elsevier, 2012, pp 45-79.
- Rosenberg D. Sodium, chloride. In Ettinger JS, Feldman EC, Côtè E (editors). Textbook of Veterinary Internal Medicine 8th edition. St. Louis, Elsevier, 2017, pp 805-821.
- Ueda Y and Hopper K. Sodium and water balance. In Drobatz KJ, Hopper K, Rozanski E, Silverstein DC (editors). Textbook of Small Animal Emergency Medicine. New Jersey, Wiley Blackwell, 2019, pp 690-699.

JAUNDICE

Francesca Del Baldo

Jaundice refers to a yellow discoloration of the sclera, skin, and mucous membranes due to the deposition of bilirubin pigment. Clinically apparent jaundice does not usually occur until the serum bilirubin concentration exceeds 2 mg/dL. Jaundice is not a disease; it is rather the clinical manifestation of an underlying disease process.

Bilirubin is the terminal product of heme metabolism. Heme is liberated from hemoglobin when senescent or damaged erythrocytes are removed from the blood via the mononuclear phagocytic system of the spleen, liver, and bone marrow. Heme is cleaved by heme oxygenase in the phagocytic cells, forming the green pigment biliverdin. Biliverdin is reduced by the biliverdin reductase to bilirubin, which is then excreted into the blood. Free bilirubin is insoluble in water and is carried in plasma to the hepatocytes, reversibly bound to albumin. Additionally, some aging red blood cells are destroyed intravascularly, and hemoglobin is released directly into the blood. Free hemoglobin is bound to haptoglobin and delivered as a complex to the hepatic reticuloendothelial system for degradation to unconjugated bilirubin. Lipophilic bilirubin is processed and conjugated into a water-soluble form within the hepatocytes via glucuronidation. The conjugated bilirubin is excreted into the bile canaliculi, incorporated into the bile, stored in the gallbladder, and excreted into the duodenum via the common bile duct. Within the intestinal tract, bilirubin is converted by the intestinal flora into urobilinogen, urobilin, stercobilinogen, and finally stercobilin, which produces the normal brown fecal color. In normal homeostasis, the liver and biliary system process and excrete all the bilirubin produced via heme metabolism. If any aspect of this system becomes overwhelmed or deranged, jaundice may result.

Jaundice can be categorized as follows: prehepatic: increased bilirubin production exceeding the capacity for hepatic excretion; hepatic: abnormal uptake, conjugation, or excretion by hepatocytes; posthepatic: obstruction of either intra- or extrahepatic biliary excretion or biliary tract rupture.

Determining the cause of jaundice requires a systematic approach targeted at classifying jaundice as prehepatic, hepatic, or posthepatic.

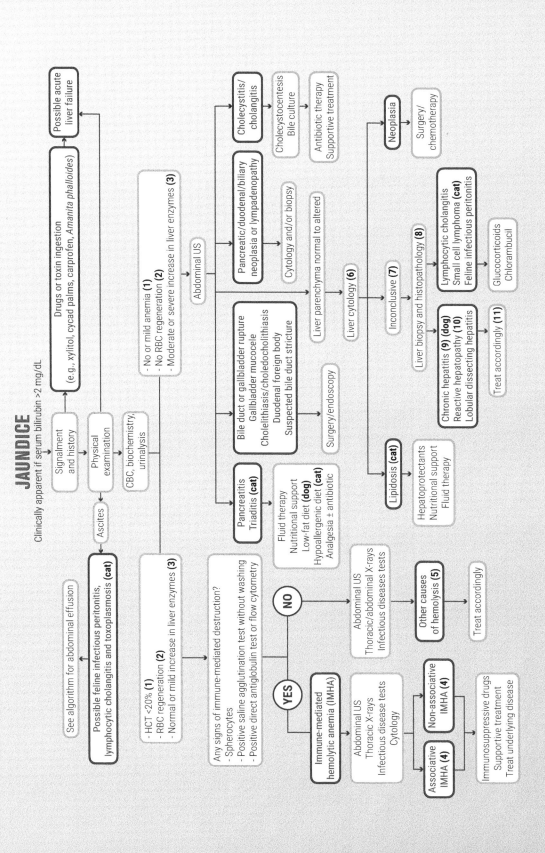

JAUNDICE

Clinically apparent if serum bilirubin >2 mg/dL

Signalment and history

Physical examination

CBC, biochemistry, urinalysis

Drugs or toxin ingestion
(e.g., xylitol, cycad palms, carprofen, *Amanita phalloides*)

Possible acute liver failure

Ascites

See algorithm for abdominal effusion

Possible feline infectious peritonitis, lymphocytic cholangitis and toxoplasmosis **(cat)**

- No or mild anemia **(1)**
- No RBC regeneration **(2)**
- Moderate or severe increase in liver enzymes **(3)**

Abdominal US

Cholecystitis/ cholangitis

Cholecystocentesis
Bile culture

Antibiotic therapy
Supportive treatment

Pancreatic/duodenal/biliary neoplasia or lympadenopathy

Cytology and/or biopsy

Bile duct or gallbladder rupture
Gallbladder mucocele
Cholelithiasis/choledocholithiasis
Duodenal foreign body
Suspected bile duct stricture

Surgery/endoscopy

Pancreatitis
Triaditis **(cat)**

Fluid therapy
Nutritional support
Low-fat diet **(dog)**
Hypoallergenic diet **(cat)**
Analgesia ± antibiotic

Liver parenchyma normal to altered

Liver cytology **(6)**

Inconclusive **(7)**

Liver biopsy and histopathology **(8)**

Neoplasia

Surgery/ chemotherapy

Lymphocytic cholangitis
Small cell lymphoma **(cat)**
Feline infectious peritonitis

Glucocorticoids
Chlorambucil

Chronic hepatitis **(9) (dog)**
Reactive hepatopathy **(10)**
Lobular dissecting hepatitis

Treat accordingly **(11)**

Lipidosis **(cat)**

Hepatoprotectants
Nutritional support
Fluid therapy

- HCT <20% **(1)**
- RBC regeneration **(2)**
- Normal or mild increase in liver enzymes **(3)**

Any signs of immune-mediated destruction?
- Spherocytes
- Positive saline agglutination test without washing
- Positive direct antiglobulin test or flow cytometry

NO

Abdominal US
Thoracic/abdominal X-rays
Infectious diseases tests

Other causes of hemolysis **(5)**

Treat accordingly

YES

Immune-mediated hemolytic anemia (IMHA)

Abdominal US
Thoracic X-rays
Infectious disease tests
Cytology

Associative IMHA **(4)**

Non-associative IMHA **(4)**

Immunosuppressive drugs
Supportive treatment
Treat underlying disease

DIAGNOSTIC PROTOCOL

1. As a general rule, if severe anemia is not present and there are no signs of red blood cell (RBC) regeneration, a prehepatic cause of jaundice can be ruled out.

2. Lack of regeneration does not completely rule out immune-mediated hemolytic anemia (IMHA) since approximately 30% of dogs have non-regenerative anemia at presentation.

3. Hypoxia may cause some increase in liver-specific enzymes (ALT, AST) which may be misleading; however, if the hematocrit is normal or there is only mild anemia, jaundice, and liver enzyme elevation, they are not likely to be of hemolytic origin. Liver enzyme activity does not help differentiate between hepatic and posthepatic jaundice. In fact, posthepatic icterus can cause secondary hepatocellular damage, and in order to differentiate these conditions, diagnostic imaging and/or surgical evaluation are usually needed.

6. If ultrasound fails in identifying the cause of jaundice and hepatic jaundice is suspected, cytology using ultrasound-guided liver fine-needle aspiration is recommended. Cytology is mainly useful for diagnosing diffuse infiltrative neoplasias and hepatic lipidosis.

7. If clinical signs are acute at onset and the clinical history suggests potential exposure to hepatotoxic drugs (e.g., carprofen, acetaminophen, azathioprine) or hepatotoxins (e.g., mycotoxin, *Amanita* mushrooms, xylitol, cycad palm) or infectious agents, such as *Leptospira* spp., consider acute liver failure. In this case, supportive treatment consisting of fluid therapy, antiemetics, analgesics, antibiotics, and antioxidant drugs (e.g., ursodeoxycholic acid, N-acetylcysteine, SAMe) should be carried out before considering a hepatic biopsy.

8. Wedge liver biopsy (with laparoscopy or celiotomy) may be recommended if the cytology results are inconclusive. In dogs with suspected chronic hepatitis, a minimum of five biopsy specimens from at least two liver lobes should be obtained for histopathology (three samples), aerobic and anaerobic culture (one sample), and quantitative copper analysis (one sample).

DIAGNOSIS

4. Immune-mediated hemolytic anemia (IMHA) is the most common cause of prehepatic jaundice in dogs. If IMHA is suspected, thoracic X-rays, abdominal ultrasound, and tests for infectious diseases (e.g., *Babesia* spp., *Anaplasma phagocytophilum*, *Ehrlichia canis*, *Leishmania infantum* in dogs, or *Mycoplasma haemofelis*, *Babesia felis*, FeLV infection in cats) should be carried out to search for potentially underlying neoplastic, infectious and for inflammatory diseases associated with the hemolytic process. If comorbidities are identified, the IMHA is defined as associative. Non-associative IMHA is that in which comorbidities are not identified in the diagnostic evaluation.

5. Other causes of hemolysis are infectious diseases (*Mycoplasma* spp., *Babesia* spp., *Cytauxzoon* felis); Heinz body anemia (acetaminophen, onion, zinc, hepatic lipidosis); envenomation (e.g., snake bite); hypophosphatemia (refeeding syndrome, insulin therapy); hereditary RBC defects; microangiopathic RBC fragmentation (DIC, vasculitis, hemangiosarcoma); neonatal isoerythrolysis (in cats).

9. Chronic hepatitis (CH) can be secondary to drugs (phenobarbital, primidone, lomustine, phenytoin), toxins (copper), infectious agents (leptospirosis, leishmaniasis, mycobacteria, histoplasmosis, protozoal), metabolic conditions (alpha-1-antitrypsin deficiency), and immune causes.

10. Reactive hepatopathies occur due to a primary disease process elsewhere in the body, often involving the splanchnic circulation that damages the liver. In this case, inflammatory changes are limited to the portal areas and are not accompanied by fibrosis or hepatocyte necrosis/apoptosis. The liver lesions do not represent the primary problem, and the presence of an extrahepatic disorder should be searched.

TREATMENT

11. Treatment of CH in dogs should target the causative agent. Unfortunately, CH is often idiopathic in dogs. If a thorough diagnostic investigation fails to disclose a plausible etiology, treatment with nonspecific hepatoprotective agents with or without a trial of immunosuppressive treatment may then be indicated. Immunosuppressive interventions (prednisolone 2 mg/kg sid or cyclosporine 5 mg/kg bid) should be based on histological evidence of a suspected immune-mediated process. Suspected hepatotoxic drugs or supplements should be promptly discontinued, and hepatic recovery monitored by serial biochemical evaluations. In most cases, antioxidant treatment is indicated. Copper-associated hepatitis involves lifelong dietary copper restriction and removal of the copper from the liver. D-penicillamine (10-15 mg/kg bid) is the copper chelator of choice; it has mild anti-inflammatory and anti-fibrotic properties.

SUGGESTED READINGS

- Ettinger SJ, Feldman EC, Côté E (editors). Textbook of Veterinary Internal Medicine 8th edition. St. Louis, Elsevier, 2017.
- Garden OA, Kidd L, Mexas AM, Chang YM, et al. ACVIM consensus statement on the diagnosis of immune-mediated hemolytic anemia in dogs and cats. *J Vet Intern Med* 33:313-334, 2019.
- Webster CRL, Center SA, Cullen JM, Penninck DG, et al. ACVIM consensus statement on the diagnosis and treatment of chronic hepatitis in dogs. *J Vet Intern Med* 33:1173-1200, 2019.

JOINT PAIN AND JOINT SWELLING

Armando Foglia and Veronica Cola

Joint pain and joint swelling are the most common clinical signs in the course of joint disease. Arthritis is the broad term encompassing the inflammatory processes concerning the joint, and several diseases could be involved in its pathogenesis. The degree of inflammation can be highly variable, and some forms are traditionally described as inflammatory and others as non-inflammatory (although some degree of inflammation is always present). Arthritis can be traumatic, degenerative, immune-mediated, or due to infectious diseases.

Joint pain and swelling can affect one or more joints, and owners may complain about specific orthopedic and/or non-specific signs, ranging from exercise intolerance, inactivity, and stiffness up to anorexia and depression.

The history should be carefully investigated to assess any predisposing factors (e.g., trauma, recent vaccination, drug administration). Subsequently, a physical examination is mandatory to identify systemic clinical signs (e.g., hyperthermia) or comorbidities (e.g., gastrointestinal diseases, neoplasia, or systemic infections).

Pain and/or swelling of one joint mainly indicate localized disease, such as septic arthritis or osteoarthritis. Nonetheless, immune-mediated polyarthritis should be considered when multiple joints are involved, and additional diagnostic investigation is required.

Diagnostic imaging of the swollen joints is crucial in identifying any signs of trauma, periarticular effusion, or degenerative joint disease (DJD); it is helpful to differentiate erosive from non-erosive polyarthritis. Subsequently, arthrocentesis is indicated to characterize the nature of arthropathy. Although synovial fluid cytology rarely yields a definitive diagnosis, it usually reveals the general cellular pattern and the characteristics of the synovial fluid, allowing a broad classification of arthropathy. Arthrocentesis is also the primary method for monitoring the response to polyarthropathy therapy.

JOINT SWELLING/JOINT PAIN

History and physical examination (1)

- One joint involved
- Two or more joints involved

Imaging of the joint involved (X-ray, CT, or others) (2)

Signs of trauma or joint fracture
- Conservative or surgical treatment (7)

Periarticular effusion ± DJD signs (3)

Synovial fluid collection and cytology (4)

Hemarthrosis (5)
- CBC, PT, aPTT
- **Coagulopathy** → Investigate systemic diseases
- Blood contamination during sampling → Re-sampling

Of the single joint involved

Inflammatory

At least two joints involved

Inflammatory → Culture and sensitivity (8)
- Positive → Check for bacterial systemic infectious
- Negative → Investigate specific infectious polyarthropathies (9)

Hemarthrosis (5)
- CBC, PT, aPTT
- **Coagulopathy**
- Blood contamination during sampling

How was the X-ray? (2)

Erosion present in at least one joint

NO → Check for periosteal proliferation
- **YES** → **Periosteal proliferative polyarthritis (10)** → Immunosuppressive treatment (16)
- **NO** → **Rheumatoid arthritis, "breed-associated" (i.e., Greyhound)** → Immunosuppressive treatment (16)

YES (Erosion)

Systemic diseases
- Serum ANA
  - Positive → **SLE (11)** → Immunosuppressive treatment (16)
  - Negative

Specific breeds → **Familial Shar Pei fever, polyarthritis of adolescent Akita Inus** → Immunosuppressive treatment (16)

On-drugs for other diseases → **Drug-induced polyarthritis** → Stop drug to see if any improvement has occurred

Vaccination within 3 weeks → **Vaccine-induced polyarthritis** → Usually self-limiting, no treatment is required

Other comorbidities? (12)
- **NO** → **Type I - Idiopathic polyarthritis (15)** → Treat underlying disease and evaluate immunosuppressive treatment (16)
- **YES**

Vasculitis → **Polyarteritis nodosa (13)**

Myositis → **Polyarthritis polymyositis (13)**

Meningitis → **Polyarthritis/ meningitis (14)**

Neoplasia → **Type IV - Polyarthritis**

Gastrointestinal disease → **Type III - Polyarthritis**

Other inflammatory diseases → **Type II - Reactive polyarthritis**

Treat underlying disease and evaluate immunosuppressive treatment (16)

Traumatic lesion → Conservative or surgical treatment (7)

Hemarthrosis (5)
- CBC, PT, aPTT
- **Coagulopathies** → Investigate systemic diseases
- Blood contamination during sampling → Re-sampling

Crystals identified (urate, calcium dihydrate) → **Crystal arthropathy (very rare)** → Medical vs. surgical treatment (7)

>90% monocytes → **OA (6)**

>90% neutrophils → Culture and sensitivity (8)
- Positive → Antimicrobial therapy based on sensitivity
- Negative → Additional investigation (i.e., PCR for infectious diseases) (9)

DIAGNOSTIC PROTOCOL

1. When polyarthritis is suspected (e.g., recent vaccinations, drug administration, correct antiparasite prophylaxis, travel to areas with specific endemic diseases), investigating specific triggers is relevant. During physical examination, evaluate whether one or more joints are involved and identify other relevant clinical signs (i.e., traumatic injury, hyperthermia, lymphadenomegaly, and the severity of the lameness and the joint pain and swelling).

2. Radiographic examination can represent the first step in the diagnostic workup since it is helpful in differentiating signs of trauma (i.e., joint fracture), degenerative joint disease (DJD), osteoarthritis, or periarticular effusion, commonly associated with acute inflammatory processes. When several joints are involved, radiology is helpful in differentiating erosive from non-erosive polyarthritis. However, in the case of unclear radiographic results, advanced diagnostic imaging may be required (i.e., computed tomography, magnetic resonance imaging, ultrasound).

3. Periarticular effusion is commonly reported in inflammatory arthritis. Subsequent cytology is required.

4. Arthrocentesis consists of a sterile collection of synovial fluid. Before the procedure, clip the hair and perform surgical asepsis. Use sterile gloves and fine needles (23 gauge) to perform the arthrocentesis. When polyarthritis is suspected, at least three joints should be sampled (usually both carpi and both tarsi). A synovial fluid sampling should be carried out to avoid blood contamination and any joint injury. On cytology, DJD or trauma are associated with mononuclear inflammation (<10% neutrophils), while immune-mediated and infectious diseases are associated with >10% neutrophils.

8. Culture and sensitivity are needed when an inflammatory pattern is observed on cytology.

9. The infectious diseases to be investigated depending on species. In dogs, the most frequent infections include *Borrelia*, *Ehrlichia*, *Anaplasma*, and *Leishmania*, while in cats, mycoplasmosis or other viral infections (e.g., calicivirosis) should be considered. Nevertheless, other causes to investigate include fungal infections.

11. Serum antinuclear antibodies (ANAs) can be helpful in diagnosing systemic lupus erythematosus (SLE). The sensitivity of the ANA test is not very high, and false-negatives frequently occur.

12. Once SLE is excluded, other comorbidities that can cause immune-mediated polyarthritis should be investigated. Based on the clinical signs, additional diagnostic investigation is often necessary: CBC, biochemistry, urinalysis, abdominal ultrasound, thorax X-ray, biopsies (e.g., muscle, skin), gastrointestinal endoscopy, and cerebrospinal fluid analysis.

DIAGNOSIS

5. Hemarthrosis must be differentiated from blood contamination. Cytologically, hemarthrosis is characterized by erythrophagia, hemosiderin-laden macrophages, and hematoidin.

In addition to trauma, other causes of hemarthrosis include coagulation defects and neoplasia.

6.   Based on cell count and a differential diagnosis, osteoarthritis (OA) is commonly represented by a high percentage of monocytes.

10. Periosteal proliferative polyarthritis is more common in cats as compared to dogs.

13. Biopsy samples are necessary to confirm the diagnosis. Polyarthritis/polymyositis syndrome presents with widespread muscle atrophy up to contracture and fibrosis in the most severe cases associated with polyarthritis. Polyarteritis nodosa affects the small arteries, and subsequently, polyarthritis, polymyositis, and meningitis can occur.

14. Cerebrospinal fluid analysis shows inflammatory patterns as increased proteins, white cells, and creatine kinase levels.

15. Idiopathic polyarthritis is a diagnosis of exclusion and concerns all those cases that cannot be associated with any predisposing factor, potential triggers, or comorbidities. It is still the most common type of polyarthritis diagnosed in both dogs and cats.

TREATMENT

7.   For specific treatment, see the chapter on "Lameness".

16. Initial treatment consists of administering corticosteroids at immunosuppressant doses (prednisone [not in cats,] prednisolone, methylprednisolone 2-4 mg/kg/day) until the symptoms have resolved and for a period of not less than two weeks. Once a clinical improvement has been achieved, the dose may be gradually reduced (e.g., reduction of 25% every 2-3 weeks). Usually, a 4-month course of corticosteroid therapy is recommended to prevent possible relapse. The addition of a second-line immune-suppressant (combined protocol) should be considered if adequate control of the clinical signs is not achieved. Second-line immunosuppressive drugs which can be combined are mycophenolate mofetil (10 mg/kg twice daily), leflunomide (2-4 mg/kg once daily), azathioprine (only in dogs) (2 mg/kg once daily) and cyclosporine (2.5-5 mg/kg twice daily); in cats, chlorambucil (2 mg/cat/day) is also a good option. Repeated synovial fluid analysis is the most sensitive method for monitoring the effectiveness of treatment or the occurrence of relapse.

SUGGESTED READINGS

- Ettinger SJ, Feldman EC, Côté E (editors). Textbook of Veterinary Internal Medicine 8th edition. St. Louis, Elsevier, 2017.
- Johnston SA, Tobias KM (editors). Veterinary Surgery: Small Animal Expert Consult 2nd edition. St. Louis, Elsevier, 2018.

LAMENESS

Sara Del Magno

Lameness is a frequent problem in small animals, mostly due to orthopedic diseases; however, other causes are possible. Lameness is frequently the consequence of pain; anyhow, mechanical lameness can cause an abnormal gait without a painful sensation. Owners sometimes report only difficulty in standing up or jumping.

Age, breed, and sex are important since some diseases are only present in growing animals, while others are typical of adults. Moreover, breed predisposition is recognized for some conditions. The history of lameness is important, namely knowing when the lameness began, its progression, recent trauma, comorbidities, and response to treatment. Before starting with an orthopedic examination, a general physical examination is necessary to detect other abnormalities.

The next step is to localize the lameness using gait evaluation. For front limb lameness, the head of the animal rises when the painful limb touches the ground, while for hindlimb lameness, asymmetry of the hips is present, with the sore hip usually being higher. If multiple limbs are affected, gait evaluation and localization are more difficult, and only a stiff gait or a reluctance to walk are observed.

Visual evaluation and palpation (proximal to distal) of the limbs with the animal standing is followed by palpation and passive movements in lateral recumbency (distal to proximal) to detect asymmetries, limb malalignments, or abnormalities of the bones, joints, muscles, paws, or interdigital spaces.

A rapid neurological evaluation (including at least conscious proprioception, neck movement, axillary palpation, spinal palpation, limb reflexes) is usually performed since neurological problems can also cause lameness. An orthopedic examination to evaluate joint laxity can be completed under sedation in uncooperative animals. At the end of the examination, it is important to have localized the problem and then consider a list of differential diagnoses to determine the diagnostic protocol.

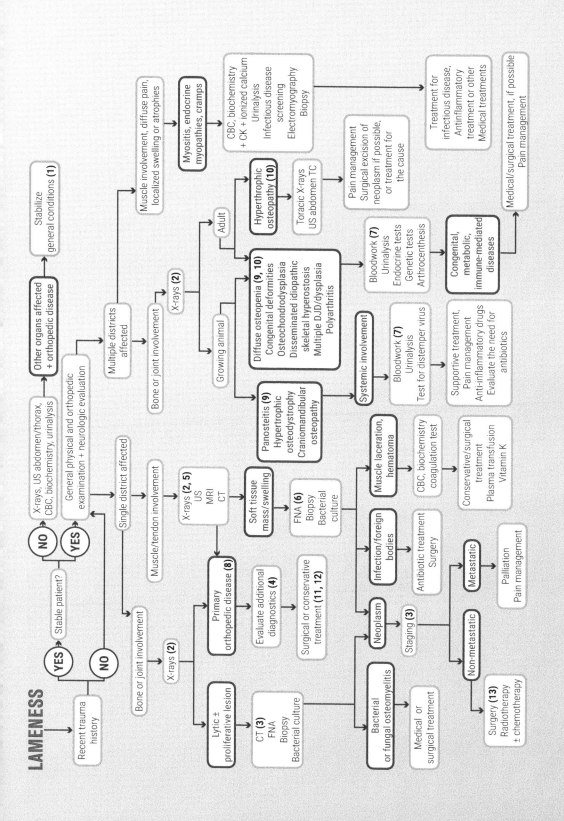

2. In the case of localization to a single osteoarticular district, radiographic examination (two orthogonal projections) is the first step in assessing or excluding bone or joint abnormalities.

3. In the case of lytic or proliferative bone lesions, fine-needle aspiration or a surgical or CT-guided biopsy should be performed for histological evaluation and bacterial culture. Staging is performed using CT or three-view thoracic radiographs and abdominal ultrasound evaluation.

4. For specific orthopedic conditions, stressed or sky-line radiographs help detect joint instability or other joint diseases (osteochondritis dissecans of the hock, shallow patellar groove). Computed tomography is useful for evaluating the presence and preoperative planning of complex fractures for elbow dysplasia, or for preoperative planning of the correction of complex angular limb deformities. Arthroscopy is an option for joint inspection/diagnosis and possibly minimally invasive treatment.

5. When X-rays exclude bone abnormalities, muscle or tendon lesions are suspected. Ultrasound or MRI are indicated for evaluating the soft tissues surrounding the joints or the nervous system, if needed.

6. In the case of a soft tissue mass, suspected myositis, nerve thickening, or synovial proliferation, fine-needle aspiration is usually performed for cytological evaluation and bacterial culture. A mass biopsy followed by histologic evaluation is usually diagnostic. In the case of hematomas, in the absence of major trauma, it is necessary to exclude coagulopathies.

7. In the case of multiple osteoarticular districts involvement, X-rays represent the first step and may lead to a diagnosis. However, to understand the cause and the treatment options, especially in the case of general malaise, additional evaluations are required, such as bloodwork, urine analysis, and specific tests for genetic, endocrine, or infectious diseases. Arthrocentesis and synovial fluid evaluation are performed to confirm inflammatory/infectious arthritis (see chapter about joint pain and swelling).

DIAGNOSIS

8. Primary orthopedic diseases localized in one limb include traumatic injuries: long bone, pelvic or spinal fractures, ligament injuries, joint luxation, muscular trauma, and tendon and/or ligament rupture; non-traumatic diseases: joint dysplasia or degenerative joint disease, patella luxation, avascular necrosis of the femoral head, slipped capital femoral epiphysis, congenital anomalies (dysostosis), bone cysts, septic arthritis, ligament lesions, tenosynovitis, muscle contracture, and myositis ossificans.

9. Diseases with multiple localizations in growing animals include inflammatory diseases (hypertrophic osteodystrophy, inflammatory arthritis, panosteitis, craniomandibular osteopathy); metabolic diseases (hypo- or hypervitaminosis D, hypo- or hypervitaminosis A, gastrointestinal disease, chronic renal failure); congenital diseases (pituitary dwarfism, congenital hypothyroidism, osteogenesis imperfecta, mucopolysaccharidosis, osteochondrodysplasia, etc.), and other diseases (multiple cartilaginous exostoses, swimmer syndrome or carpal laxity syndrome).

10. Diseases with multiple localizations in adult dogs include polyarthritis, hypertrophic osteopathy, disseminated idiopathic skeletal hyperostosis, iliopsoas muscle injury, metabolic diseases (primary, nutritional or renal secondary hyperparathyroidism), myopathies due to endocrine diseases (hypercortisolism or hypothyroidism), neurologic diseases, arterial thromboembolism, and coagulopathies causing hemarthrosis.

TREATMENT

1. In the case of major trauma, the initial evaluation should focus on the patient's general condition and life-threatening lesions. Only emergency procedures (decontamination and bandaging of an exposed fracture) should be performed.

11. Due to the large variety of the causes of lameness, therapy depends on the specific diagnosis. Rest and pain management are usually the first-line therapy for mild/moderate lameness after a normal orthopedic examination; however, if the clinical condition does not improve, additional evaluations are necessary.

12. Fractures of long bones and the pelvis are frequent, and they can be managed by surgical osteosynthesis, splinting, or conservative treatment. Severe degenerative joint diseases in adult dogs may be treated with conservative multimodal treatment, joint replacement, or excision arthroplasty. The most frequent ligament disease is cranial cruciate ligament rupture in dogs, and surgical treatment is advised.

13. In case of neoplasia of the bones and joints, amputation, or limb-sparing techniques, eventually followed by chemotherapy, can be performed after accurate staging.

SUGGESTED READINGS

- DeCamp CE, Johnston SA, Déjardin LM, Schaefer SL (editors). Brinker, Piermattei, and Flo's Handbook of Small Animal Orthopedics and Fracture Repair. St. Louis, Elsevier, 2016.
- Johnston SA, Tobias KM (editors). Veterinary Surgery: Small Animal Expert Consult 2nd edition. St. Louis, Elsevier, 2018.

LEUKOCYTOSIS

Francesco Lunetta

The number of circulating white blood cells (WBCs) depends on the production of WBCs by the bone marrow and their release into the blood, their rate of egress from the blood into the tissues, and the ratio between the circulating pool and the marginated pool (capillaries, veins, lungs, spleen, and liver) since the total WBC count only considers the circulating pool. The main causes of an increased number of leukocytes (leukocytosis) are inflammation, infection, autoimmune disease, tissue damage, and neoplasia. Since leukocytosis is a nonspecific finding, the evaluation of WBC morphology is essential by means of evaluation of the blood smear accompanied by an automatic or manual differential cell count. A complete evaluation of the patient's physical examination and history (clinical signs, drug exposure, trauma, travel, vaccinations, lifestyle) is also essential for differentiating between the various causes. Additional laboratory tests (biochemistry, urinalysis, serological or bacteriological examination, cytology, histology), diagnostic imaging (radiography, ultrasound, echocardiography, CT scan, magnetic resonance) may be necessary to localize and confirm the diagnosis of inflammation/infection. If a neoplastic disease is suspected, additional evaluation of the bone marrow (cytology or biopsy), flow cytometry, or PCR for antigen receptor rearrangement (PARR) may be required. The therapy should always be addressed to the triggering cause. However, in the case of neutrophilia and lymphocytosis in the absence of specific clinical signs (especially in young patients), an additional evaluation of the WBCs is warranted to exclude the possibility that these findings are a consequence of stress, excitement, or recent exercise.

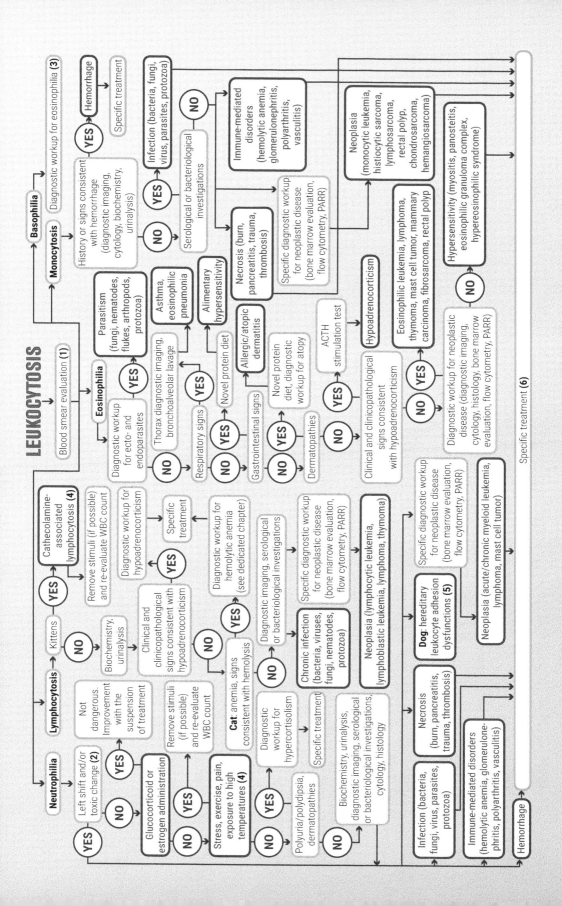

1. The total WBC count can be manually estimated in blood smears using a 10× objective lens (100× magnification) by counting the average number of leukocytes per field and multiplying it by 100-150. The percentage of each specific leukocyte is calculated (400× or 1000× magnification is recommended) and multiplied by the total WBC count to obtain the absolute differential number. In most automated cell counters, nucleated red blood cells (NRBCs) are mistakenly counted as leukocytes (often as lymphocytes). Therefore, the number of NRBCs of each 100 leukocytes counted must be evaluated, and the corrected leukocyte count (CLC) calculated using the formula: CLC = (WBCs measured × 100)/(100 + NRBCs).

2. The presence of circulating immature neutrophils indicates the presence of severe inflammatory disease, in which the demand for mature neutrophils exceeds the bone marrow storage capacity. This condition is called "left shift" and is usually characterized by circulating hyposegmented or band neutrophils. In severe cases, the presence of metamyelocytes, myelocytes, and promyelocytes can be detected, suggesting a worse prognosis. If a left shift is associated with a leukocyte count >35,000 WBCs/µL, it is considered a "leukemoid response" and must be carefully differentiated from myeloid leukemia. Toxic changes are not necessarily found with neutrophilia or left shift. They are a consequence of the neutrophil maturation defect caused by toxic endogenous or exogenous substances in the course of systemic inflammatory conditions, both infectious and non-infectious (e.g., immune-mediated anemia). They include cytoplasmic alterations, such as cytoplasmic vacuolations and basophilia, Dohle bodies, and toxic granulations. Other rare toxic changes are giant neutrophils, a ring nucleus, and karyorrhexis/karyolysis.

3. Basophilia is usually correlated with eosinophilia. In addition to the main differential diagnosis of eosinophilia, the presence of basophilia must be differentiated from basophilic leukemia or mastocytemia using blood smear evaluation. Mast cells are usually slightly bigger and present a round nucleus, unlike basophils, which have segmented nuclei. The presence of numerous basophil granules covering the nuclei can make it difficult to differentiate between the two types of cells.

DIAGNOSIS

4. A state of fright, excitement, or stress in young cats can determine a release of catecholamines that cause transient lymphocytosis and neutrophilia. Once the stimulus is removed, the leukogram returns to normal in approximately 30 minutes. Prolonged stressful conditions can determine an increased release of endogenous glucocorticoids, causing neutrophilia via the release of mature neutrophils from the bone marrow and via a shift of neutrophils from the marginated to the circulating pool. This condition can be associated with lymphopenia, eosinopenia, and, rarely, monocytosis. Neutrophils usually return to normal values within 24-48 hours after removing the stimuli.

5. Mutations of the β2 integrin adhesion molecule (Irish Setters) or kindlin-3 genes (German Shepherds) result in reduced neutrophil adhesion and bactericidal activity, causing recurring infections in these patients. The resulting neutrophilia could be a consequence of reduced chemotaxis and, consequently, reduced removal of WBCs from the circulation or a consequence of recurrent infections.

TREATMENT

6. Treatment of infectious diseases should always be carried out using the most sensitive active ingredient for the infectious agent. The majority of common ecto- and endoparasitisms (e.g., dirofilariasis, ticks, fleas) are usually avoidable with monthly prevention therapies. Bacterial infections should be treated by carrying out an antibiogram in advance in order to choose the most specific antibiotic therapy. The prolific use of broad-spectrum antibiotics predisposes to the phenomenon of antibiotic resistance, causing the development of multidrug-resistant bacterial populations and complicating the therapy of these patients. One of the most common mistakes in clinical practice is treating all patients with leukocytosis with antibiotics before a bacterial infection is identified. Although many causes of leukocytosis are related to bacterial infections, many other non-bacterial causes (e.g., immune-mediated or neoplastic) should be considered and consequently treated with specific treatments.

SUGGESTED READINGS

-   De Clue AE, Spann DR. Leukopenia, leukocytosis. In Ettinger SJ, Feldman EC, Côté E (editors). Textbook of Veterinary Internal Medicine 8th edition. St. Louis, Elsevier, 2017, pp 750-756.
-   Evaluation of leukocytic disorders. In Harvey JW (editor). Veterinary Hematology. St. Louis, Elsevier, 2012, pp 122-176.
-   Schultze AE. Interpretation of canine leukocyte responses. In Weiss DJ, Wardrop KJ (editors). Schalm's Veterinary Hematology 6th edition. Iowa, Blackwell Publishing, 2010, pp 321-344.

LEUKOPENIA

Alessandro Tirolo

Peripheral blood leukocytes, or white blood cells (WBCs), are primary components of the innate and adaptive immune system. The total quantity of WBCs is dynamic and affected by a large variety of stimuli, including infection, inflammation, autoimmune disease, tissue damage, parasitic infestation, and specific hormones. The peripheral WBC count is related to the rate of production in the bone marrow (BM), the quantity released from the BM, the proportion of WBCs in the marginated and the circulating pools, and the rate of egress of the WBCs from the blood into the tissues. Total WBC counts are higher in puppies and kittens, and the count gradually decreases throughout the lifespan; both neutrophils and lymphocytes decrease in number with advancing age. Changes in the relative ratio of the marginated pool to the central circulating pools can alter the WBC count because only the circulating pool is evaluated in a complete blood count (CBC). Neutrophils make up the largest fraction of the WBC count; therefore, leukopenia is commonly secondary to neutropenia. Neutropenia generally consists of a neutrophil count <3000 cells/μL, developing from the decreased release of neutrophils from the BM, the increased egress of neutrophils from blood to tissues, the increased destruction of neutrophils within the blood, or a shift of neutrophils from the circulating pools to the marginated pool. Lymphopenia is rarely the cause of leukopenia; however, it could contribute to a reduction in the WBC count. Lymphopenia is identified by an absolute lymphocyte count of <1500 cells/μL in adult cats and <400 cells/μL in adult dogs; it is a frequent occurrence in the latter. Lymphopenia is most commonly due to viral infection or the effect of glucocorticoids in ill animals. A decrease in circulating monocytes, eosinophils, or basophils rarely results in leukopenia because they account for a minor percentage of circulating WBCs.

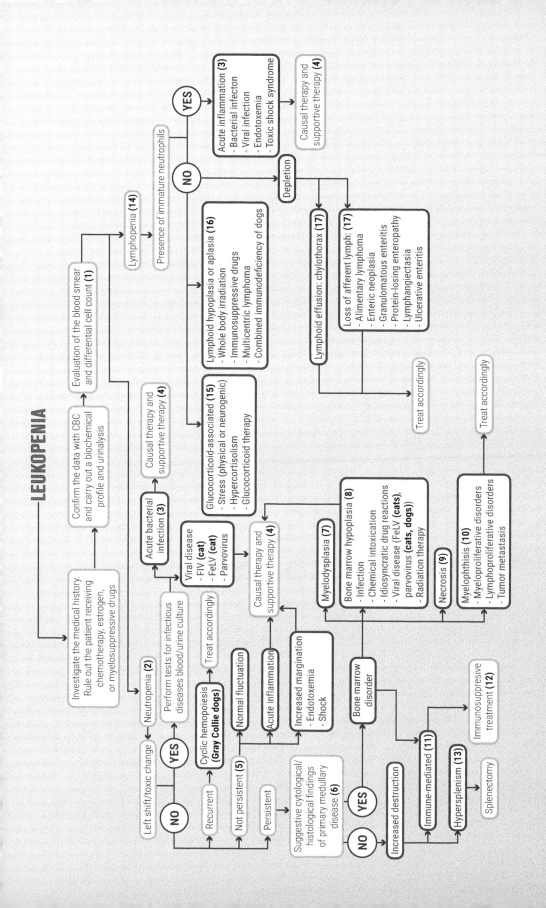

LEUKOPENIA

Confirm the data with CBC and carry out a biochemical profile and urinalysis

Investigate the medical history. Rule out the patient receiving chemotherapy, estrogen, or myelosuppressive drugs

Evaluation of the blood smear and differential cell count (1)

Neutropenia (2)

Lymphopenia (14)

Presence of immature neutrophils

YES

Acute inflammation (3)
- Bacterial infecton
- Viral infection
- Endotoxemia
- Toxic shock syndrome

NO

Causal therapy and supportive therapy (4)

Depletion

Lymphoid hypoplasia or aplasia (16)
- Whole body irradiation
- Immunosuppressive drugs
- Multicentric lymphoma
- Combined immunodeficiency of dogs

Lymphoid effusion: chylothorax (17)

Loss of afferent lymph: (17)
- Alimentary lymphoma
- Enteric neoplasia
- Granulomatous enteritis
- Protein-losing enteropathy
- Lymphangiectasia
- Ulcerative enteritis

Treat accordingly

Treat accordingly

Causal therapy and supportive therapy (4)

Acute bacterial infection (3)

Glucocorticoid-associated (15)
- Stress (physical or neurogenic)
- Hypercortisolism
- Glucocorticoid therapy

Viral disease
- FIV (cat)
- FeLV (cat)
- Parvovirus

Causal therapy and supportive therapy (4)

Myelodysplasia (7)

Bone marrow hypoplasia (8)
- Infection
- Chemical intoxication
- Idiosyncratic drug reactions
- Viral disease (FeLV (cats), parvovirus (cats, dogs))
- Radiation therapy

Necrosis (9)

Myelophthisis (10)
- Myeloproliferative disorders
- Lymphoproliferative disorders
- Tumor metastasis

Treat accordingly

Immunosuppresive treatment (12)

Left shift/toxic change

NO

YES

Perform tests for infectious diseases blood/urine culture

Recurrent

Not persistent

Persistent

Cyclic hemopoiesis (Gray Collie dogs)

Treat accordingly

Normal fluctuation

Acute inflammation

Increased margination
- Endotoxemia
- Shock

Bone marrow disorder

Not persistent (5)

Suggestive cytological/histological findings of primary medullary disease (6)

YES

NO

Increased destruction

Immune-mediated (11)

Hypersplenism (13)

Splenectomy

1. Changes in WBC counts are generally non-specific findings. Differentiating between the possible causes of leukopenia requires a comprehensive evaluation of the specific type of cells affected, clinical history, physical examination, and laboratory diagnostics. The first step should always include an overall absolute cell count, a differential cell count, and a morphologic description of the cells. Evaluation of the blood smear is an essential step in the diagnostic evaluation of any animal with leukopenia.

2. Neutropenia is classified as mild when the neutrophil count is 1500-3000 cells/µL, moderate if it is 500-1500 cells/µL, and severe if it is <500 cells/µL. Neutropenia can develop from decreased release of neutrophils from the bone marrow, increased egress of neutrophils from blood, destruction of neutrophils within the blood, or a shift of neutrophils from the circulating pool to the marginated pool.

5. Care should be taken to identify whether the leukopenia is transient or persistent by serial evaluation. Generally, the former is due to acute inflammation, and it resolves within 4-24 hours, while the latter develops either due to a shift in the leukocyte pool or when, in cases of overwhelming inflammation, the demand for leukocytes transiently exceeds the supply.

6. Bone marrow aspiration or biopsy is indicated when persistent leukopenia, bicytopenia, or pancytopenia are identified.

14. Lymphopenia in dogs is defined by a lymphocytic count <400 lymphocytes/µL; it is a frequent occurrence in this species as a common consequence of inflammation. Lymphopenia in cats is identified by a lymphocytic count <1500 lymphocytes/µL in adults or <2500 lymphocytes/µL in young patients. It is important to emphasize that lymphopenia without a decline in other cell lines rarely causes leukopenia.

DIAGNOSIS

3. Neutropenia can develop under acute inflammatory conditions when the demand for neutrophils depletes the bone marrow storage pool, and there is insufficient time to increase granulopoiesis. Neutropenia is common in overwhelming septic conditions and secondary to endotoxemia in which degenerative left shifts can also be found. Lymphopenia often accompanies neutropenia under these conditions.

7. The decreased release of neutrophils from the bone marrow can be a consequence of the decreased production of progenitor cells or an abnormal precursor cell maturation, called "dysgranulopoiesis." In some myelodysplastic syndromes, secondary myelodysplasia, FeLV infection, and FIV infection, neutrophil precursors are present in normal or increased numbers in the bone marrow; however, the release of mature neutrophils into the blood is decreased.

8. Bone marrow hypoplasia frequently involves more than one cell line. Anemia and/or thrombocytopenia are often present. In generalized marrow hypoplasia or selective neutrophil hypoplasia, a decreased production of neutrophil precursors can occur in the bone marrow. Hypoplastic bone marrow conditions include idiosyncratic drug reactions (e.g., phenylbutazone, trimethoprim/sulfadiazine, griseofulvin, cephalosporins, fenbendazole), estrogen toxicity in dogs, cytotoxic chemotherapy drugs, viral diseases (e.g., FeLV in cats is a common cause), and rickettsial diseases (e.g., *Ehrlichia canis* in dogs).

9. Bone marrow necrosis can be associated with an underlying disease or drug exposure; however, it can also be identified as idiopathic. Drugs associated with bone marrow necrosis include chemotherapeutic agents, phenobarbital, carprofen, mitotane, metronidazole, colchicine, and fenbendazole.

10. Decreased numbers of neutrophil precursors can also occur in the bone marrow when myelophthisis is present. Myelophthisic disorders are characterized by the replacement of normal hematopoietic cells with abnormal (neoplastic) cells.

11. Primary immune-mediated neutropenia is difficult to diagnose in the absence of readily available and reliable diagnostic tests. Neutrophilic precursors may be decreased or increased in the bone marrow, depending on the neutrophilic stage involved in the destruction.

13. Hypersplenism, as described in humans, is defined by four criteria: 1) cytopenias of one or more peripheral blood cell lines, 2) bone marrow hyperplasia, 3) splenomegaly, and 4) correction of cytopenia following a splenectomy. At present, however, there is no agreement regarding the specific disorders included in the category and some disorders for which there is agreement do not fulfill all four criteria.

15. Lymphopenia usually occurs in response to the endogenous or exogenous supplementation of glucocorticoids in domestic animals. This results mainly from the sequestration of lymphocytes in lymphoid organs, including bone marrow.

16. Lymphopenia can occur as a side effect of immunosuppressive drug use and radiotherapy, a consequence of lymphocyte destruction.

17. The loss of lymphocyte-rich afferent or efferent lymph results in lymphopenia. Lymphopenia can also occur when the lymph node architecture is disrupted, preventing the normal recirculation of lymphocytes.

TREATMENT

4. The treatment of bacterial infections with adequate antibiotic therapy and supportive therapies usually leads to the resolution of leukopenia. Treatment of infectious diseases should always be carried out using the most sensitive active substance for the infectious agent.

12. The treatment of immune-mediated forms should be considered when infectious causes are excluded; they require proper immunosuppressive therapy using current guidelines.

SUGGESTED READINGS

- DeClue AE, Spann DR. Leukopenia, leukocytosis. In Ettinger SJ, Feldman EC, Côté E (editors). Textbook of Veterinary Internal Medicine 8th edition. St. Louis, Elsevier, 2017, pp. 235-238.
- Harvey JW. Evaluation of leukocytic disorders. In Harvey JW (editor). Veterinary Hematology. A Diagnostic Guide and Color Atlas. St. Louis, Elsevier, 2012, pp. 122-176.
- Schultze AE. Interpretation of canine leukocyte responses. In Weiss DJ, Wardrop KJ (editors). Schalm's Veterinary Hematology 6th edition. Iowa, Wiley Blackwell, 2010, pp. 321-334.
- Valenciano AC, Decker LS, Cowell RL. Interpretation of feline leukocyte responses. In Weiss DJ, Wardrop KJ (editors). Schalm's Veterinary Hematology 6th edition. Iowa, Wiley Blackwell, 2010, pp. 335-344.

LOW SERUM T$_4$ CONCENTRATION

Andrea Corsini

Total thyroxine (T$_4$) is commonly measured in dogs as a screening test for hypothyroidism or as part of extended blood tests. Thus, a low T$_4$ concentration is a fairly common finding, and its significance must be carefully assessed.

Serum T$_4$ concentration is the sum of both protein-bound and free circulating hormone. It depends on the rate of T$_4$ synthesis by the thyroid glands, the activity of T$_4$-binding proteins, and the conversion rate of free thyroxine (fT$_4$) into the biologically more active triiodothyronine (T$_3$) and biologically inactive reverse T$_3$. Different T$_4$ assays have been validated in dogs, and only the results obtained using these validated assays should be trusted. Repeated measurements of the same patient over time should ideally be carried out using the same assay.

In the presence of typical clinical signs and clinicopathological abnormalities, low T$_4$ levels are strongly suggestive of hypothyroidism. However, other conditions can manifest with low T$_4$. Non-thyroidal diseases (especially when severe) affect the synthesis, and the metabolism of protein-bound T$_4$ by means of multifactorial mechanisms, possibly leading to low T$_4$ without clinically relevant hypothyroidism (non-thyroidal illness syndrome, NTIS). Some breeds have different reference intervals for T$_4$, which must be considered when assessing their thyroid function. There is a progressive decline in T$_4$ concentration with age; older dogs show lower T$_4$ values than puppies and young adult dogs, despite still being within the reference interval in most cases. Many drugs affect T$_4$ concentrations, leading to a mild to moderate decrease, with some drugs causing iatrogenic hypothyroidism. Finally, physiological fluctuations of T$_4$ concentrations below the lower limit of the reference interval can sometimes be detected in healthy dogs.

Low T$_4$ can occur in cats with moderate to severe concurrent diseases (NTIS), while naturally occurring hypothyroidism is extremely rare. In hyperthyroid cats receiving medical treatment with methimazole/carbimazole and/or following thyroid surgery or radioiodine therapy, low T$_4$ suggests iatrogenic hypothyroidism.

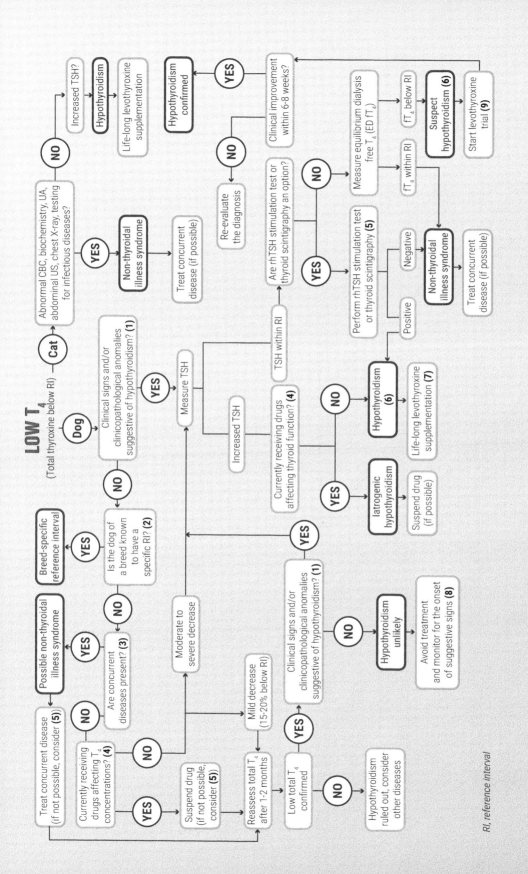

LOW T₄
(Total thyroxine below RI)

Cat

Abnormal CBC, biochemistry, UA, abdominal US, chest X-ray, testing for infectious diseases?

- **YES** → **Non-thyroidal illness syndrome** → Treat concurrent disease (if possible)
- **NO** → Increased TSH?
  - **NO** → Increased TSH? → **Hypothyroidism** → Life-long levothyroxine supplementation

Clinical improvement within 6-8 weeks?
- **YES** → **Hypothyroidism confirmed**
- **NO** → Re-evaluate the diagnosis

Are rhTSH stimulation test or thyroid scintigraphy an option?
- **YES** → Perform rhTSH stimulation test or thyroid scintigraphy **(5)**
  - Positive → **Hypothyroidism (6)**
  - Negative → **Non-thyroidal illness syndrome** → Treat concurrent disease (if possible)
- **NO** → Measure equilibrium dialysis free T₄ (ED fT₄)
  - fT₄ below RI → **Suspect hypothyroidism (6)** → Start levothyroxine trial **(9)**
  - fT₄ within RI → **Non-thyroidal illness syndrome**

Dog

Clinical signs and/or clinicopathological anomalies suggestive of hypothyroidism? **(1)**

- **YES** → Measure TSH
  - Increased TSH → Currently receiving drugs affecting thyroid function? **(4)**
    - **YES** → **Iatrogenic hypothyroidism** → Suspend drug (if possible)
    - **NO** → **Hypothyroidism (6)** → Life-long levothyroxine supplementation **(7)**
  - TSH within RI → Are rhTSH stimulation test or thyroid scintigraphy an option?

- **NO** → Is the dog of a breed known to have a specific RI? **(2)**
  - **YES** → **Breed-specific reference interval**
  - **NO** → Are concurrent diseases present? **(3)**
    - **YES** → **Possible non-thyroidal illness syndrome** → Treat concurrent disease (if not possible, consider **(5)**)
      - Currently receiving drugs affecting T₄ concentrations? **(4)**
        - **NO** →
        - **YES** → Suspend drug (if not possible, consider **(5)**)
    - **NO** → Reassess total T₄ after 1-2 months
      - Moderate to severe decrease →
      - Mild decrease (15-20% below RI) → Clinical signs and/or clinicopathological anomalies suggestive of hypothyroidism? **(1)**
        - **YES** →
        - **NO** → **Hypothyroidism unlikely** → Avoid treatment and monitor for the onset of suggestive signs **(8)**

Low total T₄ confirmed
- **NO** → Hypothyroidism ruled out, consider other diseases

RI, reference interval

DIAGNOSTIC PROTOCOL

1. The most common clinical signs of hypothyroidism are dermatological abnormalities (e.g., "endocrine" alopecia, poor quality coat, recurrent dermatitis or otitis), lethargy, exercise intolerance, and weight gain despite a normal or decreased appetite. The most common clinicopathological anomalies are hypercholesterolemia (75-80%), which is often moderate to severe, and mild non-regenerative anemia (40%). The absence of clinical or clinicopathological anomalies suggestive of the disease makes hypothyroidism extremely unlikely, despite a finding of low T_4 concentration.

2. Healthy Greyhounds and other Sighthounds (e.g., Whippets, Salukis, Sloughis) commonly show a T_4 concentration below the non-breed specific reference intervals. Breed-specific reference intervals have also been suggested for Basenjis, Dogue de Bordeauxs, Scottish Deerhounds, Irish Wolfhounds, conditioned Alaskan sled dogs, Siberian Huskies, Samoyeds, Golden Retrievers, English Setters, and Collies.

3. Non-thyroidal illness syndrome commonly leads to low T_4 values, sometimes markedly decreased. For this reason, in the case of concurrent disease, assessing thyroid function should be postponed, if possible, until resolution of the disease. Free T_4 measured with equilibrium dialysis is less influenced by non-thyroidal illness syndrome as compared with T_4. However, if thyroid function must be assessed in a dog with concurrent diseases, a recombinant human thyroid-stimulating hormone stimulation (TSH) test or thyroid scintigraphy is preferred. Notably, markedly decreased T_4 in non-thyroidal illness syndrome has been reported to be a negative prognostic factor in some canine or feline disorders.

4. Drugs known to decrease T_4 concentrations include glucocorticoids, phenobarbital, clomipramine, aspirin, sulphonamide antibiotics, and tyrosine kinase inhibitors (TKIs). Sulphonamide antibiotics can induce clinically relevant iatrogenic hypothyroidism, which manifests concurrently with increased TSH concentration. Tyrosine kinase inhibitors (e.g., toceranib) can also lead to concurrently increased TSH; however, the clinical relevance of this finding remains unclear. Numerous other drugs could potentially affect thyroid hormone concentrations, based on what has been shown in humans.

5. A recombinant human TSH (rhTSH) stimulation test and thyroid scintigraphy are considered to be the gold standards for diagnosing hypothyroidism. The stimulation test is carried out by assessing the T_4 concentration before and 6 hours after the administration of a fixed dose (75 µg) of rhTSH. A post-stimulation T_4 concentration above 1.7 µg/dL (22 nmol/L) suggests normal thyroid function, with hypothyroid dogs usually showing values below 1.3 µg/dL (17 nmol/L). This approach is also suggested to confirm hypothyroidism in dogs receiving drugs affecting the thyroid hormone concentration if treatment cannot be discontinued, in dogs with a concurrent disease which cannot be effectively treated, or when thyroid function assessment cannot be postponed.

DIAGNOSIS

6. Hypothyroidism can be congenital or acquired. Acquired primary hypothyroidism is the most common form in dogs, caused by the destruction of the thyroid glands, usually

due to lymphocytic thyroiditis. It is a progressive disease, with decreased T_4 values and clinical signs that develop when most of the thyroid tissue is no longer functional. Dogs with acquired hypothyroidism markedly improve with treatment, and the prognosis is excellent. Lack of significant improvement should lead to a re-evaluation of the diagnosis of hypothyroidism or a search for different reasons explaining the clinical signs.

TREATMENT

7. Name-brand synthetic levothyroxine approved for animal use should be started at 20 µg/kg (sid) or 10 µg/kg (bid). Optimum frequency (once or twice daily) remains controversial, also depending on the formulation administered. The gradual introduction of supplementation is recommended in dogs with relevant concurrent diseases. Therapeutic monitoring should be carried out after 6 to 8 weeks, assessing the clinical response and measuring T_4 and TSH 4 to 6 hours after levothyroxine administration.

8. Levothyroxine supplementation should be withheld if the patient shows no signs of hypothyroidism and the diagnosis is deemed unlikely.

9. A levothyroxine trial is justified if strong suspicion and suggestive clinical signs are reported; however, a definitive diagnosis cannot be reached. Response to treatment must be assessed before considering life-long supplementation.

SUGGESTED READINGS

- Corsini, A, Faroni, E, Lunetta, F, Fracassi, F. Recombinant human thyrotropin stimulation test in 114 dogs with suspected hypothyroidism: a cross-sectional study. *J Small Anim Pract* 62:257-264, 2021.
- Feldman EC, Nelson RW, Reusch CE, Scott-Moncrieff JCR, Behrend E (editors). Canine and Feline Endocrinology 4th edition. St. Louis, Elsevier, 2015.
- Mooney C. Canine hypothyroidism. In Ettinger SJ, Feldman EC, Côté E (editors). Textbook of Veterinary Internal Medicine 8th edition. St. Louis, Elsevier, 2017, pp 1731-1742.

MAGNESIUM DISORDERS

Alessandro Tirolo

Magnesium (Mg), an abundant water-soluble intracellular cation, plays a critical role in multiple cellular processes: stabilizing phosphorylation reactions, enabling glucose utilization and synthesis, supporting ion transport, and enhancing macromolecule synthesis (proteins, fats, and nucleic acids). Most magnesium-related disorders are caused by conditions that lead to total body magnesium storage depletion. The causes of hypomagnesemia include decreased intake, alteration in cellular distribution, increased renal or gastrointestinal loss, or any combination of these mechanisms. Hyperaldosteronism, hyperthyroidism, diabetic ketoacidosis, and primary hypoparathyroidism are endocrine conditions associated with hypomagnesemia. Other causes of hypomagnesemia include excessive loss secondary to lactation, myocardial infarction, acute pancreatitis, insulin administration, or an excess of catecholamine. Hypomagnesemia seems to occur with increased frequency in Bulldogs. Many drugs also play a role in developing magnesium depletion. Clinical signs of hypomagnesemia are often related to its effects on the cell membrane, resulting in a change in resting membrane potential, signal transduction, and smooth muscle tonicity. Common clinical signs associated with hypomagnesemia include cardiac arrhythmias, hypertension, coronary artery vasospasm, platelet aggregation, generalized muscle weakness, muscle fasciculations, ataxia, and seizures.

Hypermagnesemia seems to be less clinically relevant in veterinary medicine than its counterpart. However, there is a lack of information in the veterinary literature documenting the clinical signs of hypermagnesemia. Large amounts of magnesium can easily be excreted by the kidneys; therefore, it is unusual to find hypermagnesemia without azotemia. Disorders in which hypermagnesemia has been documented include renal failure, some endocrinopathies, such as hypoadrenocorticism, hyperparathyroidism, hypothyroidism, and iatrogenic magnesium overdose, especially in patients with impaired renal function. Non-specific clinical signs of hypermagnesemia include lethargy, depression, and weakness. Other clinical signs reflect the action of the electrolyte on the nervous and cardiovascular systems.

Accurate measurement of total body magnesium is a challenge due to its intracellular location and activity. The current clinical standard is to measure serum total or ionized magnesium concentrations using ion-selective electrode methods. Monitoring the biologically active serum ionized magnesium concentration is preferred over monitoring total magnesium concentration. However, determining total serum concentration is usually the most readily available technique for estimating magnesium status.

MAGNESIUM DISORDERS

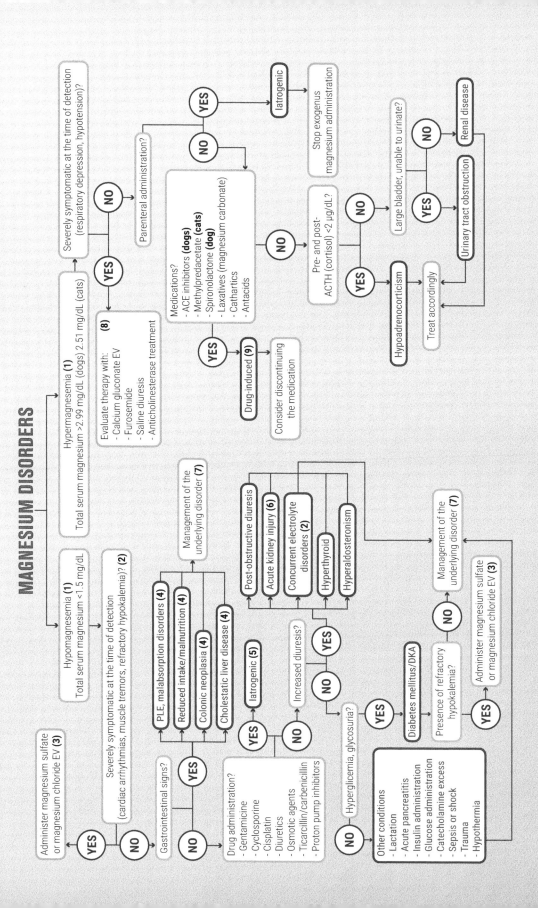

1. Magnesium deficiency should be suspected in patients predisposed to its development which exhibit clinical signs and laboratory features consistent with magnesium depletion. However, the precise clinical diagnosis of hypomagnesemia can be difficult. Since less than 1% of total body magnesium can be found in serum, serum magnesium concentration does not always reflect total body magnesium stores. Normal serum magnesium concentration does not exclude total body magnesium deficiency. However, low total serum concentration in a patient at risk for deficiency is usually consistent with real hypomagnesemia. Ionized magnesium appears to equilibrate rapidly across the cell membrane; therefore, extracellular ionized magnesium values may be more suggestive of intracellular stores. The canine reference range for ionized magnesium is 0.43 to 0.6 mmol/L, and the feline reference range is 0.43 to 0.7 mmol/L. Unlike magnesium deficiency, normal serum concentration excludes hypermagnesemia. Concentrations of ionized magnesium above 0.7 mmol/L in cats and above 0.6 mmol/L in dogs are considered to be hypermagnesemia.

2. Magnesium is necessary for the shift of sodium, potassium, and calcium across cell membranes; therefore, other clinical-pathologic abnormalities usually associated with hypomagnesemia include concurrent hypokalemia, hyponatremia, and hypocalcemia.

DIAGNOSIS

4. Decreased dietary intake, if sustained for several weeks, and prolonged diarrhea can lead to significant hypomagnesemia. This scenario occurs because the fluid from the intestinal tract contains a high concentration of magnesium and is frequently observed in inflammatory bowel disease, malabsorption syndromes, and cholestatic liver disease.

5. Diuretic agents (furosemide, thiazides, mannitol) and cardiac glycosides induce hypomagnesemia by increasing urinary excretion. Other drugs, such as aminoglycosides, amphotericin B, cisplatin, and cyclosporine, predispose to renal tubular injury and excessive magnesium loss.

6. The kidney is the primary pathway for magnesium excretion. As a consequence of glomerulonephritis or acute tubular necrosis, acute renal dysfunction is often associated with an increase in the fractional excretion of magnesium.

9. Improper dosing of magnesium replacement therapy or lack of consideration of the underlying renal function generally plays a role in iatrogenic hypermagnesemia. Drugs, such as cathartics, laxatives, and antacids, contain magnesium; therefore, care should be exercised if multiple doses are administered to a patient with underlying renal disease.

3. Supplementation with an intravenous infusion of magnesium sulfate or magnesium chloride should be considered if the total serum magnesium concentration is below 1.5 mg/dL or if there are clinical signs related to hypomagnesemia. Patients with cardiac conduction disturbances should be carefully supplemented with magnesium, and continuous electrocardiogram

(ECG) monitoring should be considered. An initial dosage of 0.5 to 1 mEq/kg q24h can be administered by constant rate infusion in 0.9% sodium chloride or 5% dextrose. A lower dosage of 0.25 to 0.5 mEq/kg q24h can be used for 3 to 5 additional days. Parenteral administration of magnesium sulfate may result in hypocalcemia because of calcium chelation with sulfate.

7. The amount and the route of magnesium replacement depend on both the degree of hypomagnesemia and the patient's clinical condition. Mild hypomagnesemia may be resolved with the management of the underlying disorder and appropriate intravenous fluid therapy.

8. Calcium is a direct antagonist of magnesium at the neuromuscular junction, and its supplementation can be beneficial in reversing the cardiovascular effects of hypermagnesemia. Calcium gluconate (10%) can be given at 0.5 to 1.5 mL/kg as an intravenous bolus, slowly administered over 20 minutes. Saline diuresis and furosemide can also be used to accelerate renal magnesium excretion if the patient is not dehydrated or hypovolemic. Hypermagnesemic patients with severely impaired renal function may require peritoneal- or hemodialysis.

SUGGESTED READINGS

- Bateman S. Disorders of magnesium: magnesium deficit and excess. In Di Bartola SP (editor). Fluid, Electrolyte, and Acid-Base Disorders in Small Animal Practice 4th edition. St. Louis, Elsevier, 2012, pp 212-229.
- Della Maggiore AM. Potassium, magnesium. In Ettinger SJ, Feldman EC, Côté E (editors). Textbook of Veterinary Internal Medicine 8th edition. St. Louis, Elsevier, 2017, 270-275.
- Humphrey S, Kirby R, Rudloff E. Magnesium physiology and clinical therapy in veterinary critical care. *J Vet Emerg Crit Care (San Antonio)* 25:210-225, 2015.
- Martin LG, Allen-Durrance AE. Magnesium and phosphate disorders. In Silverstein DC, Hopper K (editors). Small Animal Critical Care Medicine 2nd edition. St. Louis, Elsevier, 2015, pp 281-288.

MELENA/HEMATOCHEZIA

Andrea Petrelli

Melena refers to the passage of dark/black-colored stools due to hemorrhage originating from the mouth to the small intestine. The color is caused by the presence of hematin, which is oxidized to hemoglobin. The absence of melena does not rule out gastrointestinal bleeding. Hematochezia is defined as the passage of bright-red colored stools due to the presence of hemoglobin caused by a hemorrhage originating from the distal part of the large intestine (distal colon). However, the amount of time the blood spends in the intestinal tract is more important than the bleeding site. Melena can also be reported in colonic hemorrhage (if intestinal motility is decreased); hematochezia can be observed in small intestine bleeding (if intestinal motility is increased). Differentiation between melena and hematochezia is the initial step when investigating blood in the feces. Ingestion of certain substances or types of diets (e.g., raw) can either result in the dark coloration of the feces or cause the direct or indirect disruption of the mucosal barriers, causing gastrointestinal hemorrhage. Parvovirus infection should be investigated immediately using a rapid antigen test prior to admission to the clinic for all the patients with incomplete or unknown vaccination status. Apart from the gastrointestinal tract, hemorrhages can also occur in the respiratory tract; these could cause the ingestion of blood, resulting in the development of melena. The clinician should aim at differentiating the site of bleeding by means of history and physical examination to direct the investigation to the correct apparatus. Moreover, hematobiochemical exams (including a coagulation profile) may be necessary to rule out metabolic or bleeding disorders. When hematochezia is detected, anal examination and rectal palpation should always be performed since perianal lesions, or anal gland pathologies could be the reason for the presence of fresh blood in the feces.

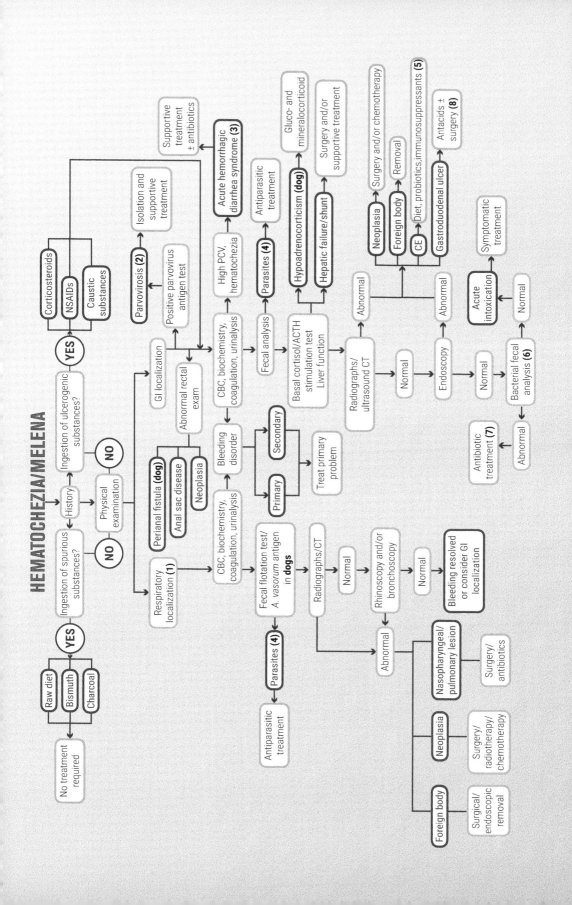

HEMATOCHEZIA/MELENA

Ingestion of spurious substances? — **YES** — Raw diet / Bismuth / Charcoal — No treatment required

Ingestion of spurious substances? — **NO**

History

Ingestion of ulcerogenic substances? — **YES** — Corticosteroids / NSAIDs / Caustic substances

Ingestion of ulcerogenic substances? — **NO**

Physical examination

Respiratory localization **(1)**

CBC, biochemistry, coagulation, urinalysis

Fecal flotation test/ *A. vasorum* antigen in **dogs** → Parasites **(4)** → Antiparasitic treatment

Radiographs/CT

Normal

Rhinoscopy and/or bronchoscopy

Normal → Bleeding resolved or consider GI localization

Abnormal → Nasopharyngeal/ pulmonary lesion → Surgery/ antibiotics

Neoplasia → Surgery/ radiotherapy/ chemotherapy

Foreign body → Surgical/ endoscopic removal

GI localization

Abnormal rectal exam

Perianal fistula **(dog)** / Anal sac disease / Neoplasia

Bleeding disorder

CBC, biochemistry, coagulation, urinalysis

Primary / Secondary → Treat primary problem

High PCV, hematochezia → Acute hemorrhagic diarrhea syndrome **(3)** → Supportive treatment ± antibiotics

Positive parvovirus antigen test → Parvovirosis **(2)** → Isolation and supportive treatment

CBC, biochemistry, coagulation, urinalysis

Fecal analysis → Parasites **(4)** → Antiparasitic treatment

Basal cortisol/ACTH stimulation test Liver function

Hypoadrenocorticism **(dog)** → Gluco- and mineralocorticoid

Hepatic failure/shunt → Surgery and/or supportive treatment

Radiographs/ ultrasound CT

Abnormal → Neoplasia → Surgery and/or chemotherapy

Foreign body → Removal

CE → Diet, probiotics, immunosuppressants **(5)**

Gastroduodenal ulcer → Antacids ± surgery **(8)**

Normal

Endoscopy

Abnormal → Acute intoxication → Symptomatic treatment

Normal

Bacterial fecal analysis **(6)**

Normal

Abnormal → Antibiotic treatment **(7)**

1. Ingestion of blood from the higher and lower respiratory tracts should always be considered in patients presenting with melena. The presence of hemoptysis or epistaxis should raise the suspicion of bleeding in the respiratory tract. Examination of the oral cavity and nostrils should always be carried out.

6. Specific enteropathogens (e.g., *Clostridium* spp., *Salmonella* spp., *Escherichia coli*, Campylobacter spp.) are associated with gastrointestinal disease in dogs and cats, leading to the development of melena/hematochezia. Since most of these bacteria are commensals and have also been isolated in healthy animals, the interpretation of a positive culture may be challenging. For this reason, it is fundamental to exclude other prior processes by carrying out a bacteriological examination of the feces, especially if the signs are chronic.

DIAGNOSIS

2. Parvovirosis is highly infective, and, therefore, patients presenting with an acute onset of hematochezia should be considered infective until proven otherwise. This is additionally supported by the presence of panleukopenia. A rapid fecal antigen test should always be carried out prior to the admission of these patients, or, if already admitted, they should be kept isolated until receiving a negative result.

3. Acute hemorrhagic diarrhea syndrome (AHDS) is defined as the sudden onset of severe bloody diarrhea, often associated with vomiting. The presence of *Clostridium perfringens* NetE and NetF toxins may play an important role in the pathogenesis; however, the diagnosis is still based on the exclusion of other causes for acute hemorrhagic diarrhea (metabolic or toxic, or coagulopathies).

4. Parasites of both the respiratory and gastrointestinal tracts can cause blood in the feces. In particular, gastrointestinal helminths, such as hookworms (e.g., *Ancylostoma* spp., *Uncinaria* spp.), canine trichuriasis (e.g., *Trichuris* spp.), and protozoans (*Cryptosporidium* spp., *Giardia* spp., *Isospora* spp.), including feline tritrichomoniasis (*Tritrichomonas foetus*) can result in severe blood loss, diarrhea, and development of either melena or hematochezia. Diagnosing helminthiasis is achieved by the microscopic visualization of eggs in the feces after fecal flotation or the visualization of adult worms in either the feces or the intestinal lumen. Regarding the diagnosis of protozoan infestations, microscopic fecal flotation is usually used as a first-line test; however, a negative result does not rule out the presence of the parasite, and additional tests (e.g., fecal IFA, fecal antigen ELISA, and fecal PCR assay) might be required.

5. The diagnosis of immunosuppressant-responsive enteropathy is usually achieved following the exclusion of the most common causes of gastrointestinal disease, including parasites, metabolic disorders, and a negative response to a novel exclusively hydrolyzed protein diet. Following the acquisition of gastrointestinal biopsies (endoscopic or laparoscopic based on the location and species), starting immunosuppressive treatment can be considered. Prednisolone

at 1 mg/kg PO q12h, given for 2 to 4 weeks, and then tapered off slowly over subsequent weeks to months. However, this can be used either alone or in combination with other drugs, such as azathioprine (2 mg/kg PO q24h, [not for cats], chlorambucil (dogs: 2 to 6 mg/m^2 PO q24h; cats >4 kg: 2 mg as total dose PO q48h, cats <4 kg: 2 mg as total dose PO q72h) and cyclosporine (5 mg/kg q24h PO).

7. The use of antimicrobial treatment following a positive fecal culture should be considered carefully. Certain infective agents can also be found in healthy asymptomatic patients, and the decision to treat them with antimicrobials should not only be based on a positive culture result but also on the severity of the clinical signs and the lack of other underlying conditions.

8. In human medicine, the use of proton pump inhibitors has been shown to be superior as compared to H$_2$ receptor blockers, sucralfate, and misoprostol. Proton pump inhibitors (e.g., omeprazole 1 mg/kg PO, IV q12h) are therefore recommended as the standard of care for the medical treatment of gastroduodenal ulceration in dogs and cats.

SUGGESTED READINGS

-   Allenspach K. Bacteria involved in acute haemorrhagic diarrhoea syndrome in dogs. *Vet Rec* 176:251-252, 2015.
-   Cerquetella M, Rossi G, Suchodolski JS, et al. Proposal for rational antibacterial use in the diagnosis and treatment of dogs with chronic diarrhoea. *J Small Anim Pract* 61:211-215, 2020.
-   Marks SL, Kook PH, Papich MG, et al. ACVIM consensus statement: support for rational administration of gastrointestinal protectants to dogs and cats. *J Vet Intern Med* 32:1823-1840, 2018.
-   Washabau RJ, Day MJ. Canine and Feline Gastroenterology. St. Louis, 2012, Elsevier.

MUSCLE WASTING

Stefania Golinelli

Muscle wasting disease is increasing in both human and veterinary medicine, partly because of cachexia and sarcopenia syndromes. Cachexia is a loss of muscle or lean body mass (LBM) that occurs with a variety of chronic diseases, including congestive heart failure, cancer, chronic kidney disease, diabetes mellitus, hypercortisolism, and hyperthyroidism, as well as being associated with acute illness and injury. Sarcopenia is related to cachexia and is characterized by loss of muscle and lean body mass. However, unlike cachexia, sarcopenia is associated with aging in the absence of disease. Since most diseases associated with muscle loss are more common in aging, cachexia and sarcopenia are often concurrent problems. The loss of LBM has important negative effects on wound healing, immune function, strength, and survival. Many of the effects of cachexia and sarcopenia, such as weight loss, weakness, reduced food intake and perceived poor quality of life, are major contributing factors to an owner's decision for euthanasia. The pathogenesis of cachexia and sarcopenia is complex and multifactorial and includes inflammation, decreased concentration of growth hormone and testosterone, insulin resistance, decreased protein synthesis, reduced physical activity, and changes in the composition of muscle fibers. Cachexia and sarcopenia refer to any muscle loss ranging from mild to severe and begin with more subtle muscle loss. To recognize cachexia and sarcopenia in their earliest stages, when intervention is more likely to be successful, body weight, body condition score (BCS), and muscle condition score (MCS) should be assessed at every visit. Muscle loss, which occurs before weight loss, is a more sensitive measurement. Evaluation of muscle mass includes visual examination and palpation of the epaxial muscles, the thoracic and lumbar vertebrae, the head, scapulae, and pelvic bones. The most effective treatment for cachexia is the correction of the underlying disease. Moreover, specific nutritional recommendations can help optimize the treatment of cachexia or sarcopenia.

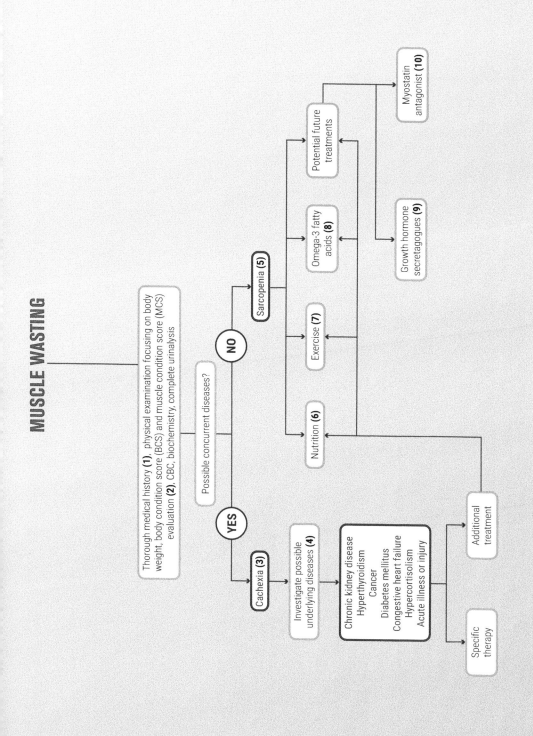

MUSCLE WASTING

Thorough medical history **(1)**, physical examination focusing on body weight, body condition score (BCS) and muscle condition score (MCS) evaluation **(2)**, CBC, biochemistry, complete urinalysis

Possible concurrent diseases?

YES

NO

Cachexia (3)

Sarcopenia (5)

Investigate possible underlying diseases **(4)**

Chronic kidney disease
Hyperthyroidism
Cancer
Diabetes mellitus
Congestive heart failure
Hypercortisolism
Acute illness or injury

Specific therapy

Additional treatment

Nutrition (6)

Exercise (7)

Omega-3 fatty acids (8)

Potential future treatments

Growth hormone secretagogues (9)

Myostatin antagonist (10)

1. When investigating the medical history of a cat or dog with muscle wasting, a complete dietary history should be carefully evaluated. The diet history should include not just the animal food but also treats, table foods, dental products, and food used to administer medications. Clinicians should ensure that the diet being eaten by the cat or the dog is nutritionally complete and balanced. Pain (e.g., dental disease) or environmental factors (e.g., multi-cat households) can negatively affect food intake and should be investigated and addressed.

2. The muscle condition score (MCS), which differs from the body condition score (BCS) because it specifically evaluates muscle mass, is based on visual examination and palpation of the muscle mass of the head, scapulae, epaxial muscles of the thoracic and lumbar vertebrae, and the pelvic bones. Typically, the epaxial muscles over the thoracic and lumbar region are the sites in which muscle loss can be identified in its earliest stages.

4. Based on the clinical signs and the clinical-pathological findings, the most appropriate diagnostic protocol should be carried out: thoracic and abdominal imaging like radiographs and ultrasonography (e.g., to investigate cancer, chronic kidney disease, congestive heart failure); echocardiography (congestive heart failure); serum T_4 (hyperthyroidism); computed tomography (cancer).

DIAGNOSIS

3. Cachexia is a complicated metabolic syndrome related to underlying illness. It is characterized by loss of muscle mass with or without the loss of fat mass.

5. Sarcopenia is a significant loss of lean body mass that occurs with aging. This loss of lean body mass, called sarcopenia, occurs in the absence of disease.

6. Careful attention must be paid to the diet composition of cats and dogs with muscle wasting. This is particularly important because reduced total caloric and protein intake may be a contributing cause of cachexia and other types of muscle wasting in these patients. Assuming an adequate caloric intake, protein is the primary macronutrient responsible for the maintenance of muscle mass.

7. Exercise may be more challenging in some of the diseases associated with cachexia in dogs (i.e., chronic heart failure), particularly in cats; however, exercise, such as walking, may provide an effective treatment for muscle loss in some diseases and in preventing sarcopenia in aging animals.

8. Omega-3 fatty acids decrease the production of inflammatory cytokines. This can reduce muscle loss and improve appetite. The optimal dosage of omega-3 fatty acids has not yet been determined; however, a dosage of fish oil to provide 40 mg/kg/day eicosapentaenoic acid (EPA) and 25 mg/kg/day docosahexaenoic acid (DHA) for animals with any degree of cachexia or sarcopenia has been recommended.

9. Growth hormone secretagogues (GHSs) are a class of small molecular compounds that stimulate the release of growth hormone (GH); they mimic ghrelin, a hormone secreted from endocrine cells in the stomach, which stimulates appetite and food intake in humans. For this reason, GHSs may be useful in the treatment of cachexia and sarcopenia. Capromorelin, an oral active ghrelin receptor agonist, has been approved as a new drug for use in dogs. Preliminary studies indicate that capromorelin also increases food intake and promotes weight gain in laboratory cats; however, only limited research studies on cats have been published to date.

10. Myostatin negatively regulates skeletal muscle mass, and myostatin mutations result in enlarged musculature. If myostatin levels are elevated, muscle loss occurs. Conversely, blocking myostatin may be beneficial in cachexia and sarcopenia by increasing muscle mass. To date, just a small study of a myostatin antagonist (activin receptor type IIB) has been carried out in dogs with naturally-occurring chronic heart failure. While no significant improvements occurred in body weight, there was a numerical, but not significant, increase in the MCS.

SUGGESTED READINGS

- Freeman LM. Cachexia and sarcopenia: emerging syndromes of importance in dogs and cats. *J Vet Intern Med* 26:3-17, 2012.
- Freeman LM. Cachexia and sarcopenia. In Feldman EC, Fracassi F, Peterson ME (editors). Feline Endocrinology. Milan, Edra, 2019, pp 627-632.
- Peterson ME, Little SE. Cachexia, sarcopenia and other forms of muscle wasting: common problems of senior and geriatric cats and of cats with endocrine disease. Proceedings of the Companion Animal Summit. Charleston, South Carolina, 2018, pp 65-73.

NASAL DISCHARGE

Rodolfo Oliveira Leal

Nasal discharge is usually a consequence of inflammation and/or infection of the nasal mucosa, being a frequent sign of local nasal disease. Less commonly, it can also reflect paranasal/sinusal, nasopharyngeal, and/or systemic disease. Nasal discharge is frequently associated with sneezing, a protective reflex triggered by subepithelial nasal receptors, activated by physical or chemical stimuli. Stertor or reverse sneezing, an exuberant inspiratory snore noise, can also be concurrently present, indicating nasopharyngeal disease.

Signalment and history help prioritize the differential diagnosis. While congenital and infectious diseases are more common in young animals, older animals are more prone to neoplasia or dental disease.

Nasal discharge can be classified according to duration, laterality, and macroscopic type. Acute nasal discharge is usually caused by either upper airway infection (namely in cats) versus foreign body inhalation (in dogs), while chronic disease is often caused by a fungal infection, neoplasia, or allergic/immune-mediated disease in both species. Bilateral discharge can occur in systemic disease, neoplasia, and inflammatory, infectious, or allergic disease. If a unilateral discharge is present, foreign bodies, neoplasia, oronasal fistulas, polyps, or dental disease are prioritized.

Nasal discharge can be serous (watery/clear – normal finding if mild), mucous/mucopurulent (white to green – common in most nasal disorders with concurrent secondary bacterial infection), blood-tinged (highlighting turbinate destruction and mucosal erosion), epistaxis (stressing local or systemic causes, such as hypertension or hemostatic disorders) or food-containing discharge (supporting congenital palate disease or an oronasal fistula). The cytology of a nasal discharge is non-specific; however, it occasionally allows the identification of parasites, fungal diseases, or neoplastic cells. Regardless of the macroscopic appearance, a nasal swab culture is of little benefit as it commonly isolates only commensal microflora.

Although useful in practice, the diagnosis of nasal disease can never be established based only on nasal discharge findings; it requires advanced complementary exams, such as computed tomography and/or rhinoscopy with nasal biopsies.

NASAL DISCHARGE

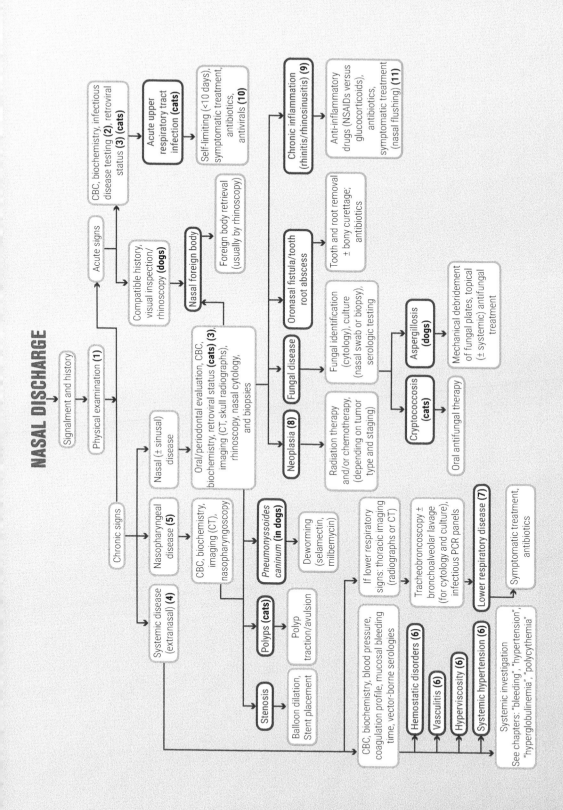

Signalment and history

Physical examination (1)

Acute signs

CBC, biochemistry, infectious disease testing (2) (cats), retroviral status (3) (cats)

Acute upper respiratory tract infection (cats)

Self-limiting (<10 days), symptomatic treatment, antibiotics, antivirals (10)

Compatible history, visual inspection/rhinoscopy (dogs)

Nasal foreign body

Foreign body retrieval (usually by rhinoscopy)

Chronic signs

Nasal (± sinusal) disease

Oral/periodontal evaluation, CBC, biochemistry, retroviral status (cats) (3), imaging (CT, skull radiographs), rhinoscopy, nasal cytology, and biopsies

Chronic inflammation (rhinitis/rhinosinusitis) (9)

Anti-inflammatory drugs (NSAIDs versus glucocorticoids), antibiotics, symptomatic treatment (nasal flushing) (11)

Oronasal fistula/tooth root abscess

Tooth and root removal ± bony curettage; antibiotics

Fungal disease

Fungal identification (cytology), culture (nasal swab or biopsy), serologic testing

Aspergillosis (dogs)

Mechanical debridement of fungal plates, topical (± systemic) antifungal treatment

Cryptococcosis (cats)

Oral antifungal therapy

Neoplasia (8)

Radiation therapy and/or chemotherapy, (depending on tumor type and staging)

Nasopharyngeal disease (5)

CBC, biochemistry, imaging (CT), nasopharyngoscopy

Pneumonyssoides caninum (in dogs)

Deworming (selamectin, milbemycin)

If lower respiratory signs: thoracic imaging (radiographs or CT)

Tracheobronchoscopy ± bronchoalveolar lavage (for cytology and culture), infectious PCR panels

Lower respiratory disease (7)

Symptomatic treatment, antibiotics

Polyps (cats)

Polyp traction/avulsion

Stenosis

Balloon dilation, Stent placement

Systemic disease (extranasal) (4)

CBC, biochemistry, blood pressure, coagulation profile, mucosal bleeding time, vector-borne serologies

Hemostatic disorders (6)

Vasculitis (6)

Hyperviscosity (6)

Systemic hypertension (6)

Systemic investigation
See chapters: "bleeding", "hypertension", "hyperglobulinemia", "polycythemia"

1. It is important to evaluate facial symmetry, tooth/periodontal disease, the nasal planum, the palate, nasal bones, retromandibular lymph nodes (if enlarged, fine-needle aspiration should be performed), and both eyes (assessing the presence of exophthalmia). Air-column permeability should be assessed for each nasal cavity. This can be done by evaluating condensation, using a cold microscope slide, or a glass in front of each nare.

2. Feline acute upper respiratory infection (URI) is often a clinically-based diagnosis. Screening for feline herpesvirus (FHV-1) and feline calicivirus (FCV) using polymerase chain reaction (PCR) should be considered; however, its value is questionable as viral status does not always correlate with clinical disease. Other organisms, such as *Chlamydia felis*, *Mycoplasma* spp., or *Bordetella* spp., can be associated with feline URI and can also be screened using PCR.

3. Testing for feline retroviruses is recommended as they can be associated with lymphoma and can induce immunosuppression which, by itself, predisposes to URI. Bacterial culture is not recommended since it could lead to isolating the commensal bacteria, for which the pathogenic role is questionable.

4. Apart from local causes, nasal discharge can also be due to lower respiratory disease (e.g., bronchopneumonia) or systemic causes (e.g., epistaxis due to clotting disorders or increased capillary fragility).

5. Nasopharyngeal disease should be prioritized in cases showing inspiratory respiratory effort with reverse sneezing and/or stertor.

DIAGNOSIS

6. Systemic causes, such as hemostatic disorders (thrombocytopathy, thrombocytopenia, von Willebrand disease, congenital or acquired coagulation factor deficiencies), increased capillary fragility due to systemic hypertension (either primary or secondary to metabolic or endocrine causes, such as kidney disease, pheochromocytoma or hyperaldosteronism), vasculitis (immune-mediated, neoplastic or secondary to vector-borne diseases, toxic, or inflammatory diseases) or hyperviscosity (either due to polycythemia or hyperglobulinemia secondary to lymphoma, ehrlichiosis, multiple myeloma or leishmaniasis), should be evaluated, especially in the case of epistaxis.

7. Lower respiratory disease can also be associated with nasal discharge, namely in aspiration pneumonia or in rare conditions, such as eosinophilic bronchopneumopathy, infectious tracheobronchitis, or primary ciliary dyskinesia. In these conditions, the microscopic changes of the lower respiratory tract can extend to the nasal epithelium.

8. Most nasal tumors are malignant and exhibit local invasive behavior. The most frequently encountered nasal neoplasia in dogs is carcinoma, while, in cats, it is nasal lymphoma.

9. In cats, chronic rhinosinusitis can affect all ages and seems to be caused by a viral infection,

secondary bacterial disease, and local immune dysregulation. In dogs, lymphoplasmacytic rhinitis (also known as allergic or immune-mediated rhinitis) commonly affects young to middle-aged, large breed, dolichocephalic dogs. A CT scan often reveals turbinate lysis in both species and increased fluid density within the nasal (± sinusal) cavities. These findings can overlap with nasal neoplasia, which is why a rhinoscopy with nasal biopsy is important for a definitive diagnosis. Rhinoscopy reveals non-specific findings (increased friability, hyperemic mucosa), and biopsies often show lymphoplasmacytic inflammation.

TREATMENT

10. Feline upper respiratory infection tends to be self-limiting over the first 10 days. If the cat shows systemic signs of disease (such as fever, anorexia, lethargy), antibiotics should be prescribed. Doxycycline is the current recommendation due to its antimicrobial spectrum (covering *Mycoplasma* spp. and *Bordetella* spp.) and its anti-inflammatory and immunomodulatory actions. Other options such as amoxicillin or amoxicillin and clavulanic acid can be considered on an individual basis. Antivirals (e.g., famciclovir) can be an option in some FHV-1/FCV-positive cats. If signs do not progressively improve, a chronic nasal respiratory disease is likely and should be appropriately investigated.

11. Either non-steroidal drugs (NSAIDs) or glucocorticoids (either orally or by metered-dose inhalation therapy) have been reported to be successful in the long-term medical management of chronic rhinitis in dogs and cats. Specifically, in cats, the use of antivirals (namely famciclovir) in suspicious cases of chronic FHV-1 is described; however, the evidence is weak. Symptomatic treatment (nasal serum flushes, mucolytics) can also be considered on an individual basis. Doxycycline or azithromycin can be prescribed in both species due to their recognized anti-inflammatory and modulator antimicrobial therapeutic effects.

SUGGESTED READINGS

- Hernandez J. Examen clinique des grands syndromes respiratoires. In Hernandez J, Poncet C (editors). Maladies respiratoires du chien et du chat. Les Éditions du Point Vétérinaire, 2012, pp 3-30.
- Johnson LR (editor). Canine and Feline Respiratory Medicine 2nd edition. Wiley Blackwell, 2020.
- Lappin MR, Blondeau J, Boothe D, et al. Antimicrobial use Guidelines for Treatment of Respiratory Tract Disease in Dogs and Cats: Antimicrobial Guidelines Working Group of the International Society of Companion Animal Infectious Diseases. *J Vet Intern Med* 31:279-294, 2017.
- Lopez J. Sneezing and nasal discharge. In Ettinger SJ, Feldman EC, Côté E (editors). Textbook of Veterinary Internal Medicine 8th edition. St. Louis, Elsevier, 2017, pp 111-115.
- Reed N. Chronic rhinitis in the cat: an update. *Vet Clin North Am Small Anim Pract* 50:311-329, 2020.

OLIGURIA/ANURIA

Erika Monari

Oliguria is defined as urine production of less than 1 mL/kg/h, whereas anuria is the absence of urine formation. In healthy patients, urine production is regulated by the kidneys by means of glomerular ultrafiltration, tubular secretion, and the reabsorption of water and electrolytes, leading to the production of concentrated urine. The kidneys can autoregulate renal blood flow (RBF) by means of tubuloglomerular feedback when systolic blood pressure values are between 80 and 180 mmHg. Changes in tubular flow rate and composition are detected by the macula densa cells, causing vasoconstriction of the afferent glomerular arteriole. For this system to be intact, systolic blood pressure should be above 80 mmHg; below this threshold, RBF decreases and follows the systolic blood pressure in a linear fashion. In healthy patients, an appropriate renal response to decreased kidney perfusion is a reduction in urine production and an increase in urine specific gravity. Instead, during acute kidney injury (AKI), due to a spectrum of diseases causing functional and/or parenchymal kidney damage, 30 to 60% of patients develop oliguria. Acute kidney injury-associated oliguria can be caused by a decreased RBF, called volume-responsive AKI, in which oliguria is caused by hypovolemia and/or hypotension and improves after volume expansion. Oliguria is also present during intrinsic AKI, in which kidney damage cannot be resolved with fluid therapy, and the persistence of oliguria and azotemia can be associated with overhydration or electrolyte and acid-base imbalances. Clinical conditions causing intrinsic AKI can develop as a consequence of hemodynamic events, such as ischemic injuries, or it can be caused by infectious, immune-mediated, neoplastic, or degenerative diseases. Furthermore, exposure to exogenous drugs or toxins (e.g., aminoglycoside antimicrobials, non-steroidal anti-inflammatory drugs) can cause a reduction in renal perfusion, inflammation, and cell death. Finally, oliguria is present in postrenal AKI, where it is caused by urinary tract rupture and/or obstruction.

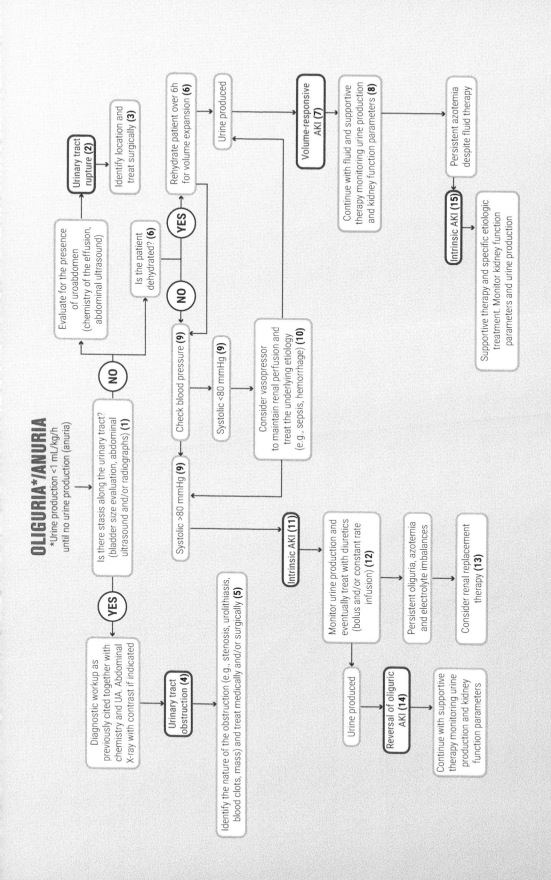

OLIGURIA*/ANURIA

*Urine production <1 mL/kg/h until no urine production (anuria)

Is there stasis along the urinary tract? (bladder size evaluation, abdominal ultrasound and/or radiographs) (1)

YES

Diagnostic workup as previously cited together with chemistry and UA. Abdominal X-ray with contrast if indicated

Urinary tract obstruction (4)

Identify the nature of the obstruction (e.g., stenosis, urolithiasis, blood clots, mass) and treat medically and/or surgically (5)

NO

Evaluate for the presence of uroabdomen (chemistry of the effusion, abdominal ultrasound)

Urinary tract rupture (2)

Identify location and treat surgically (3)

Is the patient dehydrated? (6)

YES

Rehydrate patient over 6h for volume expansion (6)

Urine produced

Volume-responsive AKI (7)

Continue with fluid and supportive therapy monitoring urine production and kidney function parameters (8)

Persistent azotemia despite fluid therapy

Intrinsic AKI (15)

Supportive therapy and specific etiologic treatment. Monitor kidney function parameters and urine production

NO

Check blood pressure (9)

Systolic <80 mmHg (9)

Consider vasopressor to maintain renal perfusion and treat the underlying etiology (e.g., sepsis, hemorrhage) (10)

Systolic >80 mmHg (9)

Intrinsic AKI (11)

Monitor urine production and eventually treat with diuretics (bolus and/or constant rate infusion) (12)

Persistent oliguria, azotemia and electrolyte imbalances

Consider renal replacement therapy (13)

Urine produced

Reversal of oliguric AKI (14)

Continue with supportive therapy monitoring urine production and kidney function parameters

1. The first step is to diagnose urinary tract stasis, evaluate bladder size, and go through urination and abdominal X-rays and/or ultrasound. The diagnostic protocol should also include blood examinations with renal function parameters and urine analysis.

6. Once urinary tract stasis, in the case of dehydration, has been excluded, the renal response after volume expansion would be the restoration of urine production. Together with hydration status, it is mandatory to check the systemic blood pressure.

9. Checking the systemic blood pressure allows for understanding whether the RBF has been maintained (systolic blood pressure above 80 mmHg) or whether there is decreased organ perfusion (systolic blood pressure below 80 mmHg).

DIAGNOSIS

2. Urinary tract rupture can cause uroabdomen and/or subcutaneous urine infiltration, resulting in the development of dermatitis at the site of the rupture. Uroabdomen can be diagnosed using effusion evaluation. Effusion chemistry with creatinine concentration analysis (which should be twice that of the blood), together with cytological evaluation in the case of a suspected septic process, is mandatory for diagnosing uroabdomen. Identifying the site/ sites of rupture allows deciding which surgical approach to use.

4. In the case of suspected urinary tract obstruction, imaging studies, together with urinalysis and, eventually, other diagnostic tests, such as fine-needle aspiration and cytologic evaluation in the case of an obstructing mass, allow identifying the nature of the obstruction (e.g., urolithiasis, masses, blood clots). Blood examinations and urine culture allow the identification of azotemia and concurrent urinary tract infection.

7. Volume-responsive AKI is defined as an increase in urine production >1 mL/kg/h over 6h and/or a decrease in serum creatinine to baseline over 48h, resulting in euvolemia. This condition can occur in azotemic patients (defined as AKI IRIS (International Renal Interest Society) grade II to grade V). Non-azotemic AKI patients (defined as AKI IRIS grade I) include animals with a 0.3 mg/dL progressive increase in creatinine concentration over 48h in the non-azotemic range.

11. Oliguria in a well-hydrated patient is a clinical sign associated with intrinsic AKI. Azotemia resulting from loss of renal function, electrolyte imbalances (above all hyperkalemia), and the presence of overhydration are clinical and laboratory findings of oliguric AKI.

14. In the case of diuretic response, the patient improves urine production, causing a reversal of oliguric AKI, together with an improvement in hyperkalemia and body weight.

15. A lack of azotemia improvement despite adequate fluid therapy points to intrinsic AKI. Parenchymal damage during intrinsic AKI cannot be solely ameliorated with fluid therapy, and treatment should address the underlying etiology, when possible, together with supportive therapy.

TREATMENT

3. Evaluate the patient's hemodynamic status and analyze abdominal effusion, urine, and other specimens (e.g., blood culture) to evaluate the risk of septic shock and to stabilize the patient before surgery.

5. The treatment of urinary tract obstruction changes according to the nature of the obstruction. With uroliths, anterograde urohydropulsion and surgical therapy for urolith retrieval allow stabilizing the patient and treating azotemia and urinary tract obstruction. Urinary tract masses should be addressed, defining their nature using fine-needle aspiration and/or biopsy and treating them accordingly. Anatomical stenosis should be treated surgically according to the site of the stenosis. The treatment of obstructing blood clots should be carried out by treating the underlying process, together with the use of spasmolytic drugs and increasing diuresis.

8. Fluid therapy is the mainstay of volume responsive AKI treatment, together with supportive and etiologic therapy (if an etiological diagnosis is available).

10. Once hypotension and then renal hypoperfusion refractory to crystalloid therapy have been identified, the use of vasopressors (e.g., norepinephrine, 0.1-2 µg/kg/min in both dogs and cats) and/or positive inotropes (e.g., dobutamine 5-20 µg/kg/min in both dogs and cats), together with etiologic therapy (such as antibiotics in the case of sepsis), can improve renal perfusion and urine production, converting oliguric AKI to non-oliguric AKI.

12. In the case of oliguric AKI, monitoring urine production and body weight allows assessing fluid balance and treating the oliguria with diuretics, thus promoting diuresis. In general, loop diuretics (e.g., furosemide) are used, and they can be administered using boluses (1 to 6 mg/kg as a single bolus or as a series in both dogs and cats) and/or constant rate infusion (in dogs and cats 0.25 to 1 mg/kg/h).

13. The persistence of oliguria, azotemia, and electrolyte imbalances, despite diuretic administration, are indications for renal replacement therapies.

SUGGESTED READINGS

-   Cowgill LD, Langston C. Acute kidney insufficiency. In Bartges J, Polzin DJ (editors). Nephrology and Urology of Small Animals. Ames, Wiley Blackwell, 2011, pp 472-523.
-   Haskins SC. Catecholamines. In Silverstein DC, Hopper K (editors). Small Animal Critical Care Medicine 2nd edition. St. Louis, Elsevier, 2015.
-   International Renal Interest Society (IRIS). Grading of acute kidney injury. Available from http://www.iris-kidney.com/pdf/4_ldc-revised-grading-of-acute-kidney-injury.pdf, 2016.
-   Langston CE. Acute kidney injury. In Ettinger SJ, Feldman EC, Côté E (editors). Textbook of Veterinary Internal Medicine 8th edition. St. Louis, Elsevier, 2017, pp 4650-4685.
-   Villiers E, Ristić J (editors). BSAVA Manual of Canine and Feline Clinical Pathology 3rd edition. British Small Animal Veterinary Association, 2016.

PAIN

Roberta Troìa and Federico Fracassi

Pain is a complex, unpleasant experience involving sensory and emotional components associated with actual or potential tissue damage. Pain is complex, unique, and individual in humans and animals. In non-verbal patients, including animals, behavioral changes, and knowledge of likely causes of pain are used to guide and manage it. The experience of pain is mediated by a complex nociceptive sensory system activated by thermal, chemical, or mechanical stimuli perceived as noxious. Two main types of neurons are involved: C-fibers (slow, dull pain) and δ-fibers (fast, sharp pain). These fibers enter the dorsal horn of the spinal cord and interact with other spinal nociceptive neurons and neurotransmitters to produce the perception of the pain stimulus in the brain. Pain can be classified as acute or chronic.

Acute pain is generally associated with tissue inflammation and damage (e.g., post-surgical pain) and represents an adaptive response to avoid or minimize tissue damage and optimize healing conditions. It can vary in severity from mild to moderate to severe. Peculiar clinical responses to pain due to peripheral or central sensitization can occur in the presence of tissue injury or inflammation, such as hyperalgesia (exaggerated response to a noxious stimulus) or allodynia (pain response to a low-intensity or an innocuous stimulus). Unlike acute pain, chronic pain persists beyond the normal time of tissue healing or persists because tissue healing does not occur. It represents a maladaptive response of the organism and can be considered a disease state. Any chronic pain condition can gradually develop a neuropathic component. Neuropathic pain is caused by a primary lesion or injury in the peripheral or central nervous system, usually characterized by hyper-responsivity to both inflammatory and innocuous stimuli (e.g., post-amputation phantom limb pain). Hyperalgesia and allodynia are frequent features of neuropathic pain. Appropriate management of acute pain is necessary to prevent the establishment of chronic or neuropathic pain.

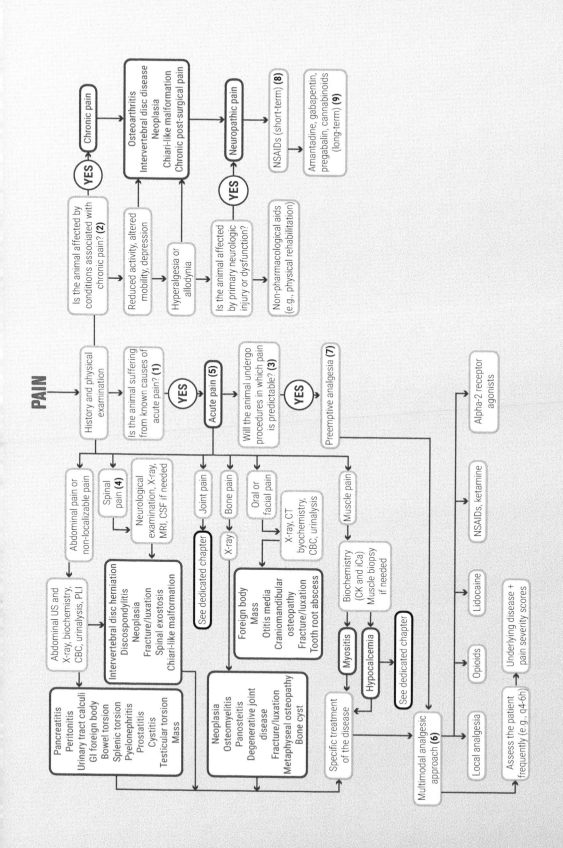

PAIN

History and physical examination

Is the animal suffering from known causes of acute pain? **(1)** → **YES** → Acute pain **(5)** → Will the animal undergo procedures in which pain is predictable? **(3)** → **YES** → Preemptive analgesia **(7)**

Is the animal affected by conditions associated with chronic pain? **(2)** → **YES** → Chronic pain

Osteoarthritis
Intervertebral disc disease
Neoplasia
Chiari-like malformation
Chronic post-surgical pain

Reduced activity, altered mobility, depression

Hyperalgesia or allodynia

Is the animal affected by primary neurologic injury or dysfunction? → **YES** → Neuropathic pain

Non-pharmacological aids (e.g., physical rehabilitation)

NSAIDs (short-term) **(8)**

Amantadine, gabapentin, pregabalin, cannabinoids (long-term) **(9)**

Abdominal pain or non-localizable pain

Spinal pain **(4)**

Neurological examination, X-ray, MRI, CSF if needed

Joint pain → See dedicated chapter

Bone pain → X-ray

Oral or facial pain → X-ray, CT byochemistry, CBC, urinalysis

Muscle pain

Abdominal US and X-ray, biochemistry, CBC, urinalysis, PLI

Intervertebral disc herniation
Discospondylitis
Neoplasia
Fracture/luxation
Spinal exostosis
Chiari-like malformation

Foreign body
Mass
Otitis media
Craniomandibular osteopathy
Fracture/luxation
Tooth root abscess

Biochemistry (CK and iCa)
Muscle biopsy if needed

Pancreatitis
Peritonitis
Urinary tract calculi
GI foreign body
Bowel torsion
Splenic torsion
Pyelonephritis
Prostatitis
Cystitis
Testicular torsion
Mass

Neoplasia
Osteomyelitis
Panosteitis
Degenerative joint disease
Fracture/luxation
Metaphyseal osteopathy
Bone cyst

Myositis

Hypocalcemia → See dedicated chapter

Specific treatment of the disease

Multimodal analgesic approach **(6)**

Alpha-2 receptor agonists

NSAIDs, ketamine

Lidocaine

Opioids

Local analgesia

Assess the patient frequently (e.g., q4-6h) → Underlying disease + pain severity scores

1. Pain assessment should always be carried out together with patient clinical examination. Some clinical findings, such as tachycardia and hypertension, could indicate pain but may be unreliable since they are also influenced by fear, stress, and environmental conditions. Knowing the animal's normal behavior (e.g., absence of grooming in cats) or the presence of new behaviors (a previously friendly animal becoming aggressive or hiding), as well as looking at facial expressions or resting postures, are useful subjective clues for identifying the presence of pain. Tense abdomen, vocalization, abnormal gait, or lying in abnormal positions may additionally reflect discomfort. A plethora of other unspecific signs (e.g., lethargy, loss of appetite) can be appreciated if the animal is in pain.

2. Assessment of chronic pain can be more difficult due to its gradual and subtle development. Chronic pain negatively affects the overall quality of an animal's life, usually making the animal less interactive and more depressed. Most of the time, chronic pain has a neuropathic component that can be appreciated by means of abnormal pain responses, such as hyperalgesia or allodynia.

3. Pain is an expected consequence after surgery and during numerous disease states. As such, clinicians must know the disease conditions likely causing mild to moderate to severe pain and treat them preemptively.

4. Spinal pain is detected by palpation over each dorsal spinous process, starting near the lumbosacral area and moving cranially to the caudal cervical area. In the cervical spine, palpate the lateral process of each vertebra and then gently move the neck from side to side and up and down. Avoid manipulation of the spine if trauma or atlantoaxial luxation is suspected. Thoracolumbar pain is often confused with abdominal pain and vice versa.

DIAGNOSIS

5. Acute pain is generally associated with tissue injury, damage, or inflammation (e.g., post-surgical pain). Although pain must be assessed and treated individually, there are some disease categories usually associated with mild (e.g., cystitis), moderate to severe pain (e.g., urethral obstruction, arthritis, peritonitis), up to excruciating pain (e.g., meningitis, necrotizing pancreatitis). There are some pain scales that have been validated for dogs and cats; they require recording subjective scores for pain intensity.

6. Pain management starts even before patient assessment since there are conditions (e.g., surgery) in which associated pain is 100% predictable. Overall, pain is best managed early and aggressively since, once it has been established and becomes severe, it is harder to manage. For this reason, predictable pain should be treated. This is part of preemptive pain management, consisting of the administration of pain treatment in advance of the pain stimulus and continuing analgesia for the expected duration of pain for that specific procedure or disease state. Drugs with a demonstrated preventive effect are nonsteroidal

anti-inflammatory drugs (NSAIDs) or N-methyl-D-aspartate receptor antagonists, such as ketamine.

7. The general approach for moderate to severe acute pain management is based on multimodal analgesia, whereas different classes of analgesics can be combined to optimize efficacy and limit the occurrence of side effects. The dose should be titrated to effect, with fixed dosing intervals in the initial phase, then based on patient response. Opioids (e.g., methadone 0.1-0.2 mg/kg q4h IV or IM; buprenorphine 10-20 µg/kg q6-8h IV or IM) are among the first-line drugs commonly used to manage acute painful conditions. Continuous intravenous infusion of ketamine or lidocaine can be used to control both cutaneous and visceral pain. Local anesthetics (e.g., chest tube-delivered bupivacaine after intrathoracic surgery) are additional aids for achieving good pain control and minimizing systemic analgesia.

8. Treating chronic pain is more challenging; nonsteroidal anti-inflammatory drugs (NSAIDs) are often used to manage acute exacerbation of chronic pain. Of the different options available, clinicians should prefer selective COX-2 inhibitors (e.g., meloxicam) since they tend to have fewer systemic side effects. Their short-term use should be considered on a case-by-case basis, considering patient characteristics, comorbidities, and susceptibility to NSAID gastrointestinal and renal adverse effects.

9. Gabapentin (GABA receptor modulator, 5-10 mg/kg q12h) or amantadine (N-methyl-D-aspartate receptor antagonist, 3-5 mg/kg q24h) could be additional choices for the long-term management of chronic pain having a neuropathic component.

SUGGESTED READINGS

-   Maddison JE, Page SW, Church DB (editors). Small Animal Clinical Pharmacology 2nd edition. Edinburgh, Saunders Elsevier, 2008.
-   Mathews K, Kronen PW, Lascelles D, et al. Guidelines for recognition, assessment and treatment of pain. *J Small Anim Pract* 55:E10-68, 2014.

PARAPLEGIA/TETRAPLEGIA

Antonella Gallucci

Paralysis or plegia is defined as a complete loss of voluntary movement in the hindlimbs (paraplegia) or all four limbs (tetraparalysis or tetraplegia). Recumbent patients showing some voluntary limb movement when assisted are defined as non-ambulatory paraparetic or tetraparetic. After a general physical examination, a complete neurological examination should be carried out to localize the lesion anatomically. In the case of acute external trauma, every effort should be made to confirm the stability of the vertebral column before performing the neurological examination.

Usually, a lesion affecting the forebrain does not induce significant motor deficits in dogs and cats. Depending on the severity of the injury, paresis or paralysis can be observed when a lesion affects the mid-caudal brain stem or, more frequently, the spinal cord. Differentiating a brain stem from a spinal cord lesion is quite simple since spinal cord lesions do not result in abnormal mentation or cranial nerve deficits.

The clinician should be able to differentiate between a spinal cord lower motor neuron (LMN) and an upper motor neuron (UMN) lesion. Clinical signs of LMN disease are induced by a lesion involving the ventral horn of the spinal cord and its lower motor neurons. A lesion of the cervical (C6-T2) or lumbosacral (L4-S3) intumescence is characterized by flaccid paralysis, hyporeflexia/areflexia, and hypotonia of the thoracic or pelvic limbs, respectively.

In patients with tetraplegia due to severe generalized LMN disease, muscle tone and spinal reflexes are reduced/absent in all four limbs. Thus, in the presence of generalized hypo-atonia and hypo-areflexia, the clinician should be able to anatomically localize the lesion at the level of the neuromuscular system.

Lesions involving the C1-C5 or T3-L3 spinal cord segments induce clinical signs of UMNs in the affected limbs, such as complete or partial lack of voluntary movement and normo- to hypertonia and normo- to hyperreflexia.

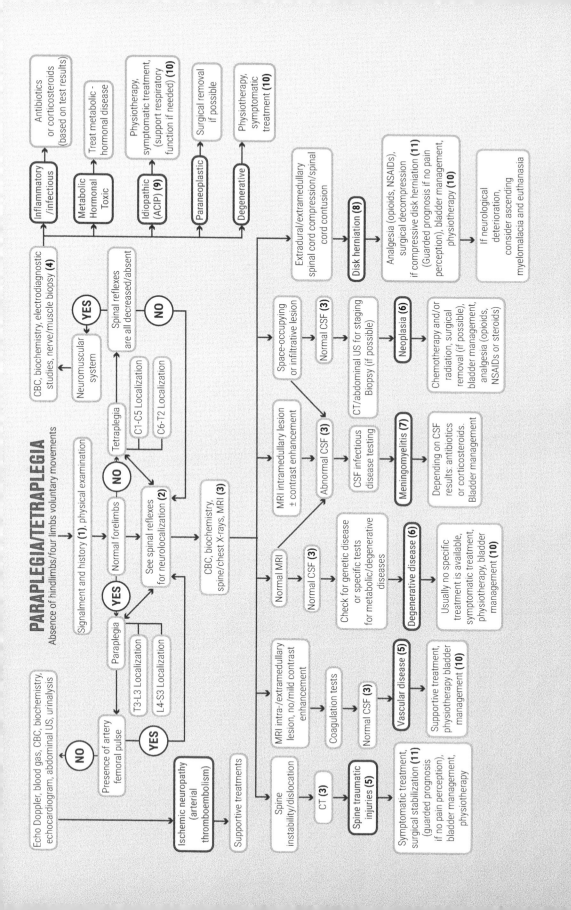

DIAGNOSTIC PROTOCOL

1. Developing a comprehensive list of differential diagnoses is dependent on appropriate neurologic localization in addition to considering the patient's signalment and history information.

2. The spinal reflexes should be tested in order to localize the lesion in the spinal cord:

    C1-C5: normal/increased spinal reflexes and muscle tone in all limbs (UMN).
    C6-T2: decreased/absent spinal reflexes and muscle tone in the forelimbs (LMN), and normal increased spinal reflexes and muscle tone in the pelvic limbs (UMN).
    T3-L3: normal/increased spinal reflexes and muscle tone in the pelvic limbs (UMN); normal forelimbs.
    L4-S1: decreased/absent spinal reflexes and muscle tone in the pelvic limbs (LMN); normal forelimbs.

3. A complete blood count (CBC) and biochemistry are useful for evaluating underlying disease and potential risks in the case of an anesthetic procedure. Survey radiographs may show displaced fractures or luxations, vertebral tumors, or chest metastasis. Computed tomography (CT) provides better bone visualization. Magnetic resonance imaging (MRI) is better suited for imaging the spinal cord, nerve roots, and intervertebral discs. Cerebrospinal fluid (CSF) analysis is indicated in the case of suspected inflammatory disease. Other tests (e.g., PCR, serology, bacterial culture) may be indicated.

4. In the case of neuromuscular disorders, electrodiagnostic studies and nerve/muscle biopsies may be useful.

DIAGNOSIS

5. Vascular and traumatic disorders have peracute onsets and often do not progress. Ischemic myelopathy is a non-painful condition, although, at initial onset, some patients may show discomfort. Spinal trauma can be detected by X-rays; however, CT provides superior details for bone and surgical planning. Vascular diseases are better evaluated using MRI scans, and in the case of hemorrhage, coagulation tests should be carried out.

6. Neoplastic and degenerative disorders often show an insidious onset of clinical signs with slower progression. Some neoplasms may be painful, and, in some cases, onset can be acute with fast progression (as in lymphoma). Neoplasm staging with chest X-rays, abdominal US, or total body CT should be considered to evaluate the extent of spread of the tumor and the possibility of performing a biopsy/surgery. Degenerative diseases are not painful, and the presumptive diagnosis is by excluding other myelopathies. A definitive diagnosis is only reached using histopathology, which is usually carried out post-mortem.

7. Inflammatory disorders tend to have acute onsets with rapid progression if not appropriately treated. Pain can be present, and blood tests can be normal. Magnetic resonance imaging usually detects a spinal lesion with or without meningeal involvement: however, CSF analysis represents a helpful exam for detecting inflammatory myelopathy. In addition

to CSF analysis, additional tests for infectious agents can be carried out. Non-infectious inflammatory disorders (meningomyelitis of unknown origin, MUO) are commonly observed in small breeds while, in cats, the most represented inflammatory diseases are feline infectious peritonitis (FIP) and toxoplasmosis. Myelitis is less common and can result from discospondylitis and/or osteomyelitis (mainly in large breed dogs).

8. Disk extrusions may have a painful acute onset with or without rapid deterioration of the neurological signs, while disk protrusion may have an insidious onset with slower progression and mild/moderate pain. They are usually easily diagnosed using MRI.

9. The most common generalized polyneuropathy in dogs is acute idiopathic polyradiculoneuritis (ACIP). It is characterized by the acute onset of flaccid paraparesis, which usually progresses rapidly to tetraparesis/tetraplegia. The diagnosis is mainly based on history and neurological and electrophysiological features. Blood test results are usually unremarkable, and CSF may show an albuminocytologic dissociation, defined as increased total protein concentration with a normal total nucleated cell count.

TREATMENT

10. Physiotherapy can play an important role in restoring motor function, modeling, and promoting neuroplasticity. The most common ways to manage the bladder are manual bladder expression or using intermittent catheterization or a Foley catheter. Medication can also be used to relax the urinary sphincter (e.g., phenoxybenzamine) or to contract the bladder (e.g., bethanechol). If respiratory paresis occurs in the case of severe neuromuscular disease, mechanical ventilation is suggested using a tracheostomy tube.

11. Surgical stabilization and decompression of the spinal cord are the most important procedures for treating acute spinal cord injuries. They should be performed quickly, and in the case of absence of pain perception, the prognosis is guarded. Worsening of the clinical condition despite treatment could be a sign of progressive myelomalacia, leading to euthanasia in case of respiratory failure.

SUGGESTED READINGS

- De Lahunta A, Glass E, Kent M (editors). Veterinary Neuroanatomy and Clinical Neurology 5th edition. Philadelphia, Saunders Elsevier, 2021.
- Dewey CW, Da Costa RC. Myelopathies: disorders of the spinal cord. In Dewey CW, Da Costa RC, editors. Practical Guide to Canine and Feline Neurology. Chichester, West Sussex, Wiley Blackwell, 2016, pp 379-381.
- Frank LR, Roynard PFP. Veterinary Neurologic Rehabilitation: The Rationale for a Comprehensive Approach. *Topics Companion Anim Med* 33:49-57, 2018.
- Skerrit G (editor). King's Applied Anatomy of the Central Nervous System of Domestic Mammals 2nd edition. Wiley Blackwell, 2018, pp 145-173.

PERICARDIAL EFFUSION

Francesco Porciello and Domenico Caivano

Pericardial effusion is characterized by the abnormal accumulation of fluid within the pericardial sac in dogs and cats. The fluid can be serous, hemorrhagic, fibrinous, or purulent, depending on the underlying causes. In dogs, neoplastic diseases (hemangiosarcomas, heart base chemoreceptor cell tumors, or mesotheliomas) are the most common causes. Idiopathic pericarditis is the second most common cause in dogs. Occasionally, pericardial effusion occurs following perforation of the left atrium in association with the myxomatous degeneration of the mitral valve, as well as uremic pericarditis, right heart failure, or coagulopathies due to rodenticide poisoning. Anecdotal descriptions of purulent pericarditis are reported as a consequence of foreign bodies (e.g., grass awn migration), penetrating wounds, systemic infection, or the extension of local infection in dogs and cats. The most common cause of pericardial effusion in cats is congestive heart failure (CHF), secondary to myocardial disease. Congenital conditions (peritoneal-pericardial-diaphragmatic hernia), lymphoma, or feline infection peritonitis may also result in pericardial effusion in cats.

The volume of the fluid collection and the rate of accumulation within the pericardial space determine the hemodynamic effects and clinical signs. When it is slow, fluid accumulation in the pericardial sac may initially be tolerated until the increased intrapericardial pressure results in compression of the right atrium and ventricle. The latter condition is known as cardiac tamponade. Rapid accumulation of pericardial fluid causes acute tamponade even if the total volume is relatively low. Cardiac tamponade is characterized by decreased cardiac output, arterial hypotension, and right-sided CHF. Constrictive pericardial disease occurs in dogs and cats when the pericardial wall becomes thickened and rigid because of recurrent idiopathic pericardial effusion, pericardial infections, traumatic pericardial hemorrhages, or intrapericardial tumors.

Dogs with chronic pericardial effusion show progressive clinical signs secondary to right-sided CHF (lethargy, exercise intolerance, respiratory effort, and abdominal distention). Dogs with acute pericardial effusion typically present with a history of acute collapse or weakness (anterograde heart failure).

PERICARDIAL EFFUSION

```
                                    History
                            Collapse, weakness (acute)
                            Right-sided CHF signs (chronic)
```

- Acute onset of anterograde heart failure
- Physical examination (1)
- CBC and biochemistry (4)
- Thoracic radiographs (3)
- Echocardiography (5)

- Electrocardiogram (2)
- Sinus tachycardia, low voltage QRS complexes associated or not with electric alternans

- Supraventricular and ventricular tachyarrhythmias
- Consider treatment with antiarrhythmics (13)

- Secondary pericardial effusion (9)
  - Treatment of the primary disease (13)

- Constrictive pericardial disease (8)
  - Pericardiocentesis (10)
  - Pericardiectomy (12)

- Cardiac tamponade (6)
  - Pericardiocentesis (11)

- Mass lesions (7)
  - Pericardiocentesis (11)
  - Pericardiectomy (12)
  - Chemotherapy (14)

- Idiopathic pericarditis (no other causes identified)
  - Pericardiocentesis (11)
  - Pericardiectomy (12)
  - Corticosteroids (15)

- Pericardial fluid analysis (10)

DIAGNOSTIC PROTOCOL

1. Physical examination may show jugular venous distension/pulsation, decreased palpable precordial impulse, abdominal enlargement with a ballotable fluid wave, and respiratory distress secondary to pleural effusion. Arterial pulse is small in amplitude (sometimes not easily detectable), frequent, weak, and sometimes paradoxus (excessively variable with respiration, especially when cardiac tamponade is present). Heart sounds are typically muffled or poorly audible. Most of these clinical signs are unusual in cats since large amounts of effusion, and cardiac tamponade rarely occur. The so-called Beck's triad is the combination of signs of arterial hypotension with a narrowed pulse pressure, jugular venous distention, and muffled heart sounds.

2. Electrocardiographic examination shows low voltage QRS complexes in dogs; however, this finding may be observed in various diseases, such as obesity, pleural effusion, or hypothyroidism. Variation in the height of the QRS complexes with alternate beats, referred to as electrical alternans, is common in animals with large pericardial effusion. Arrhythmias may be detected, arising from different ectopic sites (atrial or ventricular premature beats), or resulting from sinus hyperstimulation secondary to arterial hypotension (sinus tachycardia).

3. Radiographic examination shows a more spherical cardiac shape with loss of the normal chamber contours. If right-sided CHF is present, caudal vena cava distension, hepatomegaly and ascites may be observed.

4. Blood laboratory tests (blood cell counts and biochemistry) may show mild hypoproteinemia and elevated liver enzymes (right-sided CHF), poorly regenerative anemia (chronic disease), mild prerenal azotemia (poor cardiac output), increased troponin I (myocardial inflammation/damage), granulocytosis and neutrophilia (infection).

5. Echocardiography allows the visualization of pericardial effusion as a hypoechoic area surrounding the heart. If pleural effusion is also present, the pericardium can be visualized as a hyperechoic line separating the pleural space from the intrapericardial space.

10. Pericardiocentesis may be useful as a diagnostic test for pericardial fluid analysis. The type of effusion may be an exudate, transudate, modified transudate, hemorrhagic or neoplastic fluid. Cytology may not be helpful in diagnosing neoplastic effusions, and histopathology/immunohistochemistry of the pericardium is recommended when mesotheliomas or idiopathic pericarditis are suspected.

DIAGNOSIS

6. Cardiac tamponade is characterized by the diastolic collapse of the right atrial wall. Severe tamponade may lead to right ventricular wall collapse and an apparent increase in the left ventricular wall thickness (pseudohypertrophy), clearly visualized by echocardiography.

7. Mass lesions, detectable with echocardiography, may be visualized more easily if pericardial effusion is present. Hemangiosarcomas frequently arise from the right atrial wall. Heart

base tumors are localized around the aorta and pulmonary artery. Mesotheliomas or small cardiac tumors may not be visualized by echo study.

8. Constrictive pericardial disease is ultrasonographically characterized by a very thickened pericardial wall with mild pericardial effusion.

9. Secondary pericardial effusion is characterized by a small volume of fluid. In some cases, the fluid visualized by echo study may have a cloudy aspect when cells and fibrin aggregates are present (e.g., purulent and inflammatory pericarditis). In acute hemorrhage, it is possible to visualize blood clots floating in the effusion and/or adhering to the bleeding site.

TREATMENT

11. Pericardiocentesis is the only effective treatment for cardiac tamponade. Removal of even a small quantity of pericardial effusion in the case of constrictive pericardial disease results in a marked reduction in intrapericardial pressure.

12. Subtotal pericardiectomy is the most common surgical treatment, especially in animals with recurrent pericardial effusion. Thoracoscopic partial pericardiectomy or percutaneous balloon pericardiotomy are alternative options.

13. Secondary pericardial effusions rarely cause cardiac tamponade and can be managed conservatively using appropriate drugs (antibiotics, anti-inflammatory, antiarrhythmic, antihemorrhagic drugs).

14. Chemotherapy for pericardial effusion secondary to neoplasia varies based on the nature of the tumor.

15. Corticosteroids (anti-inflammatory doses) may be used to treat idiopathic pericarditis.

SUGGESTED READINGS

- Cohn L, Côté E (editors). Clinical Veterinary Advisor: Dogs and Cats 3rd edition. St. Louis, Elsevier, 2015.
- Kittleson MD, Kienle RD (editors). Small Animal Cardiovascular Medicine Textbook. Online edition. Davis, Veterinary Information Network (VIN) Inc., 2005.
- Porciello F, Birettoni F, Caivano D, Giorgi ME (editors). Ecocardiografia nel cane, nel gatto e nel cavallo 2nd edition. Milan, Poletto Editore, 2019.

PERIPHERAL EDEMA

Matteo Petini

Approximately two-thirds of the total body water is intracellular, and one-third is extracellular. Of the latter, approximately one-fourth is in the plasma, and the remainder is the interstitial fluid. Edema is the consequence of a clinically evident excess of interstitial fluid within tissues. The composition of the interstitial matrix creates flexible and elastic tissue. Therefore, edema does not become clinically apparent until the interstitial volume is markedly increased. Depending on the cause, edema can occur with a localized or generalized distribution.

Fluid movement between the vascular and the interstitial space is mainly controlled by two opposing forces: the intravascular hydrostatic pressure and the colloid osmotic pressure generated by plasma proteins. In addition to these two forces, lymphatic drainage and vascular permeability play a role in maintaining fluid homeostasis. Collectively, the interactions between these various forces are described by Starling's law. Under normal circumstances, excess fluid filtered into the interstitial spaces does not accumulate but is reabsorbed into venous blood by local lymphatic drainage. In general, the mechanisms involved in the formation of peripheral edema are: a) increased intravascular hydrostatic pressure (either from increased plasma volume or venous obstruction); b) decreased colloid osmotic pressure (due to reduced serum albumin levels secondary to its loss or reduced production); c) increased capillary permeability (due to local or systemic inflammatory diseases); and d) impaired lymphatic drainage (due to lymphatics or lymph node diseases). Edema secondary to reduced colloid osmotic pressure does not usually become evident until serum albumin concentrations fall below 1.5 g/dL. Conditions associated with extensive edema are characterized by a reduction in plasma volume, which produces renal hypoperfusion and, consequently, a reduction in renal sodium excretion and fluid retention by activating the renin-angiotensin system. This aggravates edema formation. Determining the etiology of the interstitial fluid accumulation is mandatory for achieving resolution of the edema.

PERIPHERAL EDEMA

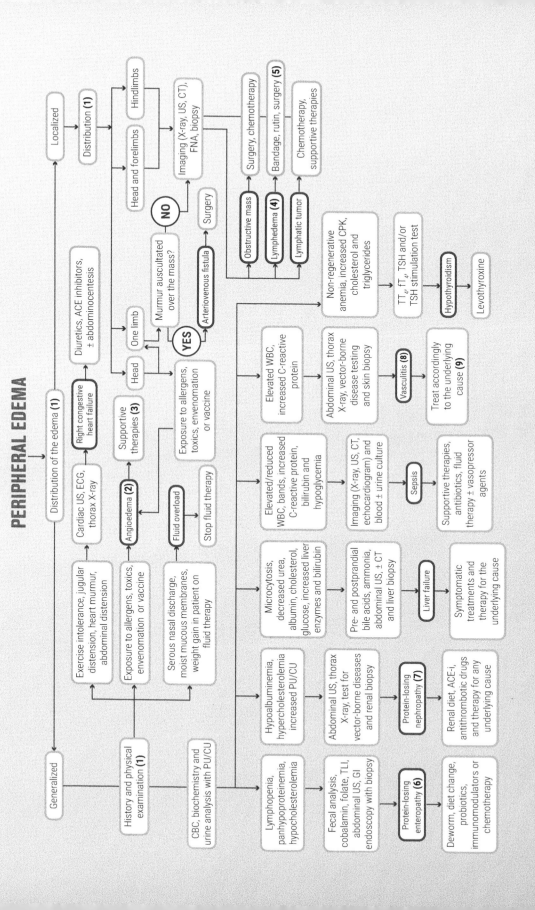

DIAGNOSTIC PROTOCOL

1. First, edema should be assessed regarding its localization. Generalized peripheral edema is commonly seen in a setting of volume overload state, decreased colloid osmotic pressure, or systemic inflammatory response. On the contrary, peripheral edema, which is localized, is usually the result of a venous or lymphatic flow abnormality. Moreover, based on the persistence or loss of skin depression after palpation, the clinician can differentiate edema in pitting (after pressure is applied to a small area, the indentation persists after the release of the pressure) or non-pitting, respectively. Thus, pitting edema is, for the most part, secondary to increased vascular permeability, venous obstruction, or lymphatic abnormalities. Non-pitting edema is usually caused by angioedema, post-surgical edema, chronic lymphedema, lymphangiosarcoma, and myxedema.

   The diagnostic workup must be planned depending on the history and physical examination of the patient. For example, historical findings can help diagnose angioedema secondary to exposure to external allergens. Similarly, some clinical findings (e.g., serous nasal discharge, jugular distension) can allow the clinician to detect a state of volume overload. Laboratory analyses are particularly required to evaluate the presence of protein-losing states, liver insufficiency, or the presence of a generalized inflammatory state. Thyroid function should be screened when myxedema is suspected. Diagnostic imaging techniques are required for both generalized or localized edema, especially when obstructive bases must be ruled out (e.g., in case of front or rear limb edema). Advanced imaging techniques (e.g., computed tomography, magnetic resonance, scintigraphy) might be necessary for evaluating the lymphatic system or to additionally characterize the masses discovered. Finally, a biopsy can be required to confirm or characterize a disease process (e.g., vasculitis, glomerular disease, intestinal disease).

DIAGNOSIS

2. Angioedema is usually caused by an acute hypersensitivity reaction with a subsequent increase in vascular permeability. Edema caused by envenomation due to biting or stinging arthropods can be generalized, as well as localized.

4. Lymphedema can generally be classified as primary or secondary. Primary lymphedema consists of a morphological or functional abnormality of the lymphatic vessels or lymph nodes. Secondary lymphedema can be caused by neoplasia, surgery, trauma, or infection.

6. Intestinal lymphangiectasia, inflammatory bowel disease, and alimentary lymphoma (AL) are three important intestinal causes of protein-losing enteropathy. This syndrome is more common in dogs as compared to cats, in which it is most often secondary to AL.

7. Glomerular diseases, as the cause of a urinary loss of protein, are more common in dogs as compared to cats, with immune complex glomerulonephritis, amyloidosis, and glomerulosclerosis more commonly diagnosed. Renal biopsy is useful for identifying the type and severity of renal lesions but also for determining whether the glomerular disease is immune-mediated or not.

8. Vasculitis can be a primary immune-mediated event, or it can occur secondary to a variety of

medications, infections, neoplastic conditions, and other diseases. Cutaneous vasculitis can appear with various clinical manifestations, and it often involves the body extremities.

TREATMENT

3. Any possible trigger should be identified and eliminated. In the case of anaphylaxis and bronchospasm, epinephrine should be administered (0.01 mg/kg IM). The dose can be repeated every 5-15 minutes. If shock is present, epinephrine should be administered by IV infusion (0.05 µg/kg/min). In mild and uncomplicated cases, a short course of glucocorticoids at an anti-inflammatory dose is appropriate.

5. In secondary lymphedema, it is mandatory to treat the underlying cause, if possible. Heavy bandages and physical therapy are indicated to promote lymphatic drainage. A local antibiotic can be used in the case of secondary cellulitis. Rutin is theoretically helpful in reducing high-protein lymphedema. Surgical interventions can facilitate lymphatic drainage.

9. In the case of an infectious etiology, antimicrobial therapy is needed. Vasculitis secondary to drug reactions requires the discontinuation of all medications. Vasculitis due to neoplastic conditions needs therapies directed against the tumor. Immunosuppressive drugs are often required once when a primary condition is suspected.

SUGGESTED READINGS

-   Ettinger SJ, Feldman EC, Côté E (editors). Textbook of Veterinary Internal Medicine 8th edition. St. Louis, Elsevier, 2017.
-   Hall JE, Hall ME. Regulation of body fluid compartments: extracellular and intracellular fluids; edema. In Hall JE, Hall ME (editors). Guyton and Hall Textbook of Medical Physiology 14th edition. Philadelphia, Elsevier, 2021, pp 305-319.

PETECHIAE AND ECCHYMOSES

Kateryna Vasylyeva

Petechiae (<3 mm in diameter) and ecchymoses (3-10 mm in size) are red or purple discolorations of the skin or mucous membranes resulting from small blood vessel bleeding (capillary and small arterioles and venules, respectively). Signalment, history, clinical findings, and characterization of the bleeding are important for planning a diagnostic workup, interpreting the test results, and establishing a final diagnosis. Petechiae and ecchymoses are mainly suggestive of defective primary hemostasis; however, they are rarely due to a secondary hemostatic problem or combined disorders. The pathogenesis of a primary hemostatic disorder relates to a severe deficiency in platelet number (thrombocytopenia), abnormal platelet function (thrombocytopathy), von Willebrand disease (vWD), or vascular diseases (e.g., primary or secondary immune-mediated vasculitis). Inherited disorders of secondary hemostasis are caused by various genetic alterations that result in decreased, absent or abnormal coagulation factors. Acquired coagulation defects more often have complex pathogenesis that involves more hemostatic processes simultaneously (primary hemostasis, secondary hemostasis [coagulation], and fibrinolysis).

Patient history can include previous occasional or recurrent bleeding tendency (e.g., during the loss of deciduous teeth, spaying or castration, estrus), suggesting a congenital defect in young animals. Acquired disorders involving platelets are frequently autoimmune, associated with underlying diseases, drug administration, or toxin exposure, and are more commonly observed in elderly animals.

Hemostatic processes can be assessed using group or specific tests. Recently, global hemostatic tests (e.g., thromboelastography/thromboelastometry) that can measure multiple coagulation pathways simultaneously, including the contribution of cells (platelets, erythrocytes) have also been evaluated. Required specimens for coagulation tests should be collected prior to therapeutic intervention. Appropriate specimen collection, correct sample containers (anticoagulant K^+-EDTA for a complete blood count and platelet count; sodium citrate anticoagulant for most coagulation assays), and timely processing are essential for a correct interpretation of the results.

PETECHIAE AND ECCHYMOSES

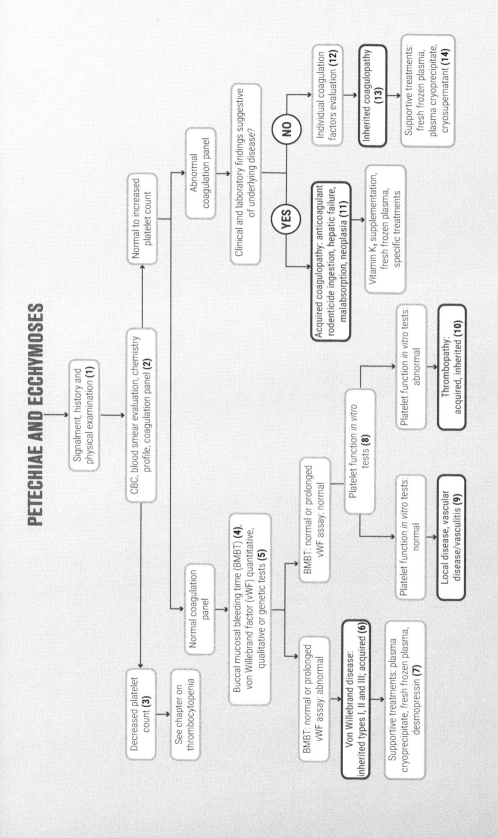

DIAGNOSTIC PROTOCOL

1. Details regarding breed, age, familial and travel history, the ingestion of toxin (e.g., anticoagulant rodenticide) or drug administration (e.g., non-steroidal anti-inflammatory drugs), and vaccination are essential for defining the hemostatic disorder (inherited or acquired) and in the diagnostic workup. Congenital bleeding disorders have been identified in several breeds (e.g., vWD in Bernese Mountain Dogs, Dachshunds, Shetland Sheepdogs, German Shepherds, and Doberman Pinschers) and are mainly diagnosed in young animals. Thrombocytopenia has been reported in vector-borne diseases or is frequently associated with viral infections in cats (e.g., FeLV, FIV, FIP). Drug-induced thrombocytopenia can be associated with any medication; however, antimicrobials (e.g., sulfonamides, cephalosporins), anti-inflammatory, chemotherapeutic drugs, or phenobarbital are the most common.

2. A CBC and coagulation panel are mandatory in patients with bleeding. Clinical chemistry and other etiological tests should also be considered since many systemic diseases can be associated with these signs.

3. Thrombocytopenia is the most common cause of petechiae and ecchymoses. Thrombocytopenia can be due to increased destruction, consumption, sequestration, or lack of production of platelets (See the chapter on thrombocytopenia).

4. In a patient with normal platelet count and coagulation panel, buccal mucosal bleeding time (BMBT) can be useful to evaluate the presence of thrombopathies or vWD; BMBT is determined by measuring the time passing between mucosal incisions and cessation of bleeding. Unfortunately, BMBT sensitivity and specificity are low; therefore, additional tests should be used.

5. A quantitative assay for plasma von Willebrand factor (vWF) antigen (vWF:Ag) concentration is considered the first step for vWD diagnosis and is used to detect type 1 and type 3 vWD. The results are reported as %, and a vWF:Ag concentration below 50% is considered abnormal. Functional assays measure the ability of the vWF to interact with platelets, collagen, or factor VIII and are used for the diagnosis of type 2 vWD. The acquired form of vWD can be secondary to other systemic disorders. Genetic tests validated for specific breeds are also available.

8. Platelet aggregation and function can be evaluated *in vitro* using different assays. The platelet function analyzer, PFA-100, can be used to screen for the presence of abnormalities in platelet function. Other more specific options are impedance, whole blood platelet aggregometry, light-transmission aggregometry, and flow-cytometry assays. There are also global hemostasis tests, such as thromboelastography/thromboelastometry. All these techniques require immediate sample processing and so cannot be shipped to the reference lab; for this reason, they are available in reference centers only or used in research settings.

12. Prolongation of PT and/or aPTT is observed in inherited coagulation factor deficiency. For a definite diagnosis, the measurement of individual coagulation factors activity is recommended.

DIAGNOSIS

6. Type 1 vWD is a partial quantitative deficiency of the vWF; the bleeding tendency can be mild to severe and is related to the severity of the decreased vWF concentration. Type 2 vWD refers to a functional deficiency in vWF. Type 3 vWD is characterized by a complete absence of plasma vWF; it is the more severe form of vWD.

9. Consider local tissue trauma or vascular diseases. Primary immune-mediated or secondary vasculitis (e.g., infectious disease, neoplasia, medications) should be considered and the underlying disease properly diagnosed. Evaluate to perform a skin biopsy.

10. Several inherited thrombopathies are recognized: Glanzmann's thrombasthenia, platelet receptors and signal transduction disorders, Chediak-Higashi syndrome, and storage pool disorders. Acquired platelet dysfunction is reported in various systemic disorders, such as neoplasia, paraproteinemia, infectious diseases, uremia, and hepatobiliary diseases.

11. The most common acquired coagulation disorders are secondary to anticoagulant rodenticide ingestion, liver disease, disseminated intravascular coagulation, and neoplasia.

13. Hemophilia A (factor VIII deficiency), the most common inherited coagulation factor deficiency, and hemophilia B (factor IX deficiency) are primarily diagnosed in males. The remaining factor deficiencies (fibrinogen, factor II, VII, X, XI, and XII) are less common in animals.

TREATMENT

7. Cryoprecipitate or fresh frozen plasma (FFP) should be used for the treatment of bleeding in dogs with vWD. A single SC administration (1-4 µg/kg) of desmopressin acetate could be used as preoperative prophylaxis for vWD-affected dogs (type 1). Desmopressin causes the release of high molecular weight multimers of vWF from the endothelial cells.

14. A transfusion of FFP can be used for the majority of coagulation factor deficiencies. Cryoprecipitate is more specific for the replacement of factor VIII; cryosupernatant can be used for treating factor IX deficiency.

SUGGESTED READINGS

-   Blois S. Petechiae ecchymoses. In Ettinger SJ, Feldman EC, Côté E (editors). Textbook of Veterinary Internal Medicine 8th edition. St. Louis, Elsevier, 2017, pp 719-725.
-   Brooks MB. Hereditary coagulopathy. In Weiss DJ, Wardrop KJ (editors). Schalm's Veterinary Hematology 6th edition. Ames, Wiley Blackwell, 2010, pp 661-667.
-   Brooks MB, Catalfamo JL. Von Willebrand disease. In Weiss DJ, Wardrop KJ (editors). Schalm's Veterinary Hematology 6th edition. Ames, Wiley Blackwell, 2010, pp 612-617.
-   Callan MB, Catalfamo JL. Immune-mediated thrombocytopenia, von Willebrand disease, and other platelet disorders. In Ettinger SJ, Feldman EC, Côté E (editors). Textbook of Veterinary Internal Medicine 8th edition. St. Louis, Elsevier, 2017, pp 2120-2136.

PIGMENTURIA

Sofia Segatore

Pigmenturia is defined as an abnormal coloration of urine. The normal yellow to amber is due to urochromes, a group of poorly defined urine pigments, one of which is riboflavin. Pale yellow urine is usually less concentrated than dark yellow urine, but not always. Gross assessment of urine is typically done with fresh, well-mixed urine. An abnormal color indicates the presence of abnormal pigments in the urine. Other parts of the urinalysis or other assays are needed to determine which pigment or pigments are present. Although concurrent pigmenturia may alter the expected color, the following are common abnormal colors and the substance that causes the color change:

- Red: erythrocytes, hemoglobin, and myoglobin.
- Red-brown: erythrocytes, hemoglobin, myoglobin, or methemoglobin.
- Brown to black: methemoglobin from hemoglobin or myoglobin.
- Yellow-orange: bilirubin.
- Yellow-green or yellow-brown: bilirubin and biliverdin.

Urine pigments may interfere with dipstick test results; therefore, a dipstick should always be performed simultaneously with the evaluation of the urinary sediment.

Test strips for heme detect intact red blood cells, hemoglobinuria, and myoglobinuria. Therefore, dipstick assessment of blood must be carried out in the context of urinary sediment evaluation, the appearance of serum, and the creatine kinase (CK) serum activity. Hematuria is common, while hemoglobinuria is less common, and myoglobinuria is rare.

Bilirubinuria with hyperbilirubinemia is expected with hemolysis, intrahepatic diseases, cholestasis, and biliary obstruction. In dogs, since the renal threshold for bilirubin is low, it may be detected in urine before hyperbilirubinemia is obvious. Canine kidneys synthesize bilirubin; thus, not all bilirubin is derived from the blood. A low bilirubin concentration may be found in concentrated urine samples from healthy male dogs.

Several conditions can cause pigmenturia. An accurate history of the patient, physical examination, bloodwork, urinalysis, and diagnostic imaging are usually required to reach a diagnosis.

The only possible therapy for pigmenturia is the identification and resolution of the underlying cause.

PIGMENTURIA

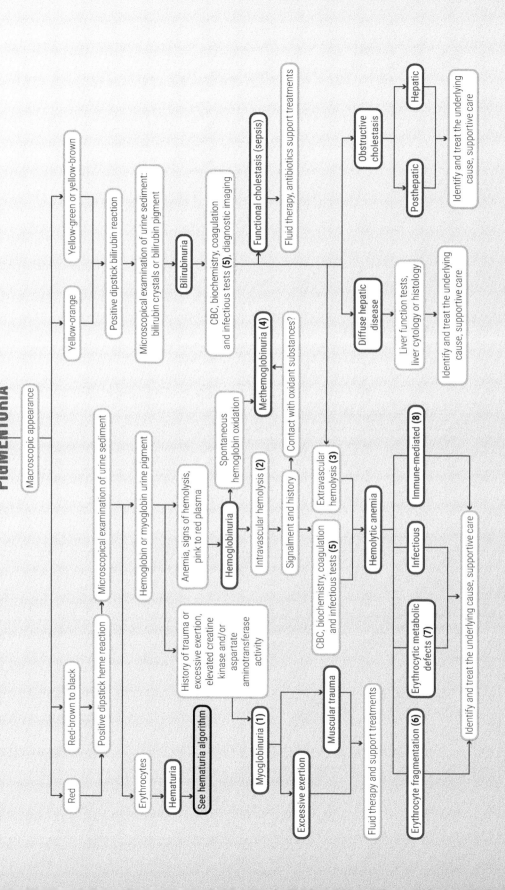

2. In intravascular hemolysis, erythrocyte destruction occurs within the blood vessels or the heart. Intravascular hemolysis does not include phagocytosis by tissue macrophages, while erythrocytes pass through sinuses of the spleen, liver, and bone marrow. It is clinically recognized when it causes hemoglobinemia and hemoglobinuria. Usually, with intravascular hemolysis, the degree of anemia is severe, the clinical symptoms acute, and regeneration usually appears after the clinical signs. Intravascular hemolysis is commonly associated with a life-threatening disease; therefore, its presence suggests a poorer prognosis, and immediate treatment and management of the case are indicated.

3. In extravascular hemolysis, the destruction of erythrocytes occurs outside the arterial-capillary-venous system. Destruction occurs in macrophages near the venular sinus of the spleen, liver, and bone marrow. Extravascular hemolysis does not cause hemoglobinemia and hemoglobinuria. The degree of anemia is usually mild to severe, clinical signs develop over days to weeks, and reticulocytosis is usually evident at the time of diagnosis.

5. Infectious hemolytic anemias:

    - Piroplasms: *Babesia* spp. (*B. canis* or *B. gibsoni*). Diagnostic procedure: cytology or PCR.
    - Hemotropic mycoplasma species: *Mycoplasma haemofelis* (more pathogenic) or *Candidatus Mycoplasma haemominutum* (typically considered an opportunist). Diagnostic procedure: cytology or PCR.
    - *Anaplasma* spp. (*A. phagocytophilum* or *A. platys*). The evidence that *Anaplasma* spp. causes hemolytic anemia is low. Diagnostic procedure: cytology, serology and/or PCR.

    Evidence that other vector-borne agents induce immune-mediated hemolytic anemia is low. For some of these organisms, such as *Leishmania* spp., Coombs' test-positive anemia is observed with infection; therefore, it is still important to exclude the presence of these infectious agents in dogs with hemolytic anemia.

DIAGNOSIS

1. Myocyte necrosis or damage can release myoglobin from the myocytes into the interstitial fluid, lymph, and finally the blood, from which the small proteins easily pass into the glomerular filtrate. If not completely resorbed by the renal tubules, myoglobin is excreted in the urine. Myoglobin is rapidly cleared from plasma, and thus pink plasma is not expected. Myoglobinuria is associated with acute myopathies caused by trauma or excessive exertion.

4. Methemoglobinuria may contribute to a positive urine heme reaction in the following situations (concurrent hemoglobinuria is expected): when hemoglobin (or hemoglobin dimer) molecules are in the urine, some of the ferrous heme undergoes spontaneous oxidation to ferric heme (forming methemoglobin); when there is intravascular hemolytic anemia caused by an overwhelming exposure to oxidants, some of the lysed erythrocytes release methemoglobin into plasma. Methemoglobin dimers can then enter the glomerular filtrate. Both metheme and heme have peroxidase activity; therefore, either molecule can give a positive heme reaction.

6. Erythrocyte damage is thought to be due to trauma caused by relatively rigid structures (fibrin) or by shear stress by high-velocity turbulent flows. Erythrocyte trauma either directly causes lysis or creates poikilocytes that have a shortened life span. Acanthocytes may form in the circulation because of membrane lipid changes; furthermore, these changes in blood flow may contribute to the accelerated fragmentation of acanthocytes. Erythrocyte damage may be caused by disseminated intravascular coagulation, vasculitis, hemangiosarcoma, caval syndrome (dirofilariasis), or cardiac valvular disease.

7. Erythrocytic metabolic defects may be acquired or inherited. The causes of metabolic defects are oxidative damage caused by Heinz body hemolytic anemia (secondary to many oxidants, e.g., acetaminophen, onions, garlic) or eccentrocytic hemolytic anemia, defects in ATP generation caused by pyruvate kinase deficiency (hereditary disorders in several breeds of dogs and cats), phosphofructokinase deficiency (recognized in the English Springer Spaniel), hypophosphatemic hemolysis (secondary to insulin administration) or L-sorbose intoxication and defects in heme synthesis that cause porphyria (described in cats).

8. Immune-mediated hemolytic anemia occurs when an animal's immune system produces antibodies that bind directly or indirectly to its erythrocytes with the consequence of erythrocyte destruction. Clinical evidence may suggest the presence of intravascular hemolysis, extravascular hemolysis, or both. Immune-mediated hemolytic anemia is considered secondary (associative) when it can be attributed to an underlying disease (e.g., infectious disease, cancer, inflammatory diseases, drugs, and toxins or vaccines) and primary (non-associative) if the cause is not found. For the diagnosis of immune-mediated hemolytic anemia, it is necessary to identify two or more signs of immune-mediated destruction (e.g., spherocytes, direct antiglobulin test, saline agglutination test) and/or one or more signs of hemolysis (e.g., hyperbilirubinemia, hemoglobinemia, hemoglobinuria, erythrocyte ghosts).

SUGGESTED READINGS

- Ettinger SJ, Feldman EC, Côté E (editors). Textbook of Veterinary Internal Medicine 8th edition. St. Louis, Elsevier, 2017.
- Garden OA, Kidd L, Mexas AM, et al. ACVIM consensus statement on the diagnosis of immune-mediated hemolytic anemia in dogs and cats. *J Vet Intern Med* 33:313-334, 2019.
- Nelson RW, Couto CG (editors). Small Animal Internal Medicine 6th edition. St. Louis, Elsevier, 2019.
- Scott MA, Stockham SL (editors). Fundamentals of Veterinary Clinical Pathology 2nd edition. Wiley Blackwell, 2013.
- Weiss DJ, Wardrop KJ (editors). Schalm's Veterinary Hematology 6th edition. Wiley Blackwell, 2011.

PLEURAL EFFUSION

Andrea Zoia

The mesothelium is a membrane composed of a monolayer of flattened squamous-like epithelial cells that form the thoracic cavity lining (pleura). The main purpose of these cells is to produce a lubricating fluid which is a low-protein plasma ultrafiltrate separating the visceral and the parietal pleurae in the thoracic cavity. This fluid also provides mechanical coupling between the chest wall and the lungs, allowing for the direct transmission of forces for normal respiration. Under normal circumstances, pleural fluid flows out from the parietal pleural capillaries and is reabsorbed by the visceral pleural capillaries and by lymphatic stoma of the parietal pleura. These stomata constitute the only way for cells and larger particles to exit the cavitary spaces, whereas proteins may also exit via active cell transport (i.e., electrolyte-coupled liquid absorption and transcytosis) and via the parietal and visceral mesothelial cells. Pleural fluid production and its removal from the pleural spaces is a continuous process. Pleural effusion develops, with different mechanisms, when more fluid enters the pleural space than is removed. Variation in the Starling forces due to an increased hydrostatic pressure gradient (i.e., increased pulmonary capillary pressure or decreased intrapleural pressure) or decreased colloid osmotic pressure causes the formation of transudative pleural effusions. In 5 to 10% of the cases, humans with decompensated liver cirrhosis and ascites may also present with transudative pleural effusions (i.e., hepatic hydrothorax), due to the movement of transudative fluid from the peritoneal space to the pleural space across small defects, for the most part, located on the right side of the diaphragmatic tendon. The movement of transudative effusion from the peritoneal space to the pleural space is considered rare in dogs. The increased permeability of the pleural membrane or pulmonary capillaries and/or impaired reabsorption from the thoracic lymphatic flow causes the formation of exudative pleural effusion. In human medicine, chylothorax and hemothorax are also considered exudative effusion.

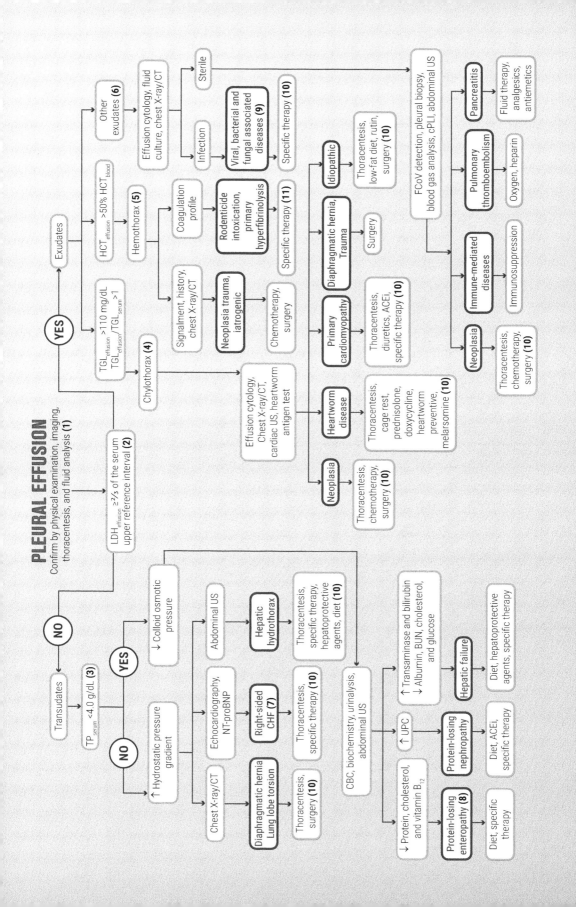

PLEURAL EFFUSION

Confirm by physical examination, imaging, thoracentesis, and fluid analysis (1)

$LDH_{effusion} \geq 2/3$ of the serum upper reference interval (2)

YES

Exudates

$TGL_{effusion} > 110$ mg/dL
$TGL_{effusion}/TGL_{serum} > 1$

Chylothorax (4)

Effusion cytology, Chest X-ray/CT, cardiac US, heartworm antigen test

Neoplasia
Thoracentesis, chemotherapy, surgery (10)

Heartworm disease
Thoracentesis, cage rest, prednisolone, doxycycline, heartworm preventive, melarsomine (10)

Primary cardiomyopathy
Thoracentesis, ACEi, diuretics, specific therapy (10)

Diaphragmatic hernia, Trauma
Surgery

Idiopathic
Thoracentesis, low-fat diet, rutin, surgery (10)

Signalment, history, chest X-ray/CT

Neoplasia trauma, iatrogenic
Chemotherapy, surgery

$HCT_{effusion} > 50\%$ HCT_{blood}

Hemothorax (5)

Coagulation profile

Rodenticide intoxication, primary hyperfibrinolysis
Specific therapy (11)

Other exudates (6)

Effusion cytology, fluid culture, chest X-ray/CT

Infection

Viral, bacterial and fungal associated diseases (9)
Specific therapy (10)

Sterile

FCoV detection, pleural biopsy, blood gas analysis, cPLI, abdominal US

Neoplasia
Thoracentesis, chemotherapy, surgery (10)

Immune-mediated diseases
Immunosuppression

Pulmonary thromboembolism
Oxygen, heparin

Pancreatitis
Fluid therapy, analgesics, antiemetics

NO

Transudates

$TP_{serum} < 4.0$ g/dL (3)

NO

↑ Hydrostatic pressure gradient

Chest X-ray/CT

Diaphragmatic hernia Lung lobe torsion
Thoracentesis, surgery (10)

Echocardiography, NT-proBNP

Right-sided CHF (7)
Thoracentesis, specific therapy (10)

YES

↓ Colloid osmotic pressure

Abdominal US

Hepatic hydrothorax
Thoracentesis, specific therapy, hepatoprotective agents, diet (10)

CBC, biochemistry, urinalysis, abdominal US

↓ Protein, cholesterol, and vitamin B_{12}

Protein-losing enteropathy (8)
Diet, specific therapy

↑ UPC

Protein-losing nephropathy
Diet, ACEi, specific therapy

↑ Transaminase and bilirubin
↓ Albumin, BUN, cholesterol, and glucose

Hepatic failure
Diet, hepatoprotective agents, specific therapy

DIAGNOSTIC PROTOCOL

1. The diagnosis of pleural effusion can be reached using clinical findings, imaging, and thoracocentesis. Rapid/shallow breathing with or without abdominal effort and muffled heart sounds are commonly present on physical examination. Radiography is the most common imaging technique used; ultrasonography is used in emergencies, while computed tomography is used less commonly. Thoracocentesis and fluid removal allow both clinical improvement and fluid analysis.

2. Classification as either a transudate or an exudate is the first step in determining its etiology. In veterinary medicine, specific gravity, fluid total protein (TP), and a fluid total nucleated cell count (TNCC) have historically been used to identify the nature of the effusion; however, the most recent adaptation of Light's criteria in both dog and cat pleural effusion have been shown to be more accurate in differentiating exudate from transudate. Light's criteria identify effusion as an exudate if one of these three conditions is met: a) pleural effusion lactic dehydrogenase (LDH) $\geq 2/3$ of the serum upper reference limit; b) pleural fluid/serum LDH ≥ 0.6; and c) pleural fluid/serum TP ≥ 0.5. If none of the above conditions are present, the effusion is a transudate. In small animals, LDH $\geq 2/3$ of the serum upper reference limit is likely to be the single most indicative Light's criteria parameter when considered alone (accuracy >90%). A pleural effusion TP >3.0 g/dL and a pleural effusion TNCC >7000/µL are most likely consistent with an exudate.

3. If pleural effusion is a transudate, a serum TP concentration ≥ 4.0 g/dL will identify a transudate formed from an increased hydrostatic pressure gradient, while a serum TP concentration <4.0 g/dL indicates a transudate from decreased colloid osmotic pressure. If a transudate is found, additional fluid analyses are not necessary, and other tests, such as bloodwork, abdominal ultrasound, echocardiography, etc., are indicated according to the suspected underlying disease.

4. Chylothorax derives from the obstruction or rupture of the intestinal lymphatic flow in the thorax and is biochemically characterized by a pleural triglyceride concentration >1.24 mmol/L (110 mg/dL), a pleural fluid cholesterol to triglyceride ratio <1, and a pleural effusion to serum triglyceride ratio >1.

5. Hemothorax occurs secondary to coagulopathy or blood vessel rupture. In veterinary medicine, no standardized definition of hemothorax exists. As the resulting hematocrit in the effusion depends on the peripheral circulating hematocrit, the human definition, which is standardized and based on this principle, can be applied. Accordingly, hemothorax is defined as any pleural effusion with a pleural fluid hematocrit >50% of the peripheral hematocrit.

6. In the case of an exudate cytological analysis of the pleural effusion, fluid culture and other tests on the effusion may be indicated. Moreover, other tests, such as bloodwork, a CT scan, or pleural or pulmonary biopsies, may be indicated.

DIAGNOSIS

7. Causes of right-sided congestive heart failure include pericardial effusion, tricuspid regurgitation, and dilated cardiomyopathy.

8. Causes of protein-losing enteropathy include inflammatory bowel disease, lymphangiectasia, intestinal lymphoma, and other neoplasias.

9. Diseases with infectious components include penetrating chest wounds, foreign body inhalation, a ruptured esophagus, a ruptured pulmonary abscess, hematogenous bacterial infection, viral infection (e.g., feline infectious peritonitis), and fungal infections.

TREATMENT

10. Therapeutic thoracentesis should be performed aseptically for large pleural effusions to relieve respiratory distress, and the volume retrieved should be recorded. While fluid removal helps an animal to breathe better, it is rarely curative. Treatment of the underlying disease is therefore required to prevent fluid re-accumulation. This could require medications or even surgery.

11. Vitamin K, with or without plasma transfusion, is recommended for rodenticide intoxication. Hemothorax due to primary hyperfibrinolysis (PHF) can occur with angystrongylosis in dogs. Coagulopathy resolution requires addressing the underlying cause; supportive treatment may require plasma, tranexamic acid, and a low dose of glucocorticoids.

SUGGESTED READINGS

- Boggs DS, Kinasewitz GT. Review: pathophysiology of the pleural space. *Am J Med Sci* 309:53-59, 1995.
- Rozanski E. Diseases of the pleural space. In Ettinger SJ, Feldman EC, Côté E (editors). Textbook of Veterinary Internal Medicine 8th edition. St. Louis, Elsevier, 2017, pp 2819-2834.
- Zoia A, Drigo M. Diagnostic value of Light's criteria and albumin gradient in classifying the pathophysiology of pleural effusion formation in cats. *J Feline Med Surgery* 18:666-672, 2016.
- Zoia A, Petini M, Righetti D, Caldin M, Drigo M. Discriminating transudates and exudates in dogs with pleural effusion: diagnostic utility of simplified Light's criteria compared with traditional veterinary classification. *Vet Rec* 187:e5, 2020.
- Zoia A, Slater LA, Heller J, Connolly DJ, Church DB. A new approach to pleural effusion in cats: markers for distinguishing transudates from exudates. *J Feline Med Surgery* 11:847-855, 2009.

POLLAKIURIA/STRANGURIA

Erika Monari

Pollakiuria refers to excessively frequent urination, whereas stranguria is defined as a painful discharge of urine; clinical signs attributable to pollakiuria and/or stranguria are suggestive of lower urinary tract disease, including the anatomical tract from the bladder to the urethra.

A complete history and physical examination are essential for any patient presenting with pollakiuria, stranguria, or both. Specifically, age at presentation, previous diagnostic procedures, medical treatment and/or surgery should be considered, whether the problem is intermittent or continuous, and, in addition, how the patient urinates, whether in drops or with a continuous urine stream. The urinary bladder should be evaluated by palpation before and after urination to confirm its size; how urine is macroscopically, whether pigmented or not, should also be evaluated. Moreover, rectal examination allows evaluation of the prostate gland, the distal urethra, and the anal tone.

If the bladder is persistently small and the frequency of urination is normal, an examination of clinical signs should be carried out in case of relapse. Instead, the persistence of these clinical signs and the presence of a large bladder should be reasons for evaluating the patient by means of a complete physical examination, rectal and vaginal, blood and urine examinations, and abdominal ultrasound and/or X-rays including a cystourethroscopy when needed.

The main differential diagnoses reached with a diagnostic workup are inflammatory infective processes, obstruction of the urinary outflow caused by masses/uroliths, or idiopathic inflammatory conditions, such as feline idiopathic cystitis (FIC). Finally, clinical signs, such as pollakiuria and/or stranguria, could be related to neurological dysfunction, for which a complete neurological examination and advanced diagnostic imaging can allow localizing the problem, usually at the level of the spinal cord and a related upper or lower motor neuron bladder.

POLLAKIURIA* / STRANGURIA§

*Excessively frequent urination
§ Painful urination

Evaluate bladder size (1)

Small bladder

Normal urination → Check clinical signs again (15)

Frequent urination (16)

- **Small volume (17)** → Diagnostic workup
Physical examination, abdominal ultrasound, urogenital examination, CBC, biochemistry, and urine examinations ± cystourethroscopy

- **Large volume (16)** → Diagnostic workup
Physical examination, abdominal ultrasound, urogenital examination, CBC, biochemistry, and urine examinations ± cystourethroscopy

→ No identifiable cause (eventual urodynamic study) (17)

→ **Detrusor urethral dyssynergia/idiopathic detrusor instability (18)**

→ Specific treatment (19)

Large bladder

Diagnostic workup
Physical exam with/without neurologic evaluation, abdominal ultrasound, urogenital examination, CBC, biochemistry and urine exams ± cystourethroscopy

- **Neurologic bladder dysfunction (12)** → Advanced imaging studies (MRI) → **Upper/lower motor neuron bladder (13)** → Medical and/or surgical treatment (14)

- **Urolithiasis (10)** → Dissolution diet and/or uroliths retrieval (11)

- **Urogenital mass (7)** → Treat based on cytological/histological diagnosis

- **Proliferative urethritis (8)** → Medical treatment, dilation with stent/balloon or laser surgery (9)

- **Active urine sediment (2)** → Urine culture (collected by cystocentesis or catheterization)
  - Negative culture → **Feline idiopathic cystitis (FIC) (5)** → Anti-inflammatory drugs, spasmolytics, wet diluted diet, environmental enrichment (6)
  - Positive culture → **Urinary tract infection/prostatitis; rule out upper urinary tract infection (3)** → Treat based on urine culture results (4)

DIAGNOSTIC PROTOCOL

1. The first diagnostic step is to evaluate bladder size after voiding.

2. An active urine sediment (e.g., presence of >5 leukocytes, or >5 red blood cells and >5 leukocytes on a ×400 high power field upon microscopic examination) should be investigated with a urine culture from a sample of urine collected in an aseptic manner.

7. Urogenital masses can be diagnosed using abdominal ultrasound or advanced diagnostic imaging modalities and with cytology and/or histopathology.

12. In the case of neurologic dysfunction, advanced diagnostic imaging modalities can better evaluate spinal cord diseases.

15. In the case of a small bladder after voiding, clinical signs should be rechecked to note the presence of stranguria and/or pollakiuria.

16. In the case of frequent urination with a large volume of urine, a diagnostic workup should include a complete physical examination, blood and urine examinations, and diagnostic imaging modalities together with cystoscopy, if needed. Polyuria/polydipsia may be present, and it should be excluded. See the chapter dedicated to polyuria/polydipsia.

17. If no identifiable causes of small bladder and frequent urination are identified, a urodynamic study (urethral pressure profilometry) can help in diagnosing neurological diseases.

DIAGNOSIS

3. An active urine sediment and a positive culture are needed to diagnose urinary tract infections (UTI). When pyelonephritis is suspected, the urinary tract should be ultrasonographically evaluated, together with inflammatory markers (e.g., leukocytes, acute-phase proteins). If there is suspicion of a mycotic UTI, a specific urine culture, together with an antimicogram, should be carried out.

5. A negative urine culture in a feline patient with lower urinary tract signs, excluding other causes of pollakiuria and/or stranguria, suggests underlying feline idiopathic cystitis.

8. Proliferative urethritis is an inflammatory and infiltrative disease that can cause complete urinary obstruction; it is often associated with urinary tract infection. The underlying etiology has not yet been established; however, it is considered secondary to an immune-mediated inflammation caused by bacteria.

10. Uroliths can be diagnosed using abdominal ultrasound together with radiographs to evaluate stone radiopacity. Urinalysis allows for visualizing crystals in the sediment and can help define the stone composition. It should be emphasized that the uroliths can be composed of different types of minerals, and the presence of crystals does not correlate with the presence of uroliths. Specific crystals (e.g., struvite crystals in dogs) can be associated with urinary tract infection, which should be diagnosed with urine culture and treated to promote stone dissolution.

13. The diagnosis of an upper/lower motor neuron bladder can be obtained with a neurologic examination, which allows for identifying a spinal cord problem. Advanced diagnostic imaging can usually identify the type and location of a spinal injury (see the chapter on urinary incontinence and retention).

18. In detrusor urethral dyssynergia, insufficient relaxation of the urethral sphincter at the time of detrusor contraction leads to functional obstruction and urine retention. Patients with idiopathic detrusor instability show detrusor hyperspasticity without underlying identifiable causes.

TREATMENT

4. A bacterial urinary tract infection (UTI) should be treated based on urine culture results, and the duration of treatment should be in accordance with the guidelines for the diagnosis and management of bacterial UTIs (ISCAID guidelines). In the case of mycotic UTIs, urine culture can help in identifying the fungal species and antifungal susceptibility.

6. Feline idiopathic cystitis (FIC), a behavioral disease, can be treated by alleviating the inflammation and the associated urethral spasms, using anti-inflammatory drugs (if kidney function parameters are within the reference range) and spasmolytics, together with environmental enrichment to decrease stressful events.

9. Urinary tract infection should be treated, when diagnosed, based on urine culture results; anti-inflammatory drugs can be administered to decrease associated clinical signs. Dilation of the urethra can be obtained, when needed, to relieve the obstruction using a balloon or metallic/silicone stenting with laser ablation.

11. Treatment should be carried out depending on the size and nature of the uroliths and whether they are causing an obstruction. In the case of non-obstructing struvite uroliths, medical dissolution with a wet diluted diet and antibiotics, in the case of an associated urinary tract infection, should be carried out. In the case of obstructing uroliths, retrograde urohydropulsion and urolith retrieval should be carried out before medical treatment. Urolith analysis is essential for optimal treatment.

14. Treatment of a neurological bladder is aimed at decreasing smooth muscle urethral sphincter tone and at optimizing bladder emptying (see the chapter on urinary incontinence and retention); surgical treatment should be considered when needed.

19. Treatment of detrusor urethral dyssynergia is aimed at smooth muscle relaxation in association with parasympathomimetics. In the case of idiopathic detrusor instability, treatment with anticholinergic drugs helps prevent the contraction of the detrusor.

SUGGESTED READINGS

- Bartges J. Clinical signs of lower urinary tract disease. In Bartges J, Polzin DJ (editors). Nephrology and Urology of Small Animals. Wiley Blackwell, 2011, pp 428-431.
- International Society for Companion Animal Infectious Diseases (ISCAID) guidelines for the diagnosis and management of bacterial urinary tract infections in dogs and cats. *Vet J* 247:8-25, 2019.
- Labato MA. Pollakiuria, stranguria and urinary incontinence. In Ettinger SJ, Feldman EC, Côté E (editors). Textbook of Veterinary Internal Medicine 8th edition. St. Louis, Elsevier, 2017, pp 666-672.
- Stilwell C, Bazelle J, Walker D, et al. Detrusor urethral dyssynergy in dogs: 35 cases (2007-2019). *J Small Anim Pract*, 62:468-477, 2021.

POLYPHAGIA

Andrea Corsini

The term polyphagia defines excessive food consumption, which can be physiologic, pathologic, or drug-induced. Food intake is regulated by different factors, such as the central nervous system (CNS), the gastrointestinal tract, and the environment. Within the CNS, food intake regulation is primarily due to the hypothalamic nuclei, which define the feeding center and the satiety center. Gastrointestinal regulation is due to gastric distension, the rate of gastric emptying, gut hormones, and nutrient absorption. Insulin and leptin are potent stimulants of the satiety center, while ghrelin acts by stimulating the feeding center. Serum concentrations of amino acids, glucose, and lipids affect hypothalamic regulation, stimulating the feeding center when they decrease.

Consequently, any condition affecting these mechanisms, either physiologic or pathologic, can result in increased food consumption. Primary polyphagia may be due to conditions that affect the CNS regulatory centers despite normal energy stores. Secondary polyphagia derives from an increased metabolic rate, a decreased energy supply, or treatment with certain drugs (e.g., glucocorticoids). The metabolic rate may increase in both physiologic (e.g., pregnancy, increased exercise) and pathologic conditions (e.g., hyperthyroidism). The decreased energy supply can be due to inadequate nutrient intake (e.g., a low-calorie diet, megaesophagus), malabsorption/maldigestion (e.g., gastrointestinal diseases or exocrine pancreatic insufficiency [EPI]), or decreased nutrient uptake within the cells (e.g., diabetes mellitus). The exact mechanisms responsible for polyphagia in certain diseases (e.g., Cushing's syndrome, liver diseases) are not completely understood.

The first step in assessing a polyphagic patient is to rule out overfeeding or gluttonous behavior by means of a thorough history. If polyphagia is the consequence of a disease, it is rarely the only clinical sign present. Establishing whether weight gain or loss has taken place is highly relevant in these patients. Weight changes and other concurrent clinical signs are usually helpful in prioritizing the steps of the diagnostic protocol. For example, polyuria/polydipsia (PU/PD) suggests endocrine diseases, such as diabetes mellitus, hyperadrenocorticism in dogs, hyperthyroidism, or acromegaly in cats, while diarrhea is more common in malabsorptive syndromes or EPI.

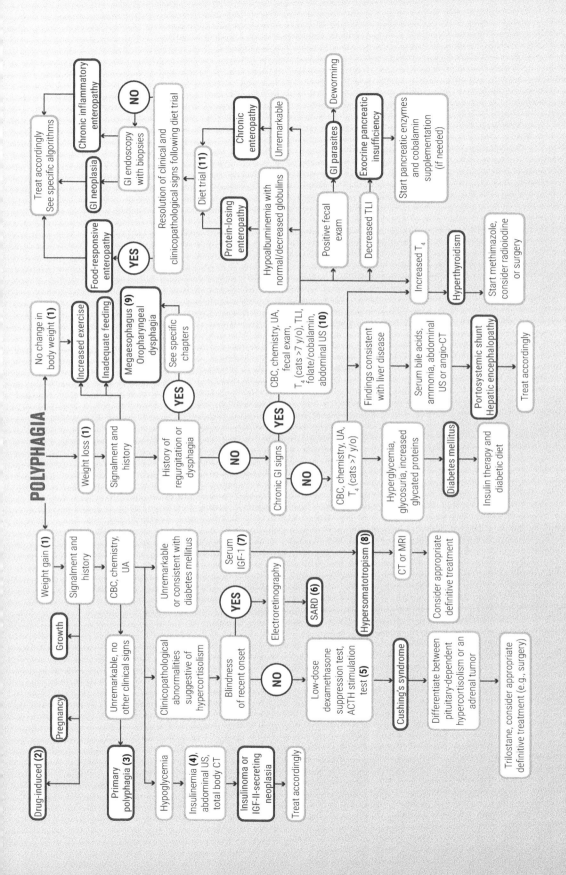

POLYPHAGIA

Weight gain (1)
- Signalment and history
  - Growth
  - Pregnancy
  - Drug-induced (2)
- CBC, chemistry, UA
  - Unremarkable or consistent with diabetes mellitus
    - Serum IGF-1 (7)
    - Electroretinography
      - Blindness of recent onset
        - YES → SARD (6)
        - NO → Low-dose dexamethasone suppression test, ACTH stimulation test (5)
          - Cushing's syndrome
            - Differentiate between pituitary-dependent hypercortisolism or an adrenal tumor
              - Trilostane, consider appropriate definitive treatment (e.g., surgery)
  - Unremarkable, no other clinical signs
    - Primary polyphagia (3)
    - Clinicopathological abnormalities suggestive of hypercortisolism
      - Hypoglycemia
        - Insulinemia (4), abdominal US, total body CT
          - Insulinoma or IGF-II-secreting neoplasia
            - Treat accordingly

Hypersomatotropism (8)
- CT or MRI
- Consider appropriate definitive treatment

Weight loss (1)
- Signalment and history
  - No change in body weight (1)
    - Increased exercise
    - Inadequate feeding
  - History of regurgitation or dysphagia
    - YES → Megaesophagus (9) Oropharyngeal dysphagia
      - See specific chapters
    - NO → Chronic GI signs
      - YES → CBC, chemistry, UA, fecal exam, T₄ (cats >7 y/o), TLI, folate/cobalamin, abdominal US (10)
      - NO → CBC, chemistry, UA, T₄ (cats >7 y/o)
        - Hyperglycemia, glycosuria, increased glycated proteins
          - Diabetes mellitus
            - Insulin therapy and diabetic diet
        - Findings consistent with liver disease
          - Serum bile acids, ammonia, abdominal US or angio-CT
            - Portosystemic shunt Hepatic encephalopathy
              - Treat accordingly
        - Increased T₄
          - Hyperthyroidism
            - Start methimazole, consider radioiodine or surgery

Food-responsive enteropathy
- Treat accordingly See specific algorithms
- GI neoplasia
  - GI endoscopy with biopsies
    - NO → Chronic inflammatory enteropathy → Treat accordingly See specific algorithms
- Resolution of clinical and clinicopathological signs following diet trial
  - YES → Diet trial (11)

Protein-losing enteropathy
- Hypoalbuminemia with normal/decreased globulins

Chronic enteropathy
Unremarkable

Positive fecal exam
- GI parasites → Deworming

Decreased TLI
- Exocrine pancreatic insufficiency
  - Start pancreatic enzymes and cobalamin supplementation (if needed)

DIAGNOSTIC PROTOCOL

1. Weight gain points to primary polyphagia or specific endocrine diseases, while weight loss is commonly associated with secondary polyphagia. However, some exceptions exist. For example, dogs with hypercortisolism can maintain a stable weight despite showing marked abdominal distension, and cats with concurrent hypersomatotropism and diabetes mellitus may sometimes gain weight. Body weight usually also remains stable in the early phase of the disease.

4. Serum insulin concentrations measured during hypoglycemia are inappropriately normal or high in dogs with insulinoma. On the contrary, low to undetectable insulin concentrations are reported in dogs with hypoglycemia due to insulin-like growth factor II (IGF-II)-secreting neoplasia or other neoplasias. Polyphagia can be triggered by chronic hypoglycemia; however, it is not a consistent finding in these patients.

5. Polyphagia is only one of the signs of hypercortisolism, albeit very common, in both dogs and cats. In order to decrease the risk of false-positive results, dogs with polyphagia should be tested for hyperadrenocorticism when other suggestive clinical (e.g., polyuria and polydipsia, abdominal distension, dermatological abnormalities) and clinicopathological (e.g., thrombocytosis, increased alkaline phosphatase, alanine transaminase, and γ-glutamyl transferase activity, hyperlipidemia, diluted urine, proteinuria) signs are present.

7. Evaluation of serum IGF-1 concentrations should be carried out in all diabetic cats, ideally after at least 6-8 weeks of insulin treatment. A result above 1000 ng/mL is strongly suggestive of hypersomatotropism; however, some cats with hypersomatotropism may have values between 800 and 1000 ng/mL or even below 800 ng/mL. In the case of strong clinical suspicion, hypersomatotropism should not be ruled out based only on the IGF-1 value. Hypersomatotropism in dogs has been described but is rare.

10. Serum cobalamin concentrations can be normal or decreased in patients with chronic enteropathy. Parenteral or oral supplementation should be started whenever serum cobalamin concentration is less than approximately 400 ng/L. Of note, hypocobalaminemia has been reported in hyperthyroid cats; however, the clinical relevance of this finding is not clear. Abdominal ultrasonography is suggested when bloodwork and fecal examinations are unremarkable and chronic enteropathy (e.g., alimentary tract lymphoma, chronic inflammatory enteropathy) is suspected. It should also be performed if the clinical signs did not improve after specific treatment for other diseases.

DIAGNOSIS

2. Glucocorticoids, phenobarbital, antihistamines, progestins, benzodiazepines, cyproheptadine, and mirtazapine are drugs capable of inducing polyphagia.

3. Primary polyphagia is usually due to the animal's gluttonous behavior, stress, or normal psychogenic behavior. It is rarely caused by diseases affecting the hypothalamic satiety center. In this case, neurological signs are usually evident.

6. Sudden acquired retinal degeneration syndrome (SARDS) is an idiopathic retinal disorder causing sudden and permanent blindness in dogs. An association between SARDS and hypercortisolism has been suggested since dogs with SARDS commonly show polyphagia, polyuria, and polydipsia. However, evidence of a connection between the two conditions is still lacking.

8. Hypersomatotropism (acromegaly) commonly leads to diabetes mellitus due to the marked diabetogenic effect of the growth hormone (GH). Feline hypersomatotropism is typically seen in middle-aged and older male cats and is caused by a GH-secreting pituitary adenoma or hyperplasia. Canine hypersomatotropism is usually due to an excess of mammary GH production induced by elevated serum progesterone concentrations. It is typically seen in females during diestrus or with mammary neoplasia or in dogs receiving exogenous progestins. Functional pituitary adenomas are reported in dogs but are extremely rare.

9. Patients with congenital megaesophagus often show polyphagia, re-eating the food after regurgitation.

TREATMENT

11. An elimination diet trial using hypoallergenic commercial diets or a home-prepared diet can be carried out in dogs and cats without protein-losing enteropathy. The response is usually assessed in the first 2-4 weeks of the trial. A diet trial in dogs with protein-losing enteropathy should be carried out by following an ultra-low fat hypoallergenic diet. Low-fat diets should contain less than 10% of fats. The serum albumin concentration and clinical signs should be reassessed after 5-7 days, and additional diagnostic evaluations (e.g., endoscopy with biopsies) are warranted if no improvement is detected.

SUGGESTED READINGS

-   Craven, MD, Washabau, RJ. Comparative pathophysiology and management of protein-losing enteropathy. *J Vet Intern Med* 33:383-402, 2019.
-   Daminet S. Polyphagia. In Ettinger SJ, Feldman EC, Côté E (editors). Textbook of Veterinary Internal Medicine 8th edition. St. Louis, Elsevier, 2017, pp 100-106.
-   Feldman EC, Nelson RW, Reusch CE, Scott-Moncrieff JCR, Behrend E (editors). Canine and Feline Endocrinology 4th edition. St. Louis, Elsevier, 2015.

POLYURIA AND POLYDIPSIA

Federico Fracassi

Polyuria/polydipsia (PU/PD) is a common clinical sign of many diseases in dogs and cats and requires a thorough and systematic medical approach. Water intake in healthy dogs and cats is variable and can be increased by the high environmental temperature, physical exercise, and the assumption of an exclusively dry diet. Most authors define polydipsia in dogs as a water intake >90-100 mL/kg/day and >45 mL/kg/day in cats. These data are easily obtained by asking the owner to measure the water consumed within 24 hours. In dogs, polyuria is defined as urine production higher than 50 mL/kg/day.

For obvious reasons, the exact amount of urine produced turns out to be difficult to objectify. The production and concentration of urine are controlled by the interaction between the kidneys, the pituitary gland, and the hypothalamus. Urine production is also influenced by baroreceptors present in the atrial and aortic arch. The antidiuretic hormone (ADH) is the main regulator of water homeostasis and is produced in the hypothalamus (supraoptic and paraventricular nuclei) and released by the neurohypophysis following adequate stimuli. Its action is carried out at the renal tubular level allowing the opening of the water channels, allowing the reabsorption of water by osmotic gradient, and influencing the concentration of urine. To obtain adequately concentrated urine, it is necessary that there is an appropriate secretion and action of ADH, that at least ⅓ of the nephrons are functioning and that there is a high osmolarity in the renal medulla. From a classification point of view, it is possible to define primary polydipsia (with secondary polyuria) or primary polyuria (with secondary polydipsia). The causes can be central (brain/pituitary) or peripheral (kidney). The causes of polyuria and polydipsia are divided into central diabetes insipidus, primary nephrogenic diabetes insipidus, secondary nephrogenic diabetes insipidus, osmotic diuresis, causes that determine a decrease in the hypertonicity of the renal medulla and other causes with a mechanism not completely known.

POLYURIA AND POLYDIPSIA

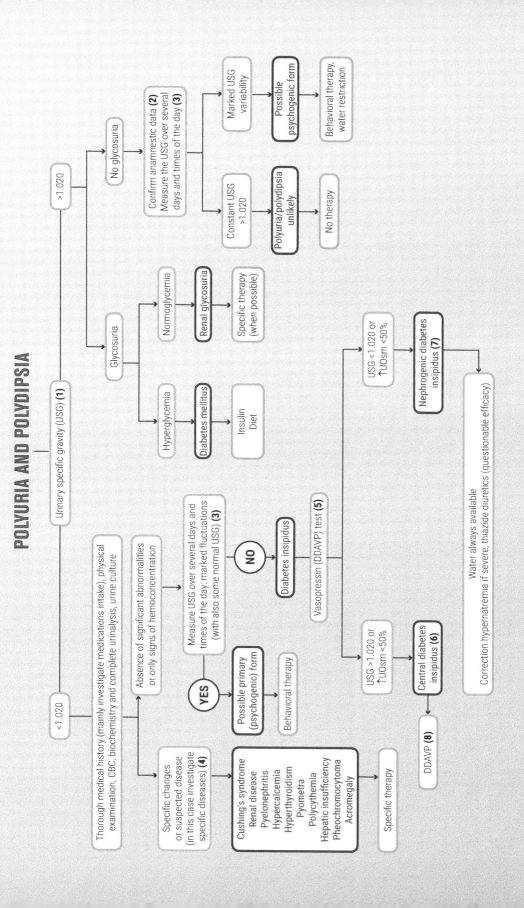

Urinary specific gravity (USG) **(1)**

>1.020

No glycosuria
- Confirm anamnestic data **(2)**
- Measure the USG over several days and times of the day **(3)**
  - Marked USG variability → **Possible psychogenic form** → Behavioral therapy, water restriction
  - Constant USG >1.020 → **Polyuria/polydipsia unlikely** → No therapy

Glycosuria
- Normoglycemia → **Renal glycosuria** → Specific therapy (when possible)
- Hyperglycemia → **Diabetes mellitus** → Insulin / Diet

<1.020

Thorough medical history (mainly investigate medications intake), physical examination, CBC, biochemistry and complete urinalysis, urine culture

- Absence of significant abnormalities or only signs of hemoconcentration
  - Measure USG over several days and times of the day: marked fluctuations (with also some normal USG) **(3)**
    - **YES** → **Possible primary (psychogenic) form** → Behavioral therapy
    - **NO** → **Diabetes insipidus** → Vasopressin (DDAVP) test **(5)**
      - USG >1.020 or ↑UOsm <50% → **Central diabetes insipidus (6)** → DDAVP **(8)**
      - USG <1.020 or ↑UOsm <50% → **Nephrogenic diabetes insipidus (7)**
        - Water always available
        - Correction hypernatremia if severe, thiazide diuretics (questionable efficacy)

- Specific changes or suspected disease (in this case investigate specific diseases) **(4)**
  - **Cushing's syndrome / Renal disease / Pyelonephritis / Hypercalcemia / Hyperthyroidism / Pyometra / Polycythemia / Hepatic insufficiency / Pheochromocytoma / Acromegaly** → Specific therapy

DIAGNOSTIC PROTOCOL

1. Urinary specific gravity (USG) is a parameter commonly used by veterinarians in routine practice. Ideally, in association with the USG, urinary osmolality could be assessed. Urinary osmolality provides more precise information, but its correlation with the USG is very good.

2. If the owner reports the presence of PU/PD but the USG, despite the absence of glycosuria, is high, it is essential to confirm the excessive water intake (>90-100 mL/kg/day in dogs and >45 mL/kg/day in cats).

3. It may be useful to ask the dog's owner (usually this test is not carried out in cats) to collect urine samples at different times of the day (up to 6-8 samples) and possibly even on consecutive days. The owner must record what the dog was doing at the time of urine collection; this can allow the association between excessive water intake and any stressful events for the animal. From the collected samples (to be kept in the refrigerator), the veterinarian assesses the USG and/or urinary osmolality. A marked fluctuation of the values (e.g., from 1.004 to 1.025) is strongly suggestive of primary (psychogenic) polydipsia, while in diseases linked to absolute or relative insufficiency of ADH, USG normally remains low (usually hypostenuria, e.g., USG <1.008).

4. Based on the clinical signs and the clinical-pathological findings, the most appropriate diagnostic protocol should be performed: thoracic and abdominal imaging, e.g., radiography, ultrasonography (tumors, pyometra, Cushing's syndrome, pheochromocytoma, pyelonephritis, kidney disease, hepatic disorders); ionized calcium (tumors, primary hyperparathyroidism, granulomatous diseases); ACTH stimulation test, LDDSt, urinary cortisol/creatinine ratio (Cushing's syndrome); serum T_4 (hyperthyroidism); urinary normetanephrine, adrenal fine-needle aspiration (pheochromocytoma); IGF-1 (acromegaly); pre- and postprandial bile acids, ammonia (liver failure); CT (tumors, Cushing's syndrome).

5. In the past, the water deprivation test was widely used; this test consists of removing water from the animal to see if the urine began to concentrate (allowing the diagnosis of psychogenic polydipsia) or not (diabetes insipidus). This is a test with a high risk of dehydration, inducing severe hypernatremia and sometimes causing a collapse of the animal. Therefore, today this test is used mainly for research purposes. At this diagnostic step, if there is no evidence of diseases that can induce polyuria/polydipsia, evaluating the response to vasopressin (DDAVP) is preferred. One or two drops of DDAVP (usually human nasal drops or ophthalmic DDAVP is used) are administered into the conjunctival sac. Alternatively, DDAVP tablets can be used (see point 8). The drops should be given q8h, and USG and/or urinary osmolality should be reassessed after 5-7 days. In central (neurogenic) diabetes insipidus, the urine becomes concentrated, while in the neurogenic form, it remains diluted.

DIAGNOSIS

6. Central (neurogenic) diabetes insipidus is due to ADH deficiency. It can be congenital or acquired. In the second case, the cause can be a brain tumor, a head injury, a granulomatous disease, or an immune-mediated process.

7. Nephrogenic diabetes insipidus can be: 1) congenital, due to agenesis of ADH receptors or aquaporins; 2) acquired, for example, as a result of toxic or infectious tubular damage (e.g., the outcome of pyelonephritis).

TREATMENT

8. DDAVP is a synthetic analog of ADH. Initial therapy includes doses of 0.05 mg PO q12h for dogs <5 kg and cats, 0.1 mg PO q12h for dogs between 5 to 20 kg, 0.2 mg PO q12h for dogs >20 kg, up to a maximum of 0.4 mg q8h. If these doses are not enough to control PU/PD, it is possible to try the administration q8h. If necessary, the conjunctival or subcutaneous route can also be used.

SUGGESTED READINGS

- Feldman EC, Nelson RW, Reusch CE, Scott-Moncrieff JCR, Behrend E (editors). Canine and Feline Endocrinology 4th edition. St. Louis, Elsevier, 2015.
- Rijnberk A, Kooistra HS. Protocols and function tests. In Rijnberk A, Kooistra HS (editors). Clinical Endocrinology of Dogs and Cats. Hannover, Schlütersche, 2010, pp 305-314.

PROSTATOMEGALY

Daniele Zambelli and Marco Cunto

Prostatic size, shape, symmetry, mobility, surface, and pain are important parameters that need to be evaluated during the physical examination; they should be correlated to history and clinical signs in order to obtain a final diagnosis. Size can be evaluated with transrectal digital palpation or more accurately with ultrasound examination. The canine prostate grows exponentially throughout adult life, showing aspects of hyperplasia that, if not symptomatic, are not considered pathologic. This aspect, as well as breed variations and the presence of diseases, can cause great variability in its size.

Prostatic volume can be calculated, using an ultrasonographic evaluation, with the following formula:

V (cm³) = [1/2.6 (length × width × height) + 1.8 (cm³)

The volume (V) should be compared with the expected prostatic volume (V1), calculated with a formula that considers body weight and age:

$V1$ (cm³) = [0.867 × body weight (kg)] + [1.885 × age (years)] + 15.88

Prostatic disorders, including benign prostatic hyperplasia (BPH), acute or chronic prostatitis (AP, CP), prostatic abscess (PA) and squamous metaplasia (SM) frequently affect non-castrated patients, over 6 years of age. Prostatic neoplasia is not very frequent and is predominantly observed in castrated dogs. Cysts are usually present secondary to other prostatic disorders or as paraprostatic cysts. Castration induces a prostatic size reduction due to the atrophy of the glandular parenchyma; however, it does not prevent all potential prostatic disorders. Only PN, cysts, and infections (prostatitis or PA) may affect neutered males. Prostatic diseases are very rare in intact or neutered cats. In cats, cases of bacterial prostatitis, prostatic abscess, squamous metaplasia, paraprostatic cysts, and neoplasia have been described.

More than one prostatic disorder can be present simultaneously; BPH, SM, or PN frequently cause aseptic prostatitis, predisposing the gland to infection. The diagnostic workup to investigate a prostatic disorder should include the evaluation of serum canine prostate-specific esterase (CPSE) concentration, a serum biochemistry profile, a complete blood count, urinalysis, and urine culture by cystocentesis or sterile catheterization, and prostatic sample collection to carry out bacteriology and cytology.

PROSTATOMEGALY

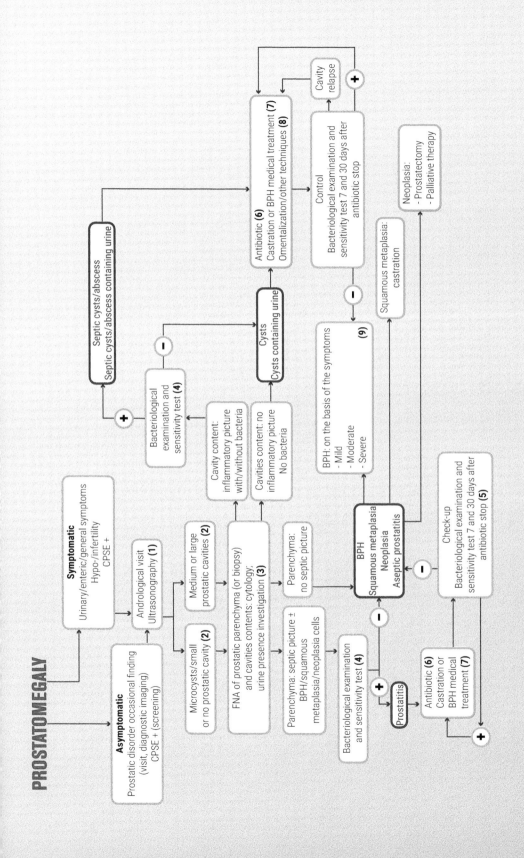

DIAGNOSTIC PROTOCOL

1. In an asymptomatic patient with prostatomegaly in which andrological visits and ultrasonography do not show pathological findings, benign prostatic hyperplasia is considered a senile modification. In these cases, no treatment is required, and patients should be monitored with an approach called "watchful waiting".

2. Benign prostatic hyperplasia (BPH) is frequently associated with retention cysts (microcysts/small, medium, or large cysts). Other cavity lesions (cysts, abscesses, or necrotic areas) can be present in other prostatic disorders; these cavity lesions frequently connect to the urethra and may contain urine, predisposing to a prostatic infection.

3. Parenchymal samples and cavity contents should be evaluated with cytology. Fluid samples of the cavities should be analyzed to investigate the presence of urine (creatinine in the fluid higher than creatinine in serum). Prostatic samples may be obtained by means of sperm collection, prostatic massage, FNA, and biopsy (if the FNA results are not diagnostic). The techniques should be chosen based on the type of lesion and clinical suspicion. Sperm collection is recommended in patients with suspicion of infection or neoplasia to avoid the possible spread of bacteria (peritonitis or septicemia) or neoplastic cells. A spread of bacteria is possible with the rupture of infected cysts/abscesses and the penetration of bacteria into the bloodstream. Performing an FNA has the risk of seeding the needle tract with bacteria/neoplastic cells, possible with prostatic massage and FNA. When it is not possible to obtain an appropriate sample by semen collection, a gentle prostate massage or ultrasound-guided FNA may be performed, carefully evaluating the risks and the pros and cons of the collection. Preputial cytology may be used to diagnose hyperestrogenism in the course of squamous metaplasia.

4. A parenchymal sample, cavities content, and urine (collected by cystocentesis) should be evaluated for bacterial culture and sensitivity.

5. Prostatitis may hide the clinical signs or the diagnostic findings of other prostatic disorders; therefore, the patient should be re-evaluated 7 and 30 days after antibiotic suspension, performing a bacteriological examination and checking for possible other prostatic disorders.

TREATMENT

6. Antimicrobial treatment is chosen based on prostatic and/or urine culture, and a sensitivity test, as well as the pharmacokinetics of the molecule, is used. The treatment should be performed only in case of positive culture and is recommended for 4 to 6 weeks with acute prostatitis and 6 to 8 weeks with chronic prostatitis and prostatic abscess, or when castration is not performed. Antimicrobials with high lipid solubility, low protein binding, and high pKa, or with zwitterion characteristics have good penetration into the prostatic parenchyma. Examples of these antibiotics are fluoroquinolone, clindamycin, and chloramphenicol.

7. Androgen stimulation may predispose to prostatic infection; therefore, castration is strongly recommended for hormonal deprivation in case of prostatitis. In dogs with valuable breeding

potential, castration may be postponed and replaced by medical treatment (e.g., finasteride, osaterone, deslorelin). This treatment should be prolonged if a second cycle of antimicrobials is required.

8. Septic or aseptic large cysts and abscessations should be surgically drained or treated by ultrasound percutaneous drainage followed by percutaneous ethanol injection; in fact, only medical treatment is rarely enough for the resolution of the problem. Surgical drainage is frequently performed with omentalization or, if not possible, with different techniques, such as placing a Penrose drain or marsupialization. Rarely, large cysts or abscessations may require partial or total prostatectomy.

9. Benign prostatic hyperplasia (BPH) may be asymptomatic or symptomatic. If clinical signs are present, the BPH is considered pathological and can be classified based on its severity as mild, moderate, or severe. Usually, no therapy is recommended in BPH asymptomatic patients (with prostatomegaly); when signs are mild or do not affect or disturb the patient, they are usually monitored with an approach called "watchful waiting". BPH therapy is based on the suppression or prevention of androgen synthesis or action by means of castration or pharmacological treatment. When BPH is associated with incontinence due to bladder hyperdistention, severe dyschezia, the presence of big retention cysts, perineal hernias, severe recurrent hematuria, urethral discharge, dysuria/acute urinary retention, or recurrent prostatitis, castration is the treatment of choice. When necessary, large cysts have to be surgically treated. In breeding dogs, in patients in which castration is not desired by owners or not possible, or in the case of mild clinical signs, pharmacological therapy may be recommended. The drugs more frequently used are 5α-reductase inhibitors (such as finasteride 1.25 mg PO q24h), progestogens/antiandrogens (osaterone acetate 0.25-0.5 mg/kg PO q24h for 7 days), GnRH analogs (deslorelin acetate 4.7 mg SC implant q6m).

SUGGESTED READINGS

-   Ettinger SJ, Feldman EC, Côté E (editors). Textbook of Veterinary Internal Medicine 8th edition. St. Louis, Elsevier, 2017.
-   Kamolpatana K, Johnston GR, Johnston SD. Determination of canine prostatic volume using transabdominal ultrasonography. *Vet Radiol Ultrasound* 41:73-77, 2000.
-   Ruel Y, Barthez PY, Mailles A, et al. Ultrasonographic evaluation of the prostate in healthy intact dogs. *Vet Radiol Ultrasound* 39:212-216, 1998.

PROTEINURIA

María C. López and Xavier Roura

Proteinuria is defined as the presence of an excessive quantity of abnormal proteins in urine. The glomerular filtration barrier, composed of the glomerular capillary endothelium, basement membrane, and epithelial podocytes, limits the passage of medium and high molecular weight proteins from the blood to the glomerular urine filtrate, with albumin (69 kDa) and larger proteins typically being retained. The glomerular filtered albumin is largely reabsorbed through the proximal convoluted tubule. However, filtered albumin is not completely reabsorbed; therefore, albumin is the major urinary protein in healthy dogs and cats as well as in those with renal proteinuria. Loss of protein in urine in normal healthy dogs and cats does not usually exceed 10-20 mg/kg/day and 30 mg/kg/day, respectively. When evidence of proteinuria is detected by urinalysis, localization of the likely source of the proteinuria is needed. Prerenal proteinuria implies that a significantly abnormal concentration of protein is being presented to the kidney in the plasma, while postrenal proteinuria implies that protein is added to the urine in the urinary tract after the kidney. In dogs and cats with persistent proteinuria, without any potential cause of pre- or postrenal proteinuria and without signs of active inflammation on urine sediment examination, renal proteinuria could be diagnosed. It could likely be either glomerular (due to changes in the structure or function of the glomerular filtration barrier) and/or tubular (reduced capacity of the proximal tubular cells to reabsorb albumin). Furthermore, determining whether proteinuria persists over time requires repeated testing, at least twice, two or more weeks apart. Finally, the use of appropriate quantitative methods such as the urine protein to creatinine ratio (UPC) to obtain reliable magnitude/quantification of the urine protein loss is crucial for clinical decision-making and for monitoring trends, including response to proteinuria treatment.

PROTEINURIA

UPC >0.5 dogs
UPC >0.4 cats **(1)**

Thorough medical history, physical examination, blood pressure, CBC, biochemistry,
serum protein electrophoresis, complete urinalysis (USG, dipstick ± culture/sensitivity)

Postrenal **(2)**

- **Lower urinary tract disease**
- **Reproductive tract disease**

→ Specific therapy

Renal

Tubular UPC ≤2

- Abdominal US
- Infectious diseases Serology/PCR → **Leptospira spp.**
- Pyelocentesis or cystocentesis with culture/sensitivity → **Pyelonephritis** → Antibiotics
- **Chronic kidney disease** → Specific therapy (IRIS guidelines)

Glomerular UPC >2 **(3)**

- Abdominal US
- Renal biopsy **(4)**
  - **Familial diseases (5)**
  - **Immune-complex glomerulonephritis (6)**
  - Glomerulosclerosis (focal segmental and global)
  - Neoplasia
  - **Amyloidosis (7)**
  → Specific therapy

- Infectious diseases Serology/PCR

DOG
- *Anaplasma* spp.
- *Borrelia burgdorferi*
- *Babesia* spp.
- *Brucella canis*
- *Ehrlichia* spp.
- *Dirofilaria immitis*
- *Hepatozoon americanum*
- *Leishmania* spp.
- *Leptospira* spp.
- *Mycoplasma* spp.
- *Rickettsia rickettsia*
- *Bartonella* spp.

→ Specific therapy

CAT
- Feline infectious peritonitis
- Feline immunodeficiency virus
- Feline leukemia virus
- *Bartonella* spp.
- *Leishmania* spp.

→ Specific therapy

Prerenal/multifactorial

Bence Jones proteins, total T$_4$,
ACTH stimulation test, low-dose
dexamethasone suppression test,
specific pancreatic lipase

- Multiple myeloma
- Systemic hypertension
- Drug reactions
- **Hyperadrenocorticism (dog)**
- Acute pancreatitis
- **Hyperthyroidism (cat)**

→ Specific therapy

Treatment for proteinuria **(8)**

Renal prescription diet **(9)** ± ACEi **(10)** ± Omega-3 fatty acid ± Angiotensin receptor blocker **(11)**

DIAGNOSTIC PROTOCOL

1. Following the International Renal Interest Society (IRIS) guidelines, dogs and cats with a UPC <0.2 are classified as non-proteinuric; dogs with a UPC of 0.2-0.5 or cats with a UPC of 0.2-0.4 as borderline; and dogs with UPC >0.5 or cats with >0.4 as proteinuric. Dogs and cats that are persistently borderline proteinuric should be reevaluated within 2 months and re-classified as appropriate.

2. Postrenal proteinuria is due to protein that is deposited in the urine distal to the kidney. Urinary or reproductive tract disorders, such as cystitis or prostatitis, are examples of postrenal causes of proteinuria. This type of proteinuria could be minimized by performing cystocentesis. However, although there are proteins present inside the red and white blood cells, only large quantities, such as macroscopic hematuria or pyuria, could produce significant postrenal proteinuria. Furthermore, postrenal proteinuria is never persistent once the underlying condition is removed; it cannot be caused by small amounts of blood contamination from cystocentesis.

3. A high degree of renal proteinuria (UPC ratio >2) could be suggestive of primary glomerular disease, particularly once kidney disease has become established. Higher values (UPC >10) could well be associated with a nephrotic syndrome. Dogs with severe proteinuria are not always azotemic when their kidney disease is diagnosed.

4. Renal biopsy is indicated only when having an accurate histological diagnosis is likely to impact patient management. Patients in which the management is most likely to be altered by the results of a renal biopsy include those with protein-losing nephropathy in chronic kidney disease (CKD) IRIS in stages 1 and 2, which does not respond to proteinuric treatment or those with acute kidney injury (AKI). Renal biopsy is generally not indicated in patients with CKD IRIS stages 3 and 4 because the results of histopathology are unlikely to change their prognosis, treatment, or outcome.

DIAGNOSIS

5. Renal dysplasia represents a group of developmental anomalies and is defined as an abnormal differentiation of the renal parenchyma. Affected breeds include Lhasa Apso, Shih Tzu, soft-coated Wheaten Terrier, Cavalier King Charles Spaniel, Bulldog, Standard Poodle, Bull Mastiff, Cairn Terrier, Alaskan Malamute, Golden Retriever, Chow Chow, Cocker Spaniel, Dutch Kooiker, Boxer, Finnish Harrier, Norwegian Elkhound, Miniature Schnauzer dogs, and the Norwegian Forest cat. Polycystic kidney disease causes a progressive development of fluid-filled cysts in the kidney. Affected breeds include Persian, Himalayan, and British Blue cats, and Bull Terrier, Cairn Terrier, and West Highland White Terrier dogs.

6. This group of disorders includes membranous glomerulonephritis, membranoproliferative glomerulonephritis, lupus nephritis, proliferative (rare), crescentic type (rare), and IgA nephropathy (rare).

7. Amyloidosis is a disease characterized by the extracellular deposition of insoluble, fibrillary proteins with a specific β-pleated sheet conformation, generally called amyloid. Amyloid

deposits can be localized, organ-limited, or generalized.

TREATMENT

8. After appropriate investigation and specific treatment of any underlying disease identified, therapeutic intervention for proteinuria, accompanied by monitoring, is recommended for proteinuric cats and dogs, and for borderline proteinuric cats.

9. Diet has a large effect on the magnitude of proteinuria, and protein-restricted diets could reduce the overall renal trafficking of protein. If circulating protein can be lowered, there is then less risk of protein overload across the filtration barrier and less tubular protein reabsorption.

10. Starting with angiotensin-converting enzyme inhibitor (ACEi), such as enalapril or benazepril at 0.5 mg/kg PO q12h, or angiotensin receptor blocker (ARB), such as telmisartan at 1 mg/kg PO q24h, reevaluate serum creatinine (tolerable increase is <30% for IRIS stages 1, 2 or 3), potassium and blood pressure in 2 weeks. If normal, reevaluate again after 4-8 weeks including UPC, and readjust the dose of ACEi or angiotensin receptor blocker.

11. If severe hyperkalemia develops or the proteinuria is not adequately controlled with an ACEi or ARB, they can be exchanged or used in combination.

SUGGESTED READINGS

-   Harley L, Langston C. Proteinuria in dogs and cats. *Can Vet J* 53:631-638, 2012.
-   International Renal Interest Society Guidelines. Available from: http://www.iris-kidney.com/guidelines/recommendations.html, 2019 (accessed January 13th 2022).
-   Lees GR, Brown SA, Elliott J, et al. Assessment and Management of Proteinuria in Dogs and Cats: 2004 ACVIM Forum Consensus Statement (Small Animal). *J Vet Intern Med* 19:377-385, 2005.
-   Roura X, Elliott J, Grauer GF. Proteinuria. In Elliot J, Grauer GF, Westropp JL (editors). British Small Animal Veterinary Association Manual of Canine and Feline Nephrology and Urology. British Small Animal Veterinary Association, 2017, pp 50-58.
-   Vaden SL. Glomerular diseases. In Ettinger SJ, Feldman EC, Côté E (editors). Textbook of Veterinary Internal Medicine 8th edition. St. Louis, Elsevier, 2017, pp 1959-1972.

PRURITUS: CATS

Silvia Colombo

Cats manifest pruritus in different ways, such as scratching, licking, biting off their fur, or shaking the head in case of auricular pruritus. To some extent, scratching and licking are part of the normal feline behavior known as grooming. However, when grooming becomes excessive (defined as overgrooming), it may represent the clinical expression of pruritus or, less commonly, pain or stress. Cats scratch with their hind paws, and its increased frequency is easily recognized by the owner, also because it usually causes excoriations on the head and neck. On the other hand, if the cat manifests pruritus by excessive licking, the owner may consider it "normal" until alopecia or erosive-ulcerative lesions become apparent. Moreover, cats often hide from the owner because they perceive their overgrooming behaviour as undesired by the owner.

An additional issue complicating the diagnostic approach to feline pruritus is the clinical presentation. Regardless of the etiology, most pruritic cats present with one (or more) of four clinical patterns: head and neck ulcerative dermatitis, self-induced alopecia, miliary dermatitis, and eosinophilic granuloma complex (eosinophilic granuloma, eosinophilic plaque, lip ulcers). These four patterns may be caused by many different conditions, including ectoparasitic diseases, dermatophytosis, allergies, autoimmune diseases, and viral, genetic, and idiopathic diseases. In some cases of self-induced alopecia, diseases of the lower urinary tract should also be considered as well as hyperthyroidism in geriatric cats. Moreover, cases of self-induced alopecia, and head and neck ulcerative dermatitis may have a behavioral etiology. Secondary infections are less common than in dogs but may make the interpretation of the clinical presentation more difficult. For these reasons, pruritus in cats is a challenging clinical sign and requires a systematic approach.

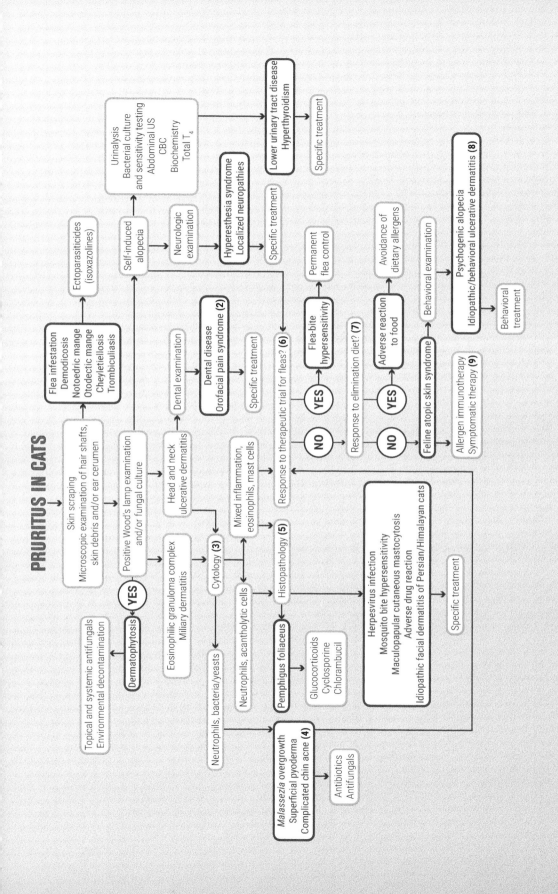

PRURITUS IN CATS

Skin scraping
Microscopic examination of hair shafts, skin debris and/or ear cerumen

Flea infestation
Demodicosis
Notoedric mange
Otodectic mange
Cheyletiellosis
Trombiculiasis

Ectoparasiticides (isoxazolines)

Positive Wood's lamp examination and/or fungal culture

Dermatophytosis ——— **YES**

Topical and systemic antifungals
Environmental decontamination

Eosinophilic granuloma complex
Miliary dermatitis

Cytology **(3)**

Neutrophils, bacteria/yeasts

Malassezia overgrowth
Superficial pyoderma
Complicated chin acne **(4)**

Antibiotics
Antifungals

Neutrophils, acantholytic cells

Pemphigus foliaceus

Glucocorticoids
Cyclosporine
Chlorambucil

Head and neck
ulcerative dermatitis

Mixed inflammation, eosinophils, mast cells

Histopathology **(5)**

Herpesvirus infection
Mosquito bite hypersensitivity
Maculopapular cutaneous mastocytosis
Adverse drug reaction
Idiopathic facial dermatitis of Persian/Himalayan cats

Specific treatment

Dental examination

Dental disease
Orofacial pain syndrome (2)

Specific treatment

Self-induced
alopecia

Urinalysis
Bacterial culture
and sensitivity testing
Abdominal US
CBC
Biochemistry
Total T$_4$

Lower urinary tract disease
Hyperthyroidism

Specific treatment

Neurologic
examination

Hyperesthesia syndrome
Localized neuropathies

Specific treatment

Response to therapeutic trial for fleas? **(6)**

NO ——— **YES**

Flea-bite
hypersensitivity

Permanent
flea control

Response to elimination diet? **(7)**

NO ——— **YES**

Adverse reaction
to food

Avoidance of
dietary allergens

Feline atopic skin syndrome

Allergen immunotherapy
Symptomatic therapy **(9)**

Behavioral examination

Psychogenic alopecia
Idiopathic/behavioral ulcerative dermatitis (8)

Behavioral
treatment

DIAGNOSTIC PROTOCOL

1. When self-induced alopecia involves the groin and abdomen, urinalysis, bacterial culture and, sensitivity testing, and abdominal ultrasound should be carried out to investigate feline lower urinary tract diseases since excessive licking of these areas may be a clinical manifestation of pain. Self-induced alopecia in an older cat may also be caused by hyperthyroidism, and it should be investigated using hematology, biochemistry, and total T_4 measurement.

3. Cytology is paramount when investigating feline pruritus. First, it may help in identifying clinical patterns, such as eosinophilic plaque/granuloma, miliary dermatitis, or support the suspicion of specific diseases characterized by eosinophilic inflammation, such as mosquito bite hypersensitivity. Second, cytology may diagnose secondary bacterial or yeast infections, which complicate the primary disease and increase the severity of the pruritus. Finally, the observation of acantholytic cells admixed with neutrophils on cytological examination may be suggestive of pemphigus foliaceus.

5. Histopathology is the confirmatory diagnostic test for some feline diseases when the clinical presentation and sometimes the cytology are suggestive of a specific condition. For example, pemphigus foliaceus is diagnosed by histopathological examination, as are other rare feline diseases, such as herpesvirus dermatitis and idiopathic facial dermatitis in Persian and Himalayan cats, mosquito bite hypersensitivity, maculopapular cutaneous mastocytosis, and adverse drug reactions.

6. In most cases of feline pruritus presenting with one of the four main clinical patterns, ectoparasites and dermatophytosis must be ruled out at the beginning of the diagnostic approach and cytological examination only shows secondary infections or eosinophilic inflammation. These cases are often caused by allergic diseases, which must be investigated systematically. The first step is a therapeutic trial for fleas that may not have been identified during the initial investigation for ectoparasites.

7. The elimination diet is the second step in the diagnostic approach to feline allergies. The diet should consist of novel protein sources or be a hydrolyzed diet and should last for a minimum of eight weeks. If the cat improves on the diet, a challenge with the previous food is required in order to diagnose an adverse reaction to food.

DIAGNOSIS

2. Cases of severe facial pruritus may occasionally require a dental examination. Orofacial pain syndrome is a rare disease observed more frequently in Burmese cats, clinically characterized by severe self-trauma to the face and oral cavity. The disease may be associated with tooth eruption, dental disease, and stress.

4. Chin acne is common in cats, and it is usually non-pruritic unless secondarily infected. Bacterial and *Malassezia* infections/overgrowth are pruritic conditions that may modify the clinical features of any dermatological disease and should always be investigated.

8. Despite applying a systematic approach, a specific cause for pruritus occasionally cannot be identified, or details from the cat's history point towards a behavioral problem. Cases presenting with self-induced alopecia or ulcerative head and neck dermatitis may be induced by stress, boredom, or other psychological disorders. In these cases, referral to a behavioral specialist is recommended.

TREATMENT

9. Treatment options for feline atopic skin syndrome (FASS) include symptomatic therapy aimed at controlling pruritus and improving the cat's quality of life and allergen-specific immunotherapy (AIT). The latter is the only treatment potentially capable of curing the disease; however, its effectiveness is unpredictable. This is mainly due to the poor reliability of serological testing, the most widely used assay to identify the causative allergens, and/or to the difficulty of carrying out intradermal testing in cats due to their thin and hard skin, and the poor quality of the wheal. Allergen-specific immunotherapy is commercially available in both subcutaneous and sublingual formulations.

    Systemic glucocorticoids, particularly prednisolone at 1-2 mg/kg orally once daily and methylprednisolone at 1-1.4 mg/kg orally once daily as starting doses, are the mainstay of symptomatic treatment in feline FASS, especially when the disease is seasonal. In cases of year-round pruritus, the best therapeutic option is cyclosporine, indicated for use in cats as a liquid oral formulation at 7 mg/kg orally once daily. Other options to control pruritus include oclacitinib and maropitant (both drugs are not registered for cats) and the less effective antihistamines, essential fatty acids, and palmitoylethanolamide.

SUGGESTED READINGS

- Colombo S. Problem-oriented approach to feline skin diseases: pruritus. In Noli C, Colombo S (editors). Feline Dermatology. Switzerland, Springer Nature, 2020, pp 161-174.
- Eckstein RA, Hart BL. The organization and control of grooming in cats. *Appl Anim Behav Sci* 68:131-140, 2000.
- Santoro D, Pucheu-Haston CM, Prost C, et al. Clinical signs and diagnosis of feline atopic syndrome: detailed guidelines for a correct diagnosis. *Vet Dermatol* 32:26-e6, 2021.

PRURITUS: DOGS

Fabia Scarampella

Itch or pruritus is defined as an "unpleasant skin sensation causing the desire to scratch". Although unpleasant, this feeling is of notable importance in nature because it is a highly effective alarm system that allows removing a series of harmful or dangerous agents. However, despite being a protective reflex, itching can cause skin damage over time.

Not all individuals perceive itch the same way. Itching is perceived only if the intensity of a given stimulus exceeds the maximum limit of tolerance or individual threshold. The "pruritic threshold" theory hypothesizes that any individual can tolerate some pruritic stimulus without becoming itchy. However, when multiple stimuli are present at the same time, and they exceed the "pruritic threshold", itching will result. This is due to the summation of the effects of different conditions.

Pruritus may occur with several diseases and is the most common complaint in canine dermatology. Itching manifests itself with particular behaviors such as scratching, licking, biting, chewing, and pathologic changes. It may be caused by primary diseases but may also be affected by modulating and/or amplifying factors, such as microbial components (bacteria and *Malassezia* spp.). The relative importance of all of these must be sorted out in each individual if successful management is to be achieved. Atopic dermatitis is by far the most common primary cause of chronic pruritus in dogs. Other allergic dermatoses (flea bite and food-induced hypersensitivity), as well as parasitic diseases (e.g., sarcoptic mange and other mite infestations), are still common causes. In the author's experience, other less common but not rare dermatologic causes of pruritus are contact dermatitis, adverse drug reactions, and epitheliotropic cutaneous T cell lymphoma. Rare conditions associated with itching are extracutaneous diseases, such as nervous system disorders (acral mutilation syndrome, Chiari-like malformation, and syringomyelia), and behavioral disorders (acral lick dermatitis).

PRURITUS IN DOGS

History and physical examination

With extracutaneous signs (1)
- Check for neurologic disease → Imaging (US, CT, MRI)
- Chiari-like malformation syringomyelia → Symptomatic treatment → Surgery
- Check and test for possible underlying causes of immunosuppression

Hypercortisolism / Hypothyroidism → Specific treatment

Recurrences → YES

Clinical remission (4) → NO

Adult/old dogs with lesions suggestive of less common differentials (biopsy) (5)
- Neoplasia (epitheliotropic lymphoma, mast cell tumor) → Antineoplastic therapy
- Pemphigus foliaceous or pemphigus foliaceous-like dermatosis → Symptomatic: lokivetmab / Corticosteroid ± azathioprine

Seasonal or recurrent itch with consistent diagnostic criteria (6) (facial, pedal, and ventral involvement and onset before 3 years of age)

YES → Flea allergy (8) → Flea control (9) / Symptomatic therapy (3)

NO → Atopic dermatitis (6)
- With consistent diagnostic criteria (6) (facial, pedal, and ventral involvement and onset before 3 years of age)
- Avoidance of flare factors
- Allergen-specific immunotherapy
- Restoring epidermal barrier (7)
- Antiallergic therapy (lokivetmab, oclacitinib, cyclosporine, corticosteroids)

Without extracutaneous signs

Skin scraping, acetate tape impression, hair examination, dermoscopy checking for mites, fleas and *Pelodera strongyloides*

Sarcoptes, Otodectes, Demodex, Cheyletiella, trombicula mites and fleas → YES → Antiparasitic treatment / Symptomatic therapy (3)

NO → Therapeutic trial with antiparasitic drugs (e.g. isoxazolines) (2)

Remission without recurrences → YES → Topical and/or systemic antimicrobial therapy

NO → Check for bacterial and yeast skin infections (cytology ± bacterial culture)

Dietary exclusion trial

Remission of pruritus and relapse with rechallenge → YES → Food allergy → Avoidance of dietary allergens

NO → Distribution compatible with contact dermatitis → YES → Avoidance and rechallenge, patch test positive → Contact dermatitis (10) → Avoidance of contact allergens / Symptomatic therapy (3)

1. When neurologic symptoms are reported in the history, a careful physical examination and specific diagnostic tests should be performed to investigate extracutaneous diseases. In particular, advanced diagnostic imaging (MRI and/or CT) is recommended in the case of Chiari-like malformation and syringomyelia.

4. Check whether the secondary infections have been resolved (dermatological examination and cytology) and determine whether the pruritus has been completely resolved or is only partially reduced. If the infection is resolved following treatment, but the pruritus persists, the main underlying causes include flea bite hypersensitivity (FBH), atopic dermatitis, cutaneous adverse food reaction, and contact allergy. If the infection and the pruritus have both been entirely resolved after antimicrobial treatment but recur shortly thereafter, an underlying cause of immunosuppression should then be ruled out. A complete blood count, biochemistry, and urinalysis should be performed, and, where indicated, specific endocrinology testing for hypothyroidism and hypercortisolism are required.

5. Biopsy should be performed if pruritus persists together with lesions compatible with less common differentials (e.g., epitheliotropic cutaneous T cell lymphoma, pemphigus foliaceous), especially in adult/old dogs.

DIAGNOSIS

6. The diagnosis of canine atopic dermatitis is based on history, clinical signs, and the exclusion of other pruritic diseases. The detection of allergen-specific immunoglobulin E (IgE) is considered a minor criterion. The distribution of skin lesions is known to vary between breeds, generally involving the face, inner aspect of the pinnae, ear canals, paws, axillae, and groin. Clinical signs of canine atopic dermatitis commonly present before 3 years of age may be either perennial or seasonal and overlap with numerous other pruritic and inflammatory skin diseases.

8. Canine flea bite hypersensitivity is characterized by pruritic, papular, crusty dermatitis, typically confined to the dorsal and lumbosacral area, caudomedial thighs, ventral abdomen, and flanks.

10. Clinical signs of contact hypersensitivity include erythematous macules, papules, lichenification, hyperpigmentation, and erosions which tend to be confined to hairless or sparsely haired areas of the skin in contact regions.

2. If ectoparasites have not been found with standard diagnostic tests, a therapeutic trial with antiparasitic drugs (e.g., isoxazolines) is recommended, especially to rule out *Sarcoptes* and *Cheyletiella* mites.

3. The management of pruritic skin diseases should always be based on a definitive diagnosis,

with therapy directed at the underlying cause. However, when the diagnosis cannot be established rapidly, antipruritic therapy is needed to prevent self-trauma and secondary infections. In the case of parasitic skin conditions, antipruritic therapy is used temporarily to provide relief to the patient while the antiparasitic agents work. Similarly, antipruritic therapy (see number 7) can be used during the first few weeks of a dietary trial or the avoidance of contact allergens.

7.   Corticosteroids have broad anti-inflammatory effects, rapid onset of activity and can still play a role in the symptomatic treatment of acute canine atopic dermatitis when prescribed judiciously and appropriately. In most cases, short courses of prednisone or prednisolone at 0.5 mg/kg twice daily for the first few days and then once daily are appropriate. Systemic corticosteroids should be avoided in the chronic management of canine atopic dermatitis whenever possible, as there are now safe, specific, and targeted therapies available, including cyclosporine A (5 mg/kg PO once daily with food), oclacitinib maleate at 0.4 to 0.6 mg/kg bid for up to 14 days of therapy and once a day thereafter for maintenance, and lokivetmab SC.

9.   In geographic regions in which fleas are endemic, all dogs with pruritus should be treated with year-round flea adulticides, combined with insect growth regulators (IGRs).

SUGGESTED READINGS

-   Hensel P, Santoro D, Favrot C, Hill P, et al. Canine atopic dermatitis: detailed guidelines for diagnosis and allergen identification. *BMC Vet Res* 11:196, 2015.
-   Miller W, Griffin C, Campbell K (editors). Muller & Kirk's Small Animal Dermatology 7th edition. St. Louis, Elsevier, 2013.

PULMONARY HYPERTENSION

Federica Marchesotti

Pulmonary hypertension is defined as a mean pulmonary artery pressure ≥25 mmHg at rest. The development of pulmonary hypertension is caused by pulmonary vascular abnormalities characterized by increased pulmonary blood flow, increased pulmonary vascular resistance, increased pulmonary venous pressure, or some combination thereof. The consequence of pulmonary hypertension is a progressive increase in right ventricle workload, which leads to right ventricle remodeling and, ultimately, dysfunction and failure, resulting in right-sided congestive heart failure (ascites), low output signs, and death.

Based on cardiac and pulmonary artery catheterization, pulmonary hypertension can be defined as precapillary, characterized by increased pulmonary vascular resistance and normal pulmonary artery wedge pressure (PAWP), or postcapillary, characterized by increased PAWP with normal (isolated postcapillary pulmonary hypertension) or increased (combined postcapillary and precapillary) vascular resistance.

Elevation of the pulmonary artery pressure is not the defining characteristic of a specific clinical condition but rather an abnormal hemodynamic state associated with numerous disorders; thus, pulmonary hypertension is classified into six distinct groups, originally developed for humans and then amended for veterinary etiologies, based on the underlying pathological process.

Signalment, history, and clinical presentation of animals with pulmonary hypertension can reflect the underlying cause. Exertional syncope, labored respiration/respiratory distress, exercise intolerance, and cardiogenic ascites are noteworthy clinical signs frequently directly attributable to pulmonary hypertension. Cough is commonly reported but, more likely, reflects an underlying respiratory disease. Cyanosis may occur secondary to primary pulmonary disease or congenital cardiac disease exhibiting right-to-left pulmonary-to-systemic shunting. Cardiac auscultation can identify heart murmurs localized to the mitral valve, tricuspid valve, or both; a diastolic heart murmur of pulmonic regurgitation is occasionally detected in patients with severe pulmonary hypertension. A split or loud second heart sound may be auscultated, particularly with severe pulmonary hypertension. According to the underlying etiology, pulmonary auscultation may identify muffled sounds, crackles, wheezes, or increased bronchovesicular sounds.

PULMONARY HYPERTENSION

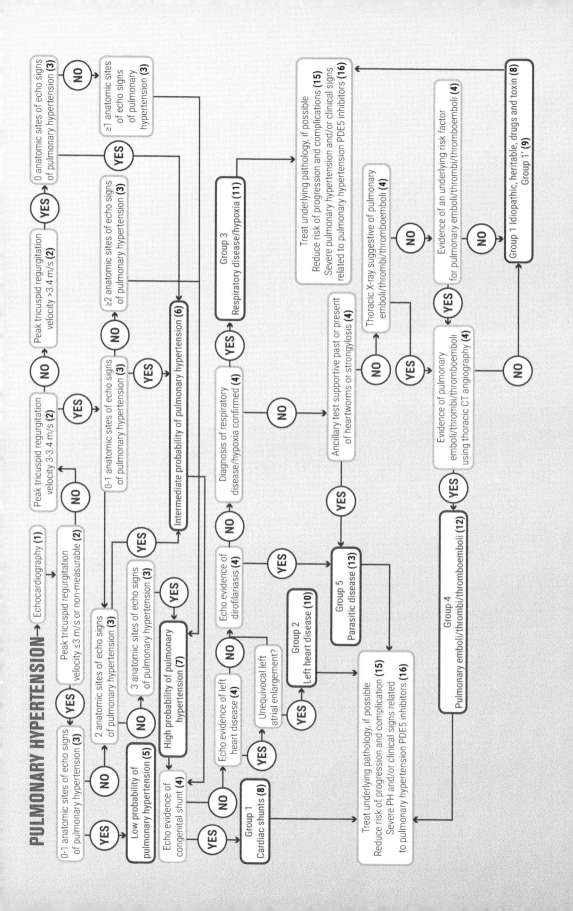

DIAGNOSTIC PROTOCOL

1. Transthoracic echocardiography is the most important non-invasive screening tool, even if the gold standard for diagnosing pulmonary hypertension is right heart and pulmonary artery catheterization.

2. In fact, peak tricuspid regurgitation velocity (PTRV) can provide a non-invasive estimate of systolic pulmonary arterial pressure.

3. In addition to PTRV, other echocardiographic signs of pulmonary hypertension can help in assessing the probability of pulmonary hypertension. These signs involve three anatomic sites: the ventricles (left ventricular underfilling, right ventricle hypertrophy, systolic flattening of the interventricular septum, and right ventricle systolic dysfunction); the pulmonary artery trunk (pulmonary artery enlargement, reduced right pulmonary artery distensibility, peak early diastolic pulmonic regurgitation velocity >2.5 m/s, and asymmetry and/or notching of the right ventricle outflow doppler acceleration), and the right atrium and caudal vena cava (right atrium and/or caudal vena cava enlargement).

4. Based on the clinical signs and the clinical-pathological findings, the most appropriate diagnostic protocol should be carried out: echocardiography (probability of pulmonary hypertension, left heart disease, cardiac shunts; parasitic diseases); CBC, biochemistry, urinalysis (parasitic diseases, systemic diseases, diseases predisposing to pulmonary thromboembolism); check the platelet count, coagulation profile, and parameters associated with hypercoagulability (e.g., D-dimer and antithrombin) (parasitic diseases, pulmonary embolism/thrombosis/thromboembolism); arterial blood gas analysis (hypoxia); *Dirofilaria immitis/Angiostrongylus vasorum* tests (parasitic diseases); cervical/thoracic imaging (e.g., radiography, fluoroscopy, computed tomography) (respiratory diseases, neoplasia, parasitic diseases, pulmonary embolism, thrombosis or thromboembolism); tracheobroncoscopy and bronchoalveolar lavage (respiratory diseases, neoplasia, parasitic diseases); pulmonary fine-needle aspiration or biopsy (pulmonary parenchymal diseases, neoplasia, parasitic diseases, pulmonary veno-occlusive disease, pulmonary capillary hemangiomatosis); contrast (e.g., microbubbles) echocardiography (right-to-left shunt).

DIAGNOSIS

Based on this approach, the probability of pulmonary hypertension can be classified as:

5. Low: PTRV ≤3 m/s or non-measurable with 0 or 1 anatomic sites having echocardiographic (echo) signs of pulmonary hypertension.

6. Intermediate: PTRV ≤3 m/s or non-measurable with 2 anatomic sites having echo signs of pulmonary hypertension; PTRV between 3.0 to 3.4 m/s with 0 or 1 anatomic sites; PTRV >3.4 m/s with 0 anatomic sites.

7. High: PTRV ≤3 m/s or non-measurable with 3 anatomic sites having echo signs of pulmonary hypertension; PTRV between 3.0 to 3.4 m/s with ≥2 anatomic sites; PTRV >3.4 m/s with ≥1 anatomic sites.

Based on the underlying disease, pulmonary hypertension can be classified into:

8. Group 1: pulmonary arterial pressure including: idiopathic; inheritable; drug and/or toxin-induced; associated with congenital cardiac shunts, pulmonary vasculitis, or pulmonary vascular amyloid deposition.

9. Group 1': pulmonary veno-occlusive disease or pulmonary capillary hemangiomatosis.

10. Group 2: left heart diseases.

11. Group 3: respiratory diseases, hypoxia, or both.

12. Group 4: pulmonary emboli (PE)/thrombi (PT)/thromboemboli (PTE).

13. Group 5: parasitic diseases (*Dirofilaria immitis* or *Angiostrongylus vasorum*).

14. Group 6: pulmonary hypertension with multifactorial or unclear mechanisms.

TREATMENT

15. Reduce the risk of progression or complication with exercise restriction, prevention of contagious respiratory pathogens, and avoidance of pregnancy, high altitude, air travel, and non-essential wellness procedures.

16. Decrease pulmonary artery pressure using phosphodiesterase-5 inhibitors (PDE5i) when clinical signs of pulmonary hypertension are present or in case of severe pulmonary hypertension. Currently, sildenafil is the only PDE5i routinely used in canine pulmonary hypertension; the therapy includes doses of 1-3 mg/kg q8-12h. Tadalafil has emerged as an appealing alternative with a longer half-life, allowing for q24h dosing. In cats, these treatment applications are speculative because published reports are scant. Thus, sildenafil can be used at an extrapolated dose of 0.25-1 mg/kg PO q8-12h. However, the use of PDE5i in some specific situations, such as in dogs with pulmonary hypertension associated with congenital cardiac shunts, pulmonary veno-occlusive disease, or secondary to left heart disease, warrants caution since it might lead to pulmonary edema.

SUGGESTED READINGS
-   Jaffey JA, Leach SB, Kong LR, et al. Clinical efficacy of tadalafil compared to sildenafil in treatment of moderate to severe canine pulmonary hypertension: a pilot study. *J Vet Cardiol* 24:7-19, 2019.
-   Reinero C, Visser LC, Kellian HB, et al. ACVIM consensus statement guidelines for the diagnosis, classification, treatment, and monitoring of pulmonary hypertension in dogs. *J Vet Intern Med* 34:549-573, 2020.
-   Williams JC. Pulmonary hypertension and pulmonary thromboembolism. In Ettinger SJ, Feldman EC, Côté E (editors). Textbook of Veterinary Internal Medicine 8th edition. St. Louis, Elsevier, 2017, pp 1131-1136.

REGURGITATION

Paolo Silvestrini

Regurgitation is the passive expulsion of food, fluid, or other material from the pharynx and/or esophagus. Diseases causing inflammation, obstruction, or hypomotility of the esophagus can alter its normal physiology and can result in regurgitation. Regurgitation must be differentiated from vomiting, oropharyngeal dysphagia, and, in some cases, expectoration using a careful history and observation of the event. With oropharyngeal dysphagia, repeated swallowing attempts occur before food or water are pushed into the proximal esophagus. Coughing usually precedes expectoration. Vomiting is usually associated with nausea, frequent swallowing, retching, and abdominal contractions. Generally, with regurgitation, no prodromic signs are recognized while retching and gagging can occur after the episode. Regurgitated material generally has a neutral or high pH unless some gastric content is refluxed into the esophagus. Patients with chronic regurgitation can have a poor body condition due to malnutrition, despite having a ravenous appetite. Following an episode of regurgitation, the patient often looks for more food and/or eats the regurgitated ingesta. Aspiration pneumonia is a frequent complication and should always be suspected in patients with a history of regurgitation, developing lethargy, anorexia, fever, cough, and/or dyspnea.

The initial evaluation consists of cervical and thoracic X-rays to check for generalized or focal esophageal dilation, foreign bodies, intra- or extraluminal masses, and aspiration pneumonia. Contrast radiography provides additional assessment if survey X-rays are non-diagnostic. The use of videofluoroscopy is beneficial to better assess esophageal motility. Endoscopy can confirm radiographic findings, provide treatment for foreign bodies or strictures, allow biopsy of mass lesions, and identify esophagitis.

Identifying the exact underlying cause of the esophageal or pharyngeal dysfunction can allow resolution of the problem (e.g., removal of an esophageal foreign body, treatment of myasthenia gravis). In some cases, it is only possible to carry out symptomatic and supportive therapy (e.g., with idiopathic megaesophagus).

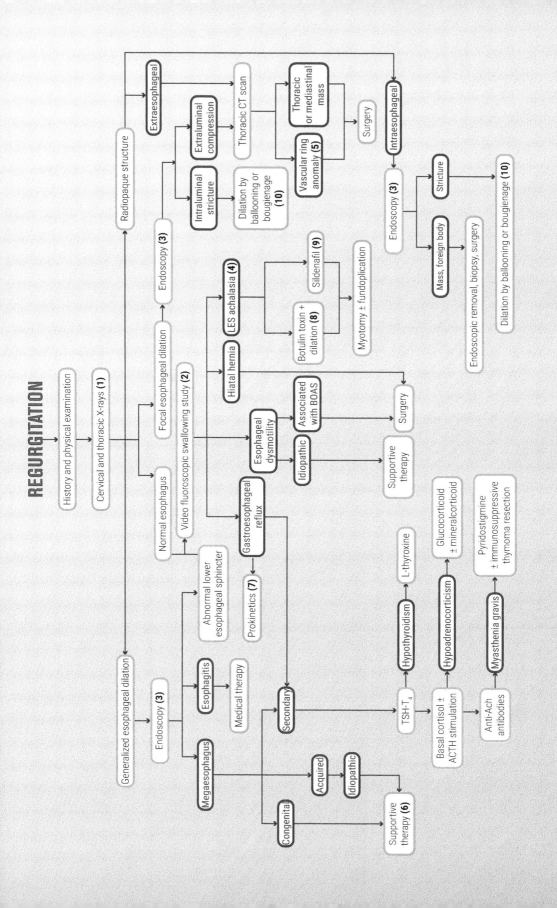

1. Cervical and thoracic X-rays: caution should be taken in patients with severe regurgitation to avoid aspiration pneumonia. In these cases, a videofluoroscopic swallowing study (VFSS) is preferred.

2. Videofluoroscopic swallowing study: patients should be offered food with different consistencies (fluid, semifluid and dry) and water.

3. Endoscopy: patients should always have a well-cuffed endotracheal tube to avoid aspiration of regurgitated/vomited material. Twelve-hour fasting is recommended, and sucralfate and barium should be avoided before the procedure. General anesthesia can result in dilation of the esophagus and opening of the lower esophageal sphincter (LES); therefore, a videofluoroscopic swallowing study is preferred when megaesophagus, gastroesophageal reflux, and LES achalasia are suspected.

DIAGNOSIS

4. Lower esophageal sphincter achalasia is diagnosed when there is evidence of a lack of lower esophageal sphincter (LES) relaxation in response to pharyngeal swallowing during a videofluoroscopic swallowing study. A "bird beak" sign is common and is due to a dilated distal esophagus terminating in an elongated taper through the LES.

5. A vascular ring anomaly is a congenital disorder of the aortic vasculature which involves complete or partial encircling of the esophagus and trachea with secondary esophageal compression. A persistent right aortic arch is one of the most common ring anomalies in dogs, with a prevalence of approximately 7%; German Shepherd dogs are overrepresented.

6. Supportive therapy for congenital and acquired idiopathic megaesophagus includes small, frequent meals and maintaining the patient in an upright position for 5-10 minutes after feeding. A Bailey chair can be useful for this purpose. Cisapride (0.1-0.5 mg/kg PO q8-12h in dogs, 2.5 mg/cat PO q12h) and bethanechol (2.5-15 mg/dog PO q8h) in dogs can increase esophageal motility and lower esophageal sphincter tone in some cases.

7. Gastroesophageal reflux (GER), leading to gastroesophageal reflux disease (GERD), in dogs and cats can occur secondary to lower esophageal sphincter (LES) incompetence, especially associated with esophageal inflammation and hypomobility, anesthesia (patient positioning and type of surgery are important factors), hiatal hernia and upper airway obstruction. The latter is important in brachycephalic breeds. Malpositioned esophageal feeding tubes which cross the LES can cause GER. Treatment ideally should be directed at the underlying causes. Since anesthesia is a common cause of GER in dogs and cats, care should be taken in positioning the patients, and administration of proton pump inhibitors (PPIs) should be considered. Administration of PPIs does not decrease gastric reflux but may prevent injury by increasing the pH of the refluxate. Prokinetic drugs, such as

metoclopramide (0.2-0.5 mg/kg PO q8h, 1-2 mg/kg q24h IV) and cisapride (0.1-0.5 mg/kg PO q8-12h) increase the pressure of the LES and enhance gastric motility. Sucralfate is a mucosal protectant that binds to inflamed and ulcerated tissue. Its efficacy in the treatment of esophagitis is questionable since sucralfate is activated in an acidic environment (the esophageal pH is generally alkaline). For the same reason, sucralfate should not be used together with PPIs, especially if these are given twice daily. Proton pump inhibitors are the most clinically effective drugs for the treatment of GER. A twice-daily administration at 1 mg/kg PO is recommended for omeprazole and pantoprazole.

8. A recent study has described the use of mechanical dilation and botulinum toxin A (BTA) injections for achalasia. Mechanical dilation is performed with balloon catheters having a diameter between 1 and 3 cm according to patient size; it is maintained for 90 seconds and repeated 2-3 times. After the dilation, BTA diluted to 40 U/mL in 0.9% sterile saline is injected at 8 sites around the LES (4 U/site) using an endoscopic injection needle. Improvement of the clinical signs is temporary (approximately 40 days) but is used to select the candidates for myotomy and fundoplication.

9. Sildenafil (1 mg/kg PO q12h) is indicated in the case of megaesophagus associated with lower esophageal sphincter achalasia.

10. The two non-surgical techniques for treating benign esophageal strictures are ballooning and bougienage. The first is performed using a catheter with an inflatable balloon which is positioned in the stricture and is then expanded with insufflated fluid or air. Bougienage involves the use of rigid instruments of different diameters pushed through the stricture. Endoscopically-guided submucosal triamcinolone (10 mg into each site in a four-quadrant pattern) should be injected before (or in some cases after) the procedure to prevent relapses. Oral feeding with watery food is restarted 24 hours post-dilation.

SUGGESTED READINGS

-   Gallagher A. Vomiting and regurgitation. In Ettinger SJ, Feldman EC, Côté E (editors). Textbook of Veterinary Internal Medicine 8th edition. St. Louis, Elsevier, 2017, pp 158-164.
-   Grobman ME, Hutcheson KD, Lever TE, et al. Mechanical dilation, botulinum toxin A injection, and surgical myotomy with fundoplication for treatment of lower esophageal sphincter achalasia-like syndrome in dogs. *J Vet Intern Med* 33:1423-1433, 2019.
-   Kook PH. Gastroesophageal reflux. In Bonagura JD, Twedt DC (editors). Kirk's Current Veterinary Therapy XV 15th edition. St. Louis, Elsevier, 2014, pp 501-504.

SHOCK

Massimo Giunti

Shock is defined as inadequate cellular energy production secondary to a reduction in effective tissue perfusion and oxygen delivery (DO_2) in relation to oxygen consumption (VO_2). Impaired tissue oxygen extraction and/or metabolic derangement (e.g., cytopathic hypoxia, hypoglycemia) might be associated with shock. Without therapeutic intervention, cellular injury, organ failure, and subsequent death are common sequelae. Classifications of shock are normally based on the pathogenesis or pathophysiology of this clinical syndrome; however, different types might coexist in the same patient. Reduction in DO_2 might be secondary to an inadequate cardiac output due to the loss of circulating blood volume (hypovolemic shock) or failure of the cardiac pump (cardiogenic shock), maldistribution of the absolute intravascular volume (distributive shock), obstruction of the great vessels or the heart itself (obstructive shock: e.g., tension pneumothorax, pericardial tamponade), and decreased arterial oxygen content (hypoxic shock: e.g., severe anemia, respiratory failure, methemoglobinemia). The recognition and classification of shock are based, for the most part, on signalment, medical history, and clinical signs of global hypoperfusion. Indices of tissue oxygenation, such as blood lactate or central venous oxygen saturation, support the suspicion of shock and be targeted in association with normalization of the clinical signs as endpoints of resuscitation. Goal-directed therapy should be instituted early in order to restore adequate DO_2, and underlying diseases need to be fixed. Large volumes of fluids may be necessary to treat a condition of hypovolemic shock and cardiovascular instability; however, individualized fluid therapy is recommended since failure to administer an adequate volume, or fluid overload can both contribute significantly to mortality. Early treatment of cardiogenic shock requires oxygen therapy, diuretics, and the administration of sedatives/tranquilizers, additionally implemented by specific drugs according to the underlying cardiac disease.

SHOCK

Inadequate cellular energy production

Clinical signs of global hypoperfusion (**dog**) (**cat**)
The shock triad (**cat**) (1)

Fluid responsiveness (2)

YES → **Hypovolemic shock**

CBC or PCV, chemistry, coagulation tests, diagnostic imaging (3)

Active hemorrhage
Severe anemia

Blood products, surgery

NO → Consider vasopressors ± active rewarming (4)

Distributive shock (5)

Acute onset following exposure to a trigger
Respiratory compromise, hypotension, gastrointestinal, dermal, ocular signs (6)

Anaphylactic shock

Epinephrine, supportive care treatment: antihistamines, glucocorticoids, bronchodilators, oxygen, fluid therapy (7)

SIRS criteria ± septic focus (8)

Cytology, samples for cultures, infectious disease testing, CBC, chemistry, lactate, coagulation, diagnostic imaging

Sepsis/septic shock

Antimicrobial treatment, removal of the septic focus, supportive care (9)

Respiratory distress

CBC, arterial blood gas analysis with co-oximeter

Hypoxemia:
PaO_2 <80 mmHg or SpO_2 <95%

Severe anemia

Packed red blood cells, whole blood

Methemoglobinemia
Carboxyhemoglobinemia

Antidotes, antioxidants,
Packed red blood cells,
O_2 therapy

Hypoxic shock

Venous admixture (12)

Moderate to severe, diffuse lung disease

O_2 therapy/continuous positive airway pressure/mechanical ventilation

Right-to-left shunts

Possible surgery

Clinical signs of forward and/or backward heart failure (10)

Pulse oximetry, ECG, arterial blood gas analysis, thoracic ultrasound, chest X-rays, and echocardiography

Tension pneumothorax, pericardial tamponade

Thoracocentesis, pericardiocentesis, IV fluid bolus

Cardiogenic shock (11)

Furosemide, pimobendan/dobutamine, O_2 therapy/continuous positive airway pressure

Responsive to treatment

NO → Mechanical ventilation

Hypercapnia:
$PaCO_2$ >60 mmHg

DIAGNOSTIC PROTOCOL

1. Clinical signs of global hypoperfusion are variable according to the body's compensatory response and include pale mucous membranes, prolonged capillary refill time, tachycardia, poor pulse quality, cold extremities, depressed mentation, oliguria, and hypotension. The unique clinical presentation of shock in cats is a triad characterized by hypothermia, bradycardia, and hypotension.

3. Hypovolemic shock is normally associated with severe dehydration due to the loss of body fluids (e.g., vomiting, diarrhea, polyuria), hemorrhage, or body cavity effusion. These additional diagnostics are helpful in characterizing the origin of the hypovolemia and in guiding additional treatment, such as point-of-care ultrasonography (TFAST and AFAST) for the rapid detection of free fluid in the thorax and abdomen, respectively.

6. Anaphylactic shock is characterized by a mixed distributive-hypovolemic pattern. Dermal and gastrointestinal signs are usually reported in dogs, including congestion in the liver and gallbladder. The respiratory tract is considered to be the "shock organ" in cats.

8. Clinical diagnosis of systemic inflammatory response syndrome (SIRS) requires at least two or three of the following criteria: fever, tachycardia or bradycardia, tachypnea, leukocytosis, or leukopenia. Major positive serum acute-phase proteins (e.g., C-reactive protein in dogs; serum amyloid-A in cats) could support a diagnosis of systemic inflammation. Non-infectious causes of SIRS (e.g., trauma, acute pancreatitis, neoplasia) need to be considered in the differential diagnosis.

10. The clinical signs of cardiogenic shock are consistent with global hypoperfusion or congestive heart failure (CHF), including common respiratory distress, tachypnea, pulmonary crackles and wheezes, cyanosis, tachycardia or arrhythmia, heart murmur or gallop. Hypothermia and pleural effusion are commonly associated with CHF in cats. Pulse oximetry, electrocardiography, blood gas analysis, thoracic point-of-care-ultrasound, chest X-rays, and echocardiography are helpful in staging patients and monitoring the response to treatment.

12. Venous admixture defines venous blood moving from the right to the left side of the circulation that is not properly oxygenated due to a mismatch in ventilation-perfusion in the lungs, diffusion impairment, or anatomic shunts.

DIAGNOSIS

5. The initial clinical signs of hyperdynamic distributive shock are hyperemic mucous membranes, tachycardia, bounding peripheral pulse, and fever in dogs. It is not usually reported in cats.

11. Cardiogenic shock commonly occurs due to an acute and abrupt reduction in cardiac output. Both systolic dysfunction or diastolic dysfunction could end up as cardiogenic shock. Dilated cardiomyopathy (the most common), myocarditis, myocardial infarction, aortic stenosis, and chordae tendineae rupture are potential causes of systolic dysfunction.

Hypertrophic cardiomyopathy, cardiac tamponade, and tachyarrhythmias could contribute to diastolic failure due to inadequate ventricular filling. Finally, bradyarrhythmias with severe bradycardia (e.g., high-grade second-degree or third-degree atrioventricular block) could result in cardiogenic shock.

TREATMENT

2. A critically unstable patient with a clinical suspicion of hypovolemic or distributive shock could benefit from a fluid challenge, defined as the administration of a fixed dose of an intravenous solution (e.g., 5-20 mL/kg in 10-15 minutes of an isotonic crystalloid solution) to assess its fluid responsiveness according to defined endpoints of resuscitation (e.g., normalization or improvement of clinical signs, metabolic indexes, echodynamics).

4. In a patient with persistent hypotension despite fluid resuscitation, vasopressors should be considered, with norepinephrine being the first choice (0.05-1 µg/kg/min IV). Early low-dose norepinephrine may be associated with fluid resuscitation in patients with a suspicion of vasoplegic shock (e.g., septic shock). Active surface and/or core rewarming to 37 °C should be carried out in a hypothermic patient.

7. Epinephrine (0.01 mg/kg IM up to a maximum of 0.5 mg) is recommended for the initial treatment. For patients in shock, constant rate infusion of epinephrine (0.05 µg/kg/min IV) should be titrated to clinical response.

9. The interventions to be instituted early (1-3 hours) include broad-spectrum antimicrobials, fluid resuscitation, or optimization of fluid therapy. Vasopressors or inotropes might be included as needed to support tissue oxygen delivery.

SUGGESTED READINGS
- Byers CG, Giunti M (editors). Feline Emergency and Critical Care Medicine. Milan, Edra, 2021.
- Silverstein DC, Hopper K (editors). Small Animal Critical Care Medicine 2nd edition. St. Louis, Elsevier, 2015.

SIALORRHEA

Andrea Petrelli

Sialorrhea or ptyalism is defined as an increase in the production of saliva (true ptyalism) or the inability to swallow it (pseudoptyalism). In some breeds of dogs (e.g., Saint Bernard, Dogue de Bordeaux, and Mastiff), excessive salivation can be considered normal. Saliva is a viscous protein-based fluid produced and secreted by the salivary tissues that are predominantly composed of glands but also occur diffusely throughout the mouth. There are four major pairs of salivary glands in cats and dogs: parotid, zygomatic, mandibular, and sublingual. In addition, cats have two other glands: the lingual molar glands. Saliva works as a lubricant, initiating the breakdown of ingesta and protecting the oral soft tissues. Both parasympathetic and sympathetic stimuli increase salivary gland secretion. Parasympathetic postganglionic cholinergic nerve fibers control the rate of salivary secretion. Sympathetic stimulation promotes saliva flow by means of muscle contractions at the salivary ducts. Sialorrhea can be caused by different conditions originating in various locations. These include the oral cavity, the esophagus, and other parts of the alimentary tract or within the salivary glands themselves. Hypersalivation can also occur due to extragastrointestinal causes, such as systemic or neurologic conditions, including contact with toxins or caustic substances.

Moreover, especially in cats, stress and bitter medications can cause profuse hypersalivation; this should be considered when collecting the history. Ptyalism can range from mild to severe as well as from intermittent to continuous. Clinical signs can occur acutely or be seen as gradual or chronic. Macroscopically, the saliva may have a clear appearance, or it can be mixed with sanguineous or purulent exudates. Other potential clinical signs, such as vomiting, regurgitation, anorexia, oral pain, and oral inflammatory lesions, may be related to the primary cause of the sialorrhea. The aim of the therapy should be to resolve the primary cause which elicited the hypersalivation. It is important to mention rabies infection, which is an important zoonosis, and animals suspected of having this condition should be isolated immediately.

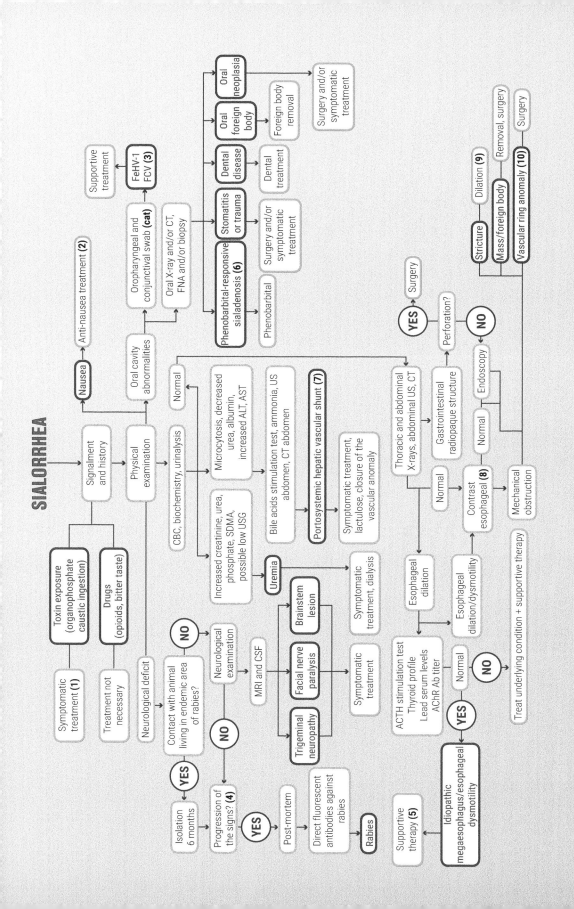

SIALORRHEA

Signalment and history → **Physical examination**

- Toxin exposure (organophosphate caustic ingestion)
  - Symptomatic treatment (1)
- Drugs (opioids, bitter taste)
  - Treatment not necessary
- Neurological deficit

Physical examination

- Nausea → Anti-nausea treatment (2)
- Oral abnormalities → Oropharyngeal and conjunctival swab (cat) → FeHV-1 FCV (3)
  - Supportive treatment
- Oral X-ray and/or CT, FNA and/or biopsy
  - Phenobarbital-responsive sialadenosis (6) → Phenobarbital
  - Stomatitis or trauma → Surgery and/or symptomatic treatment
  - Dental disease → Dental treatment
  - Oral foreign body → Foreign body removal
  - Oral neoplasia → Surgery and/or symptomatic treatment

CBC, biochemistry, urinalysis

- Normal
- Increased creatinine, urea, phosphate, SDMA, possible low USG → Uremia → Symptomatic treatment, dialysis
- Microcytosis, decreased urea, albumin, increased ALT, AST → Bile acids stimulation test, ammonia, US abdomen, CT abdomen → Portosystemic hepatic vascular shunt (7) → Symptomatic treatment, lactulose, closure of the vascular anomaly

Contact with animal living in endemic area of rabies?

- YES → Isolation 6 months → Progression of the signs? (4)
  - YES → Post-mortem → Direct fluorescent antibodies against rabies → Rabies
- NO → Neurological examination → MRI and CSF
  - Trigeminal neuropathy
  - Facial nerve paralysis → Symptomatic treatment
  - Brainstem lesion → Symptomatic treatment, dialysis

Thoracic and abdominal X-rays, abdominal US, CT

- Gastrointestinal radiopaque structure → Endoscopy
  - Perforation?
    - YES → Surgery
    - NO
      - Stricture → Dilation (9)
      - Mass/foreign body → Removal, surgery
      - Vascular ring anomaly (10) → Surgery
- Normal → Esophageal dilation → Contrast esophageal (8)
  - Normal
  - Esophageal dilation/dysmotility
    - Mechanical obstruction
    - ACTH stimulation test, Thyroid profile, Lead serum levels, AChR Ab titer
      - Normal
        - YES → Idiopathic megaesophagus/esophageal dysmotility → Supportive therapy (5)
        - NO → Treat underlying condition + supportive therapy

4. Rabies should always be suspected in animals that suddenly develop profound behavior changes or features of lower motor neuron paralysis if they live in an area endemic for rabies. Unvaccinated animals should be euthanized or put in quarantine in a secure enclosure for 6 months, avoiding contact with other animals or humans. Clinical signs usually progress rapidly over 4-7 days.

8. Esophageal dysmotility should be evaluated using contrast media mixed with food of different consistencies (dry, wet, and liquid).

DIAGNOSIS

3. The clinical signs caused by these agents are very broad; these viruses should all be considered in cats presenting with recurrent faucitis/stomatitis. Feline herpesvirus 1 (FeHV-1) causes upper respiratory tract disease with oculo-nasal discharges, conjunctivitis, sneezing, and sometimes hypersalivation and coughing. In feline calicivirus (FCV) infection, the most common sign is oral ulceration, typically located at the level of the tongue; however, other lesions may also occur elsewhere in the mouth or on the skin. Classic upper respiratory tract signs (such as sneezing, ocular and nasal discharges, and conjunctivitis) also occur commonly; however, these are generally milder as compared to that seen with FeHV-1.

6. Phenobarbital-responsive sialadenosis is a rare idiopathic disease described in dogs. Animals can be presented for retching and gulping with bilateral enlargement of the submandibular salivary glands, causing swallowing difficulties. Diagnostic examinations are required to rule out the most important systemic etiologies as there is no specific test for diagnosing this condition. Diagnosis is confirmed clinically by a rapid and dramatic improvement in clinical signs after initiating phenobarbital treatment (initial dose 2.5 mg/kg PO bid).

7. A portosystemic hepatic vascular shunt can present with different signs, including neurological, urinary, and gastrointestinal signs. The latter include vomiting, diarrhea, anorexia, pica, and/or gastrointestinal bleeding, which occur in ~30% of dogs but are less frequent in cats. On the contrary, approximately 75% of cats manifest ptyalism.

10. Vascular ring anomalies are malformations that encircle the esophagus, causing regurgitation following weaning. Persistence of the right aortic arch is the most commonly reported. Other total or partial ring anomalies can be present, such as double aortic arch or left aortic arch with right-sided ligamentum arteriosum. These disorders have been described in German Shepherds, Irish Setters, Great Danes, and German Pinschers. Vascular ring anomalies are less common in cats but have been seen.

1. In the case of organophosphate intoxication, the therapy should be aimed at preventing additional absorption (active charcoal, bath) and controlling muscarinic and nicotinic clinical signs. Atropine sulfate 0.2-0.5 mg/kg (one-fourth IV, the remainder SC or IM) is

used to control the muscarinic signs. In the case of caustic substance ingestion, the use of sucralfate (0.5-1 g PO tid), proton pump inhibitors (PPIs) such as omeprazole (1 mg/kg PO bid), and pain management is recommended.

2. Nausea can be caused by several conditions. The therapy should aim at resolving the primary cause. However, this sign can cause hyporexia/anorexia and vomiting. Starting with symptomatic treatment (e.g., maropitant 1 mg/kg IV q24h) is highly recommended while investigating the primary cause.

5. The therapy should support the animal's alimentation, reducing as much as possible any clinical signs and resolving, if possible, the primary cause if present. Affected animals should be fed a high-calorie diet, in small frequent feedings, from an elevated or upright position. Dietary consistency should be formulated based on the single individual. Sildenafil citrate can reduce the lower esophageal sphincter tone, improving the clinical signs when used at 1 mg/kg PO bid in dogs with congenital idiopathic megaesophagus.

9. Balloon dilatation can be performed by progressively increasing the diameter of the balloons. An alternative approach is the placement of an indwelling esophageal balloon dilatation feeding tube. Following the dilatation, mild to moderate mucosal hemorrhage may be present.

SUGGESTED READINGS

-   Alcoverro E, Tabar MD, Lloret A, et al. Phenobarbital-responsive sialadenosis in dogs: case series. *Top Companion Anim Med* 29:109-112, 2014.
-   Quintavalla F, Menozzi A, Pozzoli C, et al. Sildenafil improves clinical signs and radiographic features in dogs with congenital idiopathic megaoesophagus: a randomised controlled trial. *Vet Rec* 22 180:404, 2017.
-   Scansen BA, Cober RE, Bonagura JD. Congenital heart disease. In Bonagura JD, Twedt DC (editors). Kirk's Current Veterinary Therapy XV 15th edition. St Louis, Elsevier, 2014, pp 756-761.
-   Weisse C, Berent AC. Hepatic vascular anomalies. In Ettinger SJ, Feldman EC, Côté E (editors). Textbook of Veterinary Internal Medicine 8th edition. St. Louis, Elsevier, 2017, pp 1639-1657.

STOMATITIS: CATS

Emma Bellei

Stomatitis is the inflammation of the oral mucosa. It can be localized in the caudal part of the mouth, gingiva (gingivitis), mucosa of the cheek/lip (mucositis), and the tongue/palate (glossitis/palatitis). Oral inflammation is a common sign of many oral diseases, such as periodontitis (PD), odontoclastic resorptive lesions (ORLs), feline chronic gingivostomatitis (FCGS), granuloma eosinophilic complex (EGC), and pyogenic granuloma. Clinical symptoms are inappetence, fever (acute stomatitis), lethargy, hypersalivation (increased production and/or decreased swallowing), and pain. Clinical features are dependent on the cause; they vary from inflammation and ulcers adjacent to the teeth affected by periodontitis to more severe ulcers and ulceroproliferative lesions, which characterize feline chronic gingivostomatitis. Acute stomatitis can be caused by viruses, chemical agents, and thermal, electrical, and mechanical injury. Feline chronic gingivostomatitis is a severe idiopathic immune-mediated disease of multifactorial etiology which involves viruses, plaque bacteria, and impairment of the immune system. The main virus involved in feline chronic gingivostomatitis is feline calicivirus (FCV); however, other viruses, such as feline herpesvirus (FeHV1) and feline immunodeficiency virus/feline leukemia virus (FIV/FELV) have been considered. Plaque bacteria exacerbate the inflammation. The diagnostic protocol includes hematobiochemical analysis, urinalysis, FIV/FELV status, and oral brush (FCV/FeHV1). Hyperprotidemia and hypergammaglobulinemia are often present in feline chronic gingivostomatitis. Clinical examination reveals bilateral lesions of the caudal mucosa and palatoglossal arches (caudal stomatitis); the gingiva may also be involved. A complete oral examination is essential for diagnosing concomitant disorders (periodontitis, odontoclastic resorptive lesions, retained root tips) that could induce/maintain inflammation. In cases of monolateral lesions, histology should be performed to rule out other causes. Histopathology in feline chronic gingivostomatitis reveals lymphoplasmacytic infiltration of the affected tissue with a predominance of CD8+ T-cells over CD4 T-cells.

The treatment of stomatitis depends on the etiology. Medical treatment alone is indicated in acute stomatitis, autoimmune disease, and eosinophilic stomatitis. In feline chronic gingivostomatitis, surgical therapy is the treatment of choice, with substantial improvement/complete remission in more than 60% of cats. Medical treatment (analgesic/anti-inflammatory, immunomodulators, immunosuppressive drugs) is often necessary for a definite period of time post-extraction.

STOMATITIS (cats)

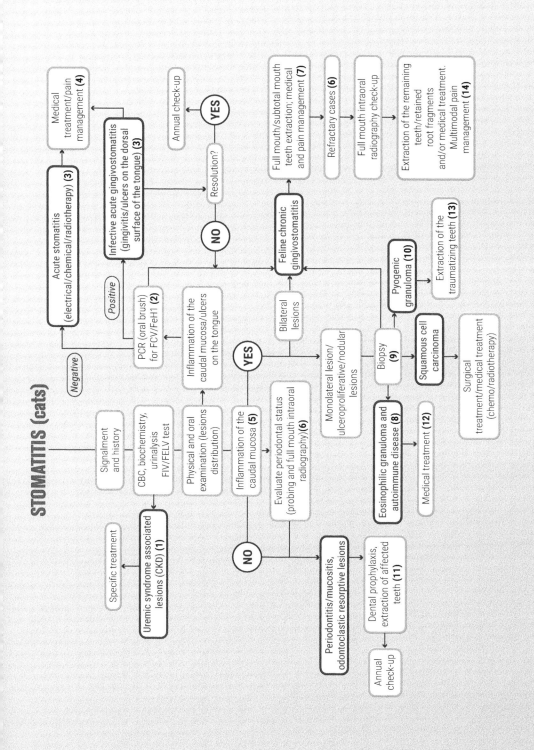

Signalment and history

CBC, biochemistry, urinalysis FIV/FELV test

Specific treatment

Uremic syndrome associated lesions (CKD) **(1)**

Physical and oral examination (lesions distribution)

Inflammation of the caudal mucosa/ulcers on the tongue

PCR (oral brush) for FCV/FeH1 **(2)**

Negative

Positive

Acute stomatitis (electrical/chemical/radiotherapy) **(3)**

Medical treatment/pain management **(4)**

Infective acute gingivostomatitis (gingivitis/ulcers on the dorsal surface of the tongue) **(3)**

Resolution?

NO

YES

Annual check-up

Inflammation of the caudal mucosa **(5)**

YES

NO

Evaluate periodontal status (probing and full mouth intraoral radiography) **(6)**

Bilateral lesions

Feline chronic gingivostomatitis

Full mouth/subtotal mouth teeth extraction; medical and pain management **(7)**

Refractary cases **(6)**

Full mouth intraoral radiography check-up

Extraction of the remaining teeth/retained root fragments and/or medical treatment. Multimodal pain management **(14)**

Monolateral lesion/ ulceroproliferative/nodular lesions

Biopsy **(9)**

Eosinophilic granuloma and autoimmune disease **(8)**

Medical treatment **(12)**

Squamous cell carcinoma

Pyogenic granuloma **(10)**

Extraction of the traumatizing teeth **(13)**

Surgical treatment/medical treatment (chemo/radiotherapy)

Periodontitis/mucositis, odontoclastic resorptive lesions

Dental prophylaxis, extraction of affected teeth **(11)**

Annual check-up

2. A PCR test for the detection of FCV/FeHV1-positive cats is indicated when ulcerative lesions are present in the dorsal surface of the tongue (acute stomatitis) and in feline chronic gingivostomatitis.

5. Bilateral inflammation of the mucosa lateral to the palatoglossal folds and the palatoglossal folds themselves is indicative of feline chronic gingivostomatitis; the mucosa of the hard palate is not involved.

6. Full mouth intraoral radiography and probing should always be performed for staging periodontal status and diagnosing periodontitis and/or odontoclastic resorptive lesions.

9. Biopsy is mandatory for reaching a final diagnosis, especially when monolateral ulcerative and/or ulceroproliferative lesions are present.

DIAGNOSIS

1. Uremic stomatitis includes erosion, ulcers, and necrosis of the oral mucosa and tongue (ventral surface) due to urea excretion.

3. Anamnesis is helpful in reaching a diagnosis. In cases of FCV/FeHV1 infection, ulcers on the dorsal surface of the tongue, hyperthermia, and respiratory symptoms are also present. Electrical/chemical trauma lesions can be localized anywhere in the mouth. Chemotherapeutic drugs and radiotherapy may predispose to the development of oral lesions.

8. Tongue, palate, and mucocutaneous junctions are the most frequent locations for oral eosinophilic granulomas. The surface of the lesions has a characteristic white/yellowish appearance. These lesions are the result of a hypersensitivity reaction to different antigens.

10. Pyogenic granuloma manifests as an ulceroproliferative lesion caused by the traumatic contact of the teeth with the oral mucosa. The most frequent location is the buccal mucosa adjacent to the mandibular molar due to contact with the cusp of the maxillary fourth premolar. Histology shows a granulation tissue with some degree of lymphoplasmacytic infiltration. These lesions should be differentiated from oral neoplasia (e.g., squamous cell carcinoma).

4. The use of local treatment in association with systemic drugs may be helpful (clean and rinse with a solution containing 0.12% chlorhexidine and/or lidocaine; eventually apply a gel containing sucralfate). Broad-spectrum antibiotics are utilized to control secondary infections. In severe cases, consider the positioning of an esophagostomy tube.

7. Full mouth (all teeth) and subtotal (all premolar and molar teeth) extraction depend upon

the distribution of the lesions. Pain management is a key point in controlling symptoms. A multimodal approach should be considered (e.g., a combination of low doses of NSAIDs, gabapentin, and/or buprenorphine or tramadol, palmitoylethanolamide [PEA]). Immunomodulatory therapy with interferon omega (daily oromucosal administration of 0.1 MU for 3 months) is also recommended.

11. Extraction of the teeth affected by periodontitis/odontoclastic resorptive lesions associated with mucosal inflammation is essential for remission of contact mucositis.

12. Identify and remove the underlying causes (e.g., food, environmental, parasitic). Immunosuppressive therapy is indicated in severe cases for a definite period (1 mg/kg prednisolone PO q12h until the remission of the lesions, then gradually tapering off the dosage to reach the lowest efficacious dose). Surgery is also performed to remove some nodular lesions.

13. Extraction of traumatized teeth and marginal excision of the granuloma. Extraction of the tooth adjacent to the lesion could be necessary if affected by periodontitis/odontoclastic resorptive lesions. Odontoplasty of the cusp of the traumatizing tooth has been reported; however, recurrence of the lesions is frequent. If odontoplasty is performed, care must be taken not to expose the pulp, and unfilled resin must be applied to seal the dentinal tubules.

14. Medical treatment is necessary in some cases for a definite period of time. A small percentage of refractory cases require lifelong therapy with medication, such as glucocorticoids and/or cyclosporine. If glucocorticoids are used, the lowest efficacious dose should be used (starting with 0.025 mg/kg q24h of prednisolone daily/every other day and increasing the dosage if necessary; carrying out frequent check-ups to evaluate clinical improvement/remission of the lesions before decreasing or withdrawing the drugs). The use of stem cells in refractory cases after tooth extraction has also been reported.

SUGGESTED READINGS

- Anderson JG, Hennet P. Management of severe oral inflammatory conditions in dogs and cats. *Vet Clin North Am Small Anim Pract* 52:159-184, 2022.
- Murphy BG, Bell CM, Soukup JW (editors). Veterinary Oral and Maxillofacial Pathology 1st edition. Hoboken, Wiley Blackwell, 2020.
- Reiter AM, Gracis M. British Small Animal Veterinary Association Manual of Canine and Feline Dentistry and Oral Surgery 4th edition. Aberystwyth, British Small Animal Veterinary Association, 2018.
- Winer JN, Arzi B, Verstraete FJM. Therapeutic Management of Feline Chronic Gingivostomatitis: A Systematic Review of the Literature. *Front Vet Sci* 3:54, 2016.

STOMATITIS: DOGS

Emma Bellei

Stomatitis is the inflammation of the oral mucosa. The inflammation can be focal or generalized and can be localized on the mucosa in contact with the teeth (vestibular mucosa, sublingual mucosa) or on the palate and the surface and lateral margin of the tongue. Inflammatory lesions of the oral cavity in dogs can result from various causes. Inflammation and ulcers in contact with the teeth are generally indicative of canine chronic ulcerative stomatitis; however, 40% of the lesions associated with this disease may involve the gingiva and edentulous areas (areas of the mouth where teeth are lacking), such as the palatal mucosa; thus, the original term "paradental stomatitis" should not be utilized. In the early stage, canine chronic ulcerative stomatitis can be asymptomatic while, in severe and advanced cases, pain, hypersalivation, dysphagia/inappetence, drooling, and halitosis are evident. Terriers and Cocker Spaniels seem to be more predisposed. A differential diagnosis of canine chronic ulcerative stomatitis includes uremic syndrome, chemo/radiotherapy, thermic, mechanical, and electrical injury, autoimmune diseases, epitheliotropic T-cell lymphoma, fungal stomatitis, drug reactions, eosinophilic stomatitis, and Wegener-like granulomatosis. Localization of the lesions can help to differentiate autoimmune disease from canine chronic ulcerative stomatitis. In autoimmune diseases (e.g., erythema multiforme, lupus erythematosus, pemphigus vulgaris, mucous membrane pemphigoid), the ulcers, the result of disruption of vesiculobullous lesions, are localized on the dorsal surface of the tongue, the hard palate, and the gingiva (keratinized epithelium), and lesions on the skin are always present. In canine eosinophilic stomatitis, inflammation (ulcerated plaque or nodules) is the result of the reaction to different stimuli (e.g., foreign bodies, bee stings). A genetic predisposition of eosinophilic granuloma is described in Cavalier King Charles Spaniels, Siberian Huskies, and German Shepherds. The lesions are localized on the palatoglossal fold, the soft/hard palate, and lateral/ventral surfaces of the tongue. Instead, Wegener-like granulomatosis is a vascular disease (vasculitis) characterized by ulcerated proliferative dark red lesions (one or more) on the gingiva/oral mucosa. Diagnosis is usually reached after excluding other pathologies and after the response to immunosuppressive therapy.

STOMATITIS (dogs)

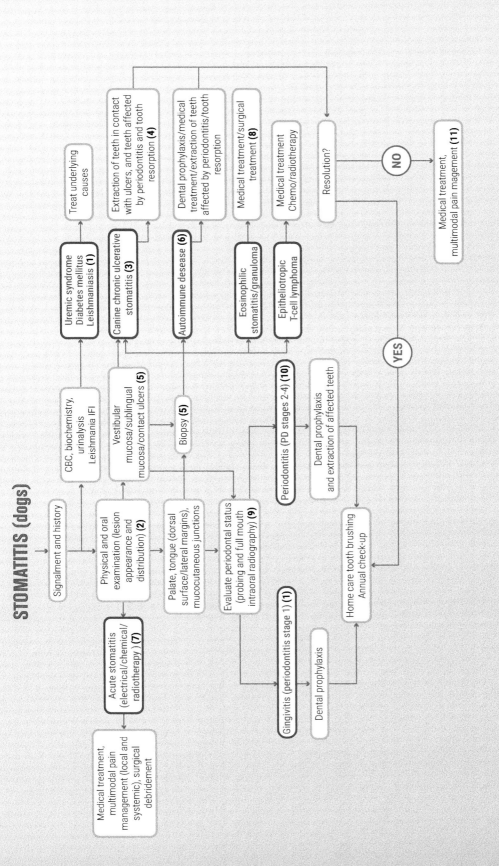

Signalment and history

Physical and oral examination (lesion appearance and distribution) (2)

Acute stomatitis (electrical/chemical/radiotherapy) (7)

Medical treatment, multimodal pain management (local and systemic), surgical debridement

CBC, biochemistry, urinalysis Leishmania IFI

Vestibular mucosa/sublingual mucosa/contact ulcers (5)

Palate, tongue (dorsal surface/lateral margins), mucocutaneous junctions

Biopsy (5)

Evaluate periodontal status (probing and full mouth intraoral radiography) (9)

Gingivitis (periodontitis stage 1) (1)

Dental prophylaxis

Periodontitis (PD stages 2-4) (10)

Dental prophylaxis and extraction of affected teeth

Uremic syndrome Diabetes mellitus Leishmaniasis (1)

Canine chronic ulcerative stomatitis (3)

Autoimmune desease (6)

Eosinophilic stomatitis/granuloma

Epitheliotropic T-cell lymphoma

Treat underlying causes

Extraction of teeth in contact with ulcers, and teeth affected by periodontitis and tooth resorption (4)

Dental prophylaxis/medical treatment/extraction of teeth affected by periodontitis/tooth resorption

Medical treatment/surgical treatment (8)

Medical treatment Chemo/radiotherapy

Resolution?

Home care tooth brushing Annual check-up

YES

NO

Medical treatment, multimodal pain magement (11)

2. Depending on the dog's age, a complete blood count and chemistry analysis, and urinalysis are recommended. The distribution of the lesions in the oral cavity should be evaluated; it is important to check for the presence of lesions on the skin and mucocutaneous junctions (MCJs).

5. Biopsy of the oral, skin, and mucocutaneous junction lesions should be performed to reach a final diagnosis; in some cases, cultures (fungal disease) and cytology could be helpful.

9. Periodontitis (PD) is the inflammatory process of periodontal tissues (gingiva, periodontal ligament, alveolar bone, cementum) induced by plaque. It can be associated with mucositis; PD is subdivided into four stages. PD1: gingivitis (the only reversible stage); PD2: 0-25% periodontal attachment loss; PD3: 25-50% attachment loss; PD4: >50 attachment loss.

DIAGNOSIS

1. Dogs with diabetes mellitus seem to be more prone to develop stomatitis and/or periodontal disease. In rare cases, plaque-like lesions may be seen in the mucocutaneous junctions and the tongue/oral mucosa in dogs affected by leishmaniasis.

3. Canine chronic ulcerative stomatitis is an immune-mediated inflammatory disease. The leucocytes involved in the process are B-cells, T-cells, CD3 negative IL17+ cells, macrophages, and mast cells. Histologically, three subtypes have been described: lichenoid stomatitis (infiltration of the inflammatory cells between the mucosal epithelium and the subepithelium connective tissue, similar to the lichen planum in humans), deep stomatitis and granulomatous stomatitis.

6. Mucous membrane pemphigoid is the autoimmune disease with the most frequent involvement of the oral cavity. With pemphigus vulgaris, 50% of the cases show oral lesions before skin lesions are evident. Erythema multiforme is a vesiculobullous and/or ulcerative autoimmune skin disease that can involve the oral mucosa in 30% of cases. Stomatitis triggered by periodontitis (canine chronic ulcerative stomatitis) can mimic erythema multiforme; however, skin lesions are not present in canine chronic ulcerative stomatitis. Mucocutaneous pyoderma and dermatitis of the lower lip secondary to drooling in dogs affected by canine chronic ulcerative stomatitis should be considered in the differential diagnosis of autoimmune diseases. Response to antibiotic therapy is indicative of this condition.

7. Anamnesis is helpful in reaching a diagnosis. In electrical trauma, the lesions can be localized anywhere in the mouth. In dogs, chemotherapy drugs cause oral lesions (ulcers) less commonly than they do in humans. Instead, radiotherapy is responsible for inducing severe mucositis, which can also result in osteoradionecrosis.

10. Periodontal status should always be evaluated by probing and full mouth intraoral radiography in order to check and treat the teeth affected by periodontitis and tooth resorption (conditions that may induce/aggravate oral inflammation).

TREATMENT

4. Treatment for canine chronic ulcerative stomatitis includes dental prophylaxis, extraction of the teeth in contact with the lesions and teeth periodontically compromised (periodontitis/ tooth resorption). In severe cases, full mouth extraction seems to be the only method for long-term control of the disease. However, more recent studies have found that the microbiomes of the lesions were different from those of the plaque of the opposite teeth, the healthy mucosa, and severe periodontitis so that, in less severe cases, healthy teeth should not be extracted. In severe cases, broad-spectrum antibiotic therapy, analgesics/ anti-inflammatory drugs, and immunosuppressive therapy should be considered. A key point for controlling canine chronic ulcerative stomatitis is daily tooth brushing. Frequent clinical check-ups are advised.

8. The lesions of eosinophilic stomatitis in dogs can be flat or proliferative granulomas (a foreign body response to degenerative collagen). The lesions respond well to glucocorticoids (e.g., prednisolone 1 mg/kg q12h until the lesions disappear, then tapered off in 6-8 weeks); spontaneous resolution has also been described. Seasonal recurrence is possible. In selective cases, surgery is recommended.

11. Analgesic drugs should be administered. In refractory cases, the use of cyclosporine and subantimicrobial doses of doxycycline, as host modulators, should be considered.

SUGGESTED READINGS

- Anderson JG, Hennet P. Management of severe oral inflammatory conditions in dogs and cats. *Vet Clin North Am Small Anim Pract* 52:159-184, 2022.
- Anderson JG, Kol A, Bizikova P, et al. Immunopathogenesis of canine chronic ulcerative stomatitis. *PLoS ONE* 15:e0227386, 2020.
- Murphy BG, Bell CM, Soukup JW (editors). Veterinary Oral and Maxillofacial Pathology 1st edition. Hoboken, Wiley Blackwell, 2020.
- Reiter AM, Gracis M. BSAVA Manual of Canine and Feline Dentistry and Oral Surgery 4th edition. Aberystwyth, British Small Animal Veterinary Association, 2018.

TENESMUS/CONSTIPATION

Fabio Procoli

Fecal tenesmus is defined as ineffective and/or difficult straining at defecating; it is usually caused by disorders of the colon and/or rectum of various natures. Tenesmus may be associated with dyschezia, defined as painful or difficult evacuation of feces from the rectum. Dyschezia is typically caused by disorders localized in the anorectal or perianal regions. Constipation is defined as the infrequent evacuation of dry and hardened feces. When constipation is particularly severe or longstanding, the feces may be so dry and hard that the dog or cat is no longer able to defecate. The absence of defecation is called obstipation; it should always be promptly investigated and medically managed to avoid a permanent loss of colonic function and motility and the development of megacolon. The large intestine has two main functions: the absorption of water and electrolytes, carried out by the ascending and transverse colon, and the storage and evacuation of feces carried out by the descending colon in coordination with the rectum and the internal and external anal sphincters. Both functions are facilitated by colonic motility consisting of non-propagating and propagating contractions. For the most part, non-propagating contractions (also called stationary contractions) occur in the ascending and transverse colon, where they mix endoluminal content, favoring the absorption of water and electrolytes. Propagating anterograde contractions are lumen-occlusive events that occur in the descending colon, propelling fecal content aborally and, ultimately, leading to defecation. Colonic muscular contractility is made possible by the presence of smooth muscular layers organized in an inner circular layer and an outer longitudinal layer. Colonic contractility is regulated by the ganglia and neurons of the intrinsic autonomic nervous system, located in the myenteric and submucosal plexuses, and by extrinsic nerves, which connect the gut to the extraintestinal ganglia and the central nervous system. Tenesmus, dyschezia, and constipation can be the result of a variety of disorders with diverse pathophysiology mechanisms, such as mucosal irritation and inflammation or obstruction (intra- or extraluminal) along the large intestine. Therefore, treatment must rely on the recognition and removal of the inciting cause and on preventing its recurrence.

FECAL TENESMUS

Ineffective straining to defecate

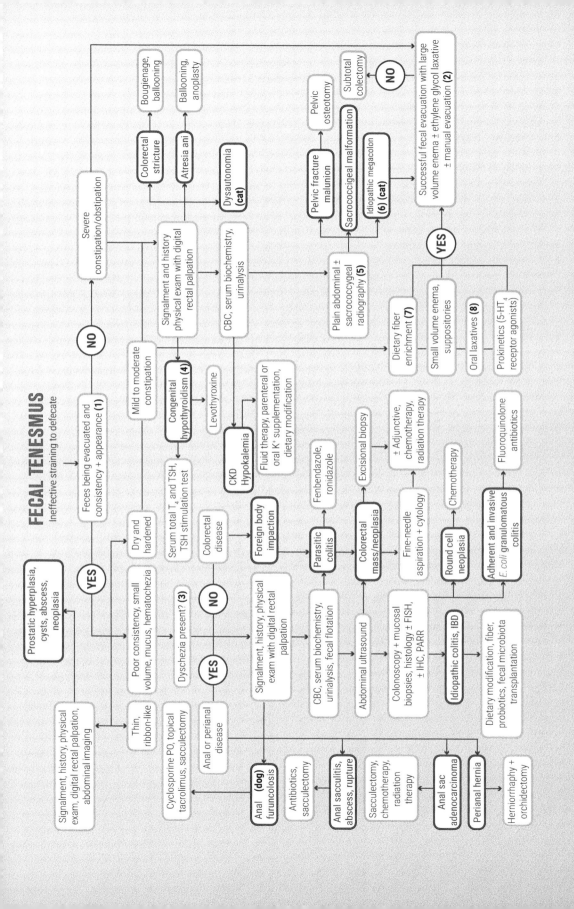

1. When presented with a dog or a cat having tenesmus, it is fundamental to determine whether feces are being evacuated or not. The absence of defecation is indicative of severe constipation or obstipation and requires hospitalization of the dog or cat to initiate supportive therapy and colonic fecal evacuation. It is equally important to determine fecal consistency and water content, the number of evacuations, and the presence or absence of mucus, fresh blood, or foreign material, as this will aid in understanding the disease pathophysiology and localization along the large intestine.

3. The presence of dyschezia associated with fecal tenesmus is highly indicative of anorectal or perianal diseases. Therefore, visual inspection of the anal and perineal region should be carried out together with conscious or sedated/anesthetized careful digital exploration of the rectum.

5. Abdominal orthogonal radiography should be performed in the case of constipation or obstipation to assess the degree and extension of the colonic fecal impaction and/or dilation, evaluate the presence of caudal abdominal organomegaly or masses, rule out pelvic bone fractures, and evaluate lumbosacral or coccygeal vertebral abnormalities. In cats, the finding of a ratio of maximal diameter of the colon to the fifth lumbar vertebral length >1.48 on lateral abdominal radiography is a good indicator of a diagnosis of idiopathic megacolon.

DIAGNOSIS

4. Congenital hypothyroidism is a rare cause of chronic constipation in young dogs and cats. Constipation is associated with other clinical signs, such as lethargy, dullness, skeletal developmental abnormalities with small disproportionate size, and hair coat abnormalities. Affected puppies and kittens may appear normal at birth; however, they usually develop clinical signs by 1-2 months of age. The causes of the central form include thyroid-stimulating hormone (TSH) deficiency (dogs only) and TSH unresponsiveness, while, for the primary form, the causes are thyroid dysgenesis, dyshormonogenesis, and iodine deficiency.

6. Feline idiopathic megacolon is the most common cause of chronic recurrent constipation in middle-aged cats. It is characterized by diffuse dysfunction of the circular and longitudinal colonic muscular layer with reduced isomeric stress in response to a neurotransmitter and membrane depolarization. The result is a progressive loss of motility, function, and dilation.

2. When presented with a severely constipated or obstipated dog or cat, fecal evacuation of the colon must be ensured in order to avoid permanent loss of colon function and motility. Prior to colonic evacuation, the patient needs to be adequately rehydrated with intravenous isotonic fluids, and any electrolyte imbalance needs to be corrected. Cats will need to be anesthetized, and the trachea intubated to avoid aspiration of the gastric content should colonic manipulation induce vomiting. For the evacuation, a large volume (10 mL/kg) of

warm isotonic crystalloid solution is instilled in the colon with a soft 12F rubber catheter. To facilitate evacuation, the fecal mass is gently broken down with both hands and is gently massaged out of the colonic and the rectum (in small dogs and cats).

7. Following the colonic evacuation of previously severely constipated or obstipated animals, or initially in mildly constipated cases, dietary modification is recommended alone or in conjunction with an oral laxative and/or prokinetics. Dietary modification is ensured either by feeding a commercial fiber-enriched diet or by adding a fiber supplement to the existing diet. Fiber exerts its beneficial effects by bulk formation, increasing fecal water content, reducing colonic transit time, and increasing the frequency of defecation. For fiber supplementation of the existing diet, psyllium (1-4 teaspoon) or pumpkin (1-4 tablespoon) can be added per meal, titrating to effect.

8. Oral laxatives promote colonic evacuation by stimulating water, electrolyte transport, and colonic propulsive motility. They include emollient laxatives (dioctyl sodium sulfosuccinate), lubricant laxatives (mineral oil), osmotic laxatives (lactulose, 0.5 mL/kg PO q8-12h), and stimulant laxatives (bisacodyl, most efficacious in cats at 5 mg/cat PO q24h). The laxatives can be used in conjunction with dietary modification and prokinetics.

SUGGESTED READINGS

-   Gaschen FP. Constipation and megacolon. In Procoli F, Allenspach K, Salavati Schmitz S (editors). Feline Gastroenterology. Milan, Edra, 2021, pp 307-318.
-   Jergens AE. Dyschezia and tenesmus. In Washabau RJ, Day MJ (editors). Canine and Feline Gastroenterology. W.B. Saunders, 2013, pp 109-113.
-   Washabau RJ. Constipation. In Washabau RJ, Day MJ (editors). Canine and Feline Gastroenterology. W.B. Saunders, 2013, pp 93-98.

THROMBOCYTOPENIA

Michele Tumbarello

Thrombocytopenia is defined as the reduction of circulating platelets; it is one of the most common acquired bleeding disorders in dogs and cats. In healthy patients, platelets range from approximately 200,000 to 500,000/µL. Thrombocytopenia is frequently observed on a routine CBC in asymptomatic patients; it should always be confirmed with a microscopic examination. When looking at the blood smear, it is important to confirm the low number of platelets (<10 platelets in 10 oil immersion fields using a 100× objective) and check platelet clumping, a common condition that causes artifactual thrombocytopenia, especially in cats. Platelet morphology and size should also be evaluated. Causes of thrombocytopenia include one or a combination of the following mechanisms: increased platelet utilization, increased destruction, and decreased platelet production. Other causes are platelet sequestration in the liver or spleen or loss of platelets. Sequestration and hemorrhage do not usually cause platelet counts to drop below 100,000/µL.

Reported clinical signs of thrombocytopenia consist of mucosal or surface bleeding (petechiae and ecchymoses, epistaxis, hematemesis, melena, hematochezia, hematuria, hyphema) and, sometimes, prolonged bleeding after venipuncture or injuries. However, clinical signs of bleeding are infrequently due to thrombocytopenia when the platelet count is >30,000/µL. Moreover, patients having a low platelet count may present clinical signs, such as lethargy, weakness, fever, or other signs related to an underlying disease. Diagnostic evaluation should then include drug and travel history, physical examination, a coagulation panel, imaging to rule out neoplastic disorders, tests for infectious diseases, and bone marrow examination. Thrombocytopenia combined with other cytopenias suggests a production defect. Abnormal coagulation results could indicate increased platelet utilization due to disseminated intravascular coagulation (DIC). If the causes of decreased platelet production or consumption of platelets are not evident, immune-mediated thrombocytopenia (IMT) should be considered; in this disorder, antibodies bind to platelet surfaces leading to their destruction. Treatment of thrombocytopenia depends on the underlying etiology. Patients with severe bleeding could be supported with transfusions. Immunosuppression is the mainstay of treating primary or idiopathic ITP.

THROMBOCYTOPENIA
(PLT <150,000/µL)

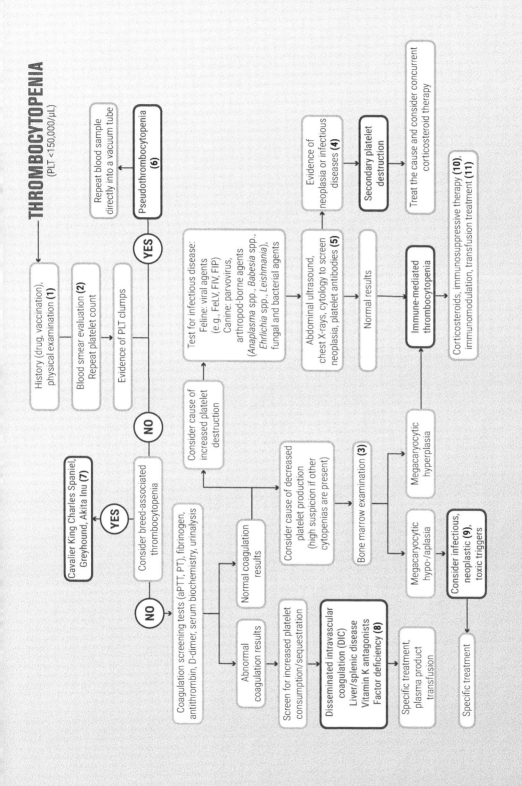

History (drug, vaccination), physical examination **(1)**

Blood smear evaluation **(2)**
Repeat platelet count

Evidence of PLT clumps

YES → Pseudothrombocytopenia **(6)** → Repeat blood sample directly into a vacuum tube

NO → Consider cause of increased platelet destruction

Test for infectious disease: Feline: viral agents (e.g., FeLV, FIV, FIP) Canine: parvovirus, arthropod-borne agents (*Anaplasma* spp., *Babesia* spp., *Ehrlichia* spp., *Leishmania*), fungal and bacterial agents

→ Evidence of neoplasia or infectious diseases **(4)** → Secondary platelet destruction → Treat the cause and consider concurrent corticosteroid therapy

Abdominal ultrasound, chest X-rays, cytology to screen neoplasia, platelet antibodies **(5)**

→ Normal results → Immune-mediated thrombocytopenia → Corticosteroids, immunosuppressive therapy **(10)**, immunomodulation, transfusion treatment **(11)**

YES → Cavalier King Charles Spaniel, Greyhound, Akita Inu **(7)**

NO → Consider breed-associated thrombocytopenia

Coagulation screening tests (aPTT, PT), fibrinogen, antithrombin, D-dimer, serum biochemistry, urinalysis

Normal coagulation results → Consider cause of decreased platelet production (high suspicion if other cytopenias are present) → Bone marrow examination **(3)**

→ Megacaryocytic hyperplasia → Immune-mediated thrombocytopenia

→ Megacaryocytic hypo-/aplasia → Consider infectious **(9)**, neoplastic, toxic triggers → Specific treatment

Abnormal coagulation results → Screen for increased platelet consumption/sequestration

Disseminated intravascular coagulation (DIC) Liver/splenic disease Vitamin K antagonists Factor deficiency **(8)** → Specific treatment, plasma product transfusion

DIAGNOSTIC PROTOCOL

1. Some drugs, e.g., sulfonamides in dogs and methimazole in cats, can induce thrombocytopenia due to an immune-mediated process. Other medications, e.g., chemotherapeutic agents, phenobarbital, and estrogen, can produce bone marrow suppression.

2. The number of circulating platelets can be estimated by evaluating a blood smear. Six to seven platelets per oil immersion field (×1000) in the monolayer region of a smear, correspond to approximately 100,000 platelets per microliter. Therefore, fewer than three or four platelets per oil immersion field represent clinically significant thrombocytopenia. A cytologic review of the blood smear is also necessary to exclude the presence of platelet aggregates and to evaluate the possible presence of cellular morphologic abnormalities (large platelets can be consistent with a regenerative response) or other cytopenias.

3. Bone marrow evaluation may be indicated to determine whether thrombocytopenia is secondary to diminished platelet production or is caused by peripheral platelet destruction. The absence of, or a decreased number of megakaryocytes, may lead to the suspicion of diminished/defective platelet production. Megakaryocytic hyperplasia is a common finding in patients with immune-mediated destruction of platelets. However, some forms of immune-mediated platelet destruction may also involve megakaryocytes and result in immune-mediated amegakaryocytic thrombocytopenia.

4. Infectious diseases, which cause thrombocytopenia due to a combination of mechanisms, are the most common cause of thrombocytopenia in cats. Hence, cats that show a low platelet count should be screened for retroviruses (FIV, FeLV, FIP) and evaluated for bacterial and fungal agents. Moreover, the main vector-borne diseases (e.g., rickettsial disease [e.g., anaplasmosis, ehrlichiosis]), protozoal infection [e.g., babesiosis]) of dogs and cats presented for thrombocytopenia should be excluded.

5. Immune-mediated thrombocytopenia (IMT) is considered the most common cause of severe thrombocytopenia in dogs. The diagnosis remains a diagnosis of exclusion of known causes of thrombocytopenia and underlying diseases and is also based on the response to immunosuppressive therapy. The finding of platelet autoantibodies using a cytofluorimetric assay additionally supports the diagnosis of IMT. This test is considered to be a sensitive but not specific tool for the diagnosis of primary IMT since the assay does not differentiate platelet autoantibodies from antibodies induced by underlying infectious diseases, neoplastic disorders, or drugs.

DIAGNOSIS

6. Pseudothrombocytopenia is an in vitro alteration resulting from platelet clumping secondary to traumatic venipuncture and inadequate blood sample mixing with subsequent platelet activation or exposure of the blood to certain anticoagulants (e.g., EDTA in dogs). It is divided into artifactual or spurious. Feline platelets are more reactive and tend to aggregate more as compared to other species.

7. Thrombocytopenia is an incidental finding in certain dog breeds (e.g., Cavalier King Charles

Spaniel, Greyhound, Akita Inu). Affected dogs are healthy and do not show evidence of a bleeding disorder. Many healthy greyhounds have platelet concentrations below typical canine reference intervals (e.g., approximately 100,000/μL). Autosomal recessive inherited thrombocytopenia occurs in approximately 50% of Cavalier King Charles Spaniels; in this breed, platelet counts can range from 30,000 to 100,000/μL, and large platelets are frequently observed.

8. Progressive platelet consumption is the main characteristic of DIC; DIC occurs secondarily to a wide variety of causes and disorders. Common processes associated with DIC include infectious or neoplastic disorders and potentially any inflammatory syndrome. Conditions that lead to splenomegaly (hypersplenism) or hepatomegaly can result in an increase in platelet sequestration.

9. Infiltrative disorders typically result in hematopoietic failure (myelophthisis). Thrombocytopenia is reported in neoplastic disorders, such as lymphoma, multiple myeloma, mast cell tumors, histiocytic hemophagocytic sarcoma, and metastatic carcinoma. Clonal expansion of dysplastic features (myelodysplasia) can induce thrombocytopenia.

TREATMENT

10. Glucocorticoids (methylprednisolone/prednisone/prednisolone 1-2 mg/kg q12h) are the first-line drugs in immune-mediated diseases due to their rapid onset of action in controlling disease, ease of administration (parenteral and oral) and low costs. Azathioprine (2 mg/kg q12h, only in dogs), cyclosporine (5 mg/kg q12h), mycophenolate mofetil (10 mg/kg q12h), and leflunomide (2 mg/kg q12h) have all been used in association with corticosteroids owing to their immunosuppressive properties. The immunomodulation properties of vincristine (0.02 mg/kg) and human intravenous immunoglobulin (hIVIG, 0.5 g/kg) have been reported in some studies regarding canine IMT.

11. Supportive care can include the use of blood products. In patients with severe bleeding and concurrent anemia, packed red blood cells are helpful in providing additional oxygen-carrying support. Conversely, platelet products are not often used since transfused platelets are rapidly destroyed following administration.

SUGGESTED READINGS

- Brooks M.B. Thrombocytopenia, thrombocytosis. In Ettinger SJ, Feldman EC, Côté E (editors). Textbook of Veterinary Internal Medicine 8th edition. St. Louis, Elsevier, 2017, pp. 757-764.
- Russell K.E. Platelet kinetics and laboratory evaluation of thrombocytopenia. In Weiss DJ, Wardrop KJ (editors). Schalm's Veterinary Hematology 6th edition. Ames, Iowa, 2010, Wiley Blackwell, pp 576-585.

TRANSIENT LOSS OF CONSCIOUSNESS

Giovanni Romito

Collapse is a generic term indicating sudden loss of postural tone, which is not necessarily accompanied by a loss of consciousness. Transient loss of consciousness is a term used to describe all conditions characterized by self-limited loss of consciousness regardless of the underlying etiology. Mechanisms resulting in transient loss of consciousness can be classified as traumatic and non-traumatic; the latter category includes syncope, epileptic seizures, and rare miscellaneous causes (e.g., endocrinological disorders). The term syncope (from the Greek "sunkopé" = to interrupt) indicates a specific pathophysiology and should be used selectively to describe a transient loss of consciousness resulting from inadequate cerebral perfusion. Cerebral hypoperfusion can result from a drop in cardiac output (e.g., reflex bradycardia, disturbances of cardiac rhythm, structural/functional cardiac diseases, inadequate venous return), total vascular resistance (e.g., reflex vasodilatation, primary/secondary/drug-induced dysfunction of the autonomic nervous system), or from both. From a classification point of view, syncope can be classified as cardiac syncope, reflex (neurally-mediated) syncope, and syncope secondary to orthostatic hypotension. The latter type is common in humans, but its occurrence is poorly described in animals, whereas the remaining two are frequently encountered in both species. Cardiac syncope results from inadequate effective cardiac output and may reflect underlying severe cardiac disease, which can be mechanical (i.e., structural/functional abnormalities affecting the cardiac chambers, valves, large vessels, and/or pericardium), electric (disturbances of cardiac rhythm), or both. Reflex syncope includes carotid sinus syndrome, situational syncope, and neurocardiogenic syncope (vasovagal syncope); the latter represents the most common type in both human and veterinary medicine. The pathophysiology of reflex syncope is complex, consisting of abnormal interaction between the autonomic systems, paradoxically favoring parasympathetic tone. This, in turn, causes disproportionate bradycardia, which may ultimately lead to cardiac arrest (cardioinhibitory syncope), hypotension (vasodepressor syncope), or both (mixed syncope). As syncope is a complex symptom with many potential causes, a logical, systematic diagnostic approach is advised in order to increase the chance of identifying the underlying etiology and providing appropriate treatment.

TRANSIENT LOSS OF CONSCIOUSNESS

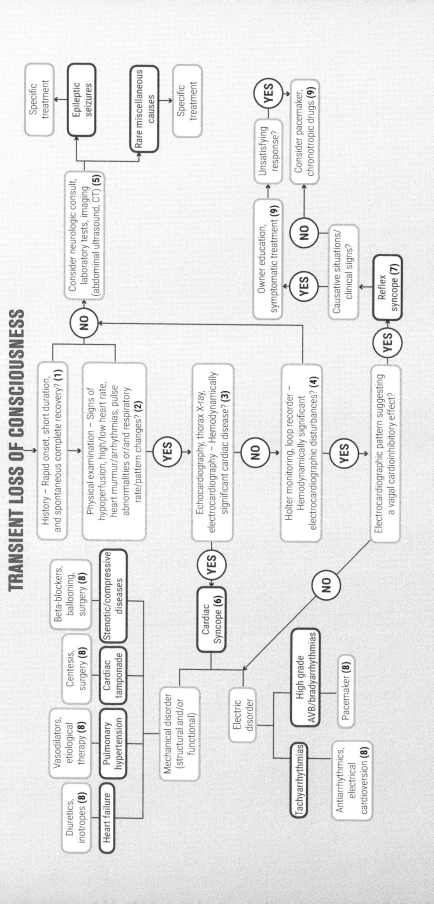

DIAGNOSTIC PROTOCOL

1. A detailed history is essential for having an accurate description of the event(s) and for formulating an appropriate diagnostic plan. However, it should be noted that there may be an overlap between the historical findings of neurological and cardiac transient loss of consciousness. Syncope is characterized by a sudden loss of consciousness and postural tone, and its typical findings include rapid onset, often under physical activity/emotional stress and without prodromes, short duration (usually <20 seconds), and complete spontaneous recovery.

2. The next step is a thorough physical examination since this, in conjunction with the history, may help rule in/out some disorders. Suspicion of a cardiac cause of transient loss of consciousness is generally strengthened by the detection of signs of peripheral hypoperfusion (e.g., pale mucous membranes, prolonged capillary refill time, cold extremities), unexpectedly high/low heart rate, heart murmur, arrhythmias, femoral pulse abnormalities (e.g., weak femoral pulse, pulse deficit), and/or abnormal respiratory rate/pattern. In contrast, patients with reflex syncope may show unremarkable findings during physical examination.

3. When historical/clinical findings suggest a cardiac etiology, the investigation should initially include widely available, non-invasive diagnostic tests, such as transthoracic echocardiography (valvular diseases, stenotic valve diseases, hypokinetic cardiomyopathies, pulmonary hypertension, compression by heart base masses, pericardial diseases); thoracic radiography (cardiomegaly, congestive heart failure, pulmonary hypertension, heart base masses); six-/ twelve-lead electrocardiogram, usually over 1-5 minutes (bradyarrhythmias, tachyarrhythmias).

4. Not infrequently, additional tests may be necessary to reach a diagnosis due to the intermittent nature of some cardiac and neutrally mediated conditions causing syncope (e.g., paroxysmal tachyarrhythmias, reflex bradycardia), including 24-hour Holter monitoring and an external/ implantable loop recorder.

5. When history and physical examination do not suggest a cardiac etiology, a laboratory database should be obtained to investigate possible extracardiac disorders. This should include at least serum biochemistry (electrolyte abnormalities, hypoglycemia) and a complete blood count (anemia, polycythemia). Additional laboratory tests (e.g., urinalysis, endocrine tests) and/or imaging (e.g., abdominal ultrasound, computed tomography) and/or a neurologic consultation may be necessary for some extracardiac conditions.

DIAGNOSIS

6. Cardiac syncope is diagnosed when hemodynamically significant echocardiographic and/ or electrocardiographic abnormalities are documented, especially in patients experiencing transient loss of consciousness under physical activity/emotional stress. In dogs, common mechanical causes include advanced myxomatous mitral valve disease, dilated/ arrhythmogenic cardiomyopathy, severe pulmonary hypertension, severe pulmonic/ subaortic stenosis, and cardiac tamponade, whereas common electric causes include high-grade atrioventricular blocks, sick sinus syndrome, and persistent atrial standstill. In cats, cardiac syncope is often due to advanced cardiomyopathies and atrioventricular blocks.

7. The diagnosis of reflex syncope is complex and often presumptive. Suspicion is raised by transient loss of consciousness occurring after situations, such as coughing, swallowing, emesis, micturition, or defecation, and is then subsequently strengthened by the detection of electrocardiographic patterns suggesting a vagal cardioinhibitory effect (e.g., progressive sinus bradycardia until sinus arrest, progressive sinus bradycardia followed by high-grade atrioventricular blocks with a concomitant decrease in sinus rate, atrial fibrillation followed by a progressive decrease in the ventricular response until ventricular arrest).

TREATMENT

8. The primary therapeutic goal is the prevention of syncope recurrence/reduction of syncopal events and, consequently, improvement in the quality of life. In cardiac syncope, this is achieved by managing the underlying disorder, either by medical (e.g., diuretics for congestive heart failure, phosphodiesterase-5 inhibitors for severe pulmonary hypertension, antiarrhythmics for tachyarrhythmias) or interventional (e.g., balloon valvuloplasty for severe pulmonic stenosis, pacemaker implantation for atrioventricular blocks/bradyarrhythmias) approaches.

9. Treatment of reflex syncope is challenging, especially in patients experiencing hypotension as a component of the abnormal vagal reflex (i.e., vasodepressor/mixed syncope). Client education and control of causative situations/clinical signs are important but are not always resolutive. Oral positive chronotropic drugs (e.g., terbutaline) are rarely effective, especially in the long term, but may act as a bridge to pacemaker implantation. The latter is a valuable strategy in patients with cardioinhibitory syncope.

SUGGESTED READINGS

-   Bright JM, Cali JV. Clinical, usefulness of cardiac event recording in dogs and cats examined because of syncope, episodic collapse, or intermittent weakness: 60 cases (1997-1999). *J Am Vet Med Assoc* 216:1110-1114, 2000.
-   Martin M. Syncope. In Ettinger SJ, Feldman EC, Côté E (editors). Textbook of Veterinary Internal Medicine 8th edition. St. Louis, Elsevier, 2017, pp 123-126.
-   Miller RH, Lehmkuhl LB, Bonagura JD, et al. Retrospective analysis of the clinical utility of ambulatory electrocardiography (Holter) recordings in syncopal dogs: 44 cases (1991-1995). *J Vet Intern Med* 13:111-122, 1999.

URINARY INCONTINENCE AND RETENTION

Marika Menchetti

The normal function of micturition consists of a storage phase and a voiding phase.

The key anatomical components of the micturition process include the detrusor muscle (smooth muscle forming the body and neck of the bladder), the internal urethral sphincter (smooth muscle), and the external urethral sphincter (striated muscle).

The urine storage and voiding process occur under the control of the hypogastric nerve (sympathetic: L1-L4 in dogs, L2-L5 in cats), which induces detrusor muscle relaxation and internal urethral sphincter contraction, the pelvic nerve (parasympathetic: S1-S3) which causes detrusor muscle contraction and the pudendal nerve (somatic: S1-S3) which induces contraction/relaxation of the external urethral sphincter.

The coordinated micturition mechanism requires a complex interaction between the somatic and autonomic nervous systems as well as the normal function of the anatomical components and supraspinal centers.

Urinary incontinence is defined as the involuntary leakage of urine, and it can appear as intermittent or continuous dribbling of urine, representing a disorder of the storage phase.

Neurogenic causes of incontinence involve the lumbosacral (L4-S3) spinal cord segments and/or cauda equina, leading to "lower motor neuron" bladder signs. Typically, neurologic diseases are traumatic or degenerative in origin.

Non-neurogenic causes are associated with anatomical or functional disorders of the urinary tract. Many causes of urinary retention can result in "false" or "paradoxical" urinary incontinence, also called overflow incontinence. This type of false incontinence is actually a voiding disorder.

Urinary retention is defined as the inability to completely empty the bladder, representing a disorder of the voiding phase. Animals with urinary retention may make frequent attempts to void with partial or no urine emission. Sometimes, accessory signs are associated (e.g., stranguria/dysuria).

Neurogenic causes of retention involve the segments between the pons and the L7 segment of the spinal cord (most commonly the T3-L3 segments), leading to signs of "upper motor neuron" bladder. Quite frequently, these diseases are more degenerative in nature. The non-neurogenic causes of retention are mainly associated with anatomical or functional obstruction.

URINARY INCONTINENCE AND URINARY RETENTION

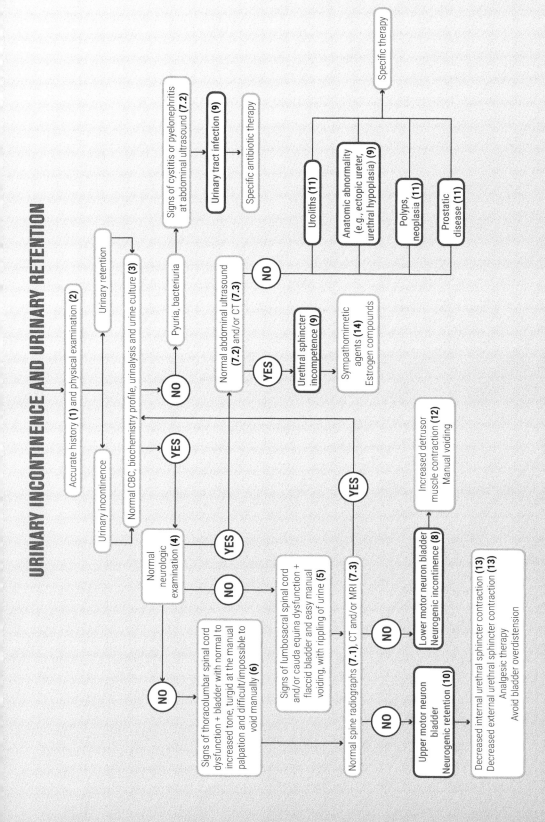

1. An accurate history should be obtained to determine whether the problem is urinary incontinence (involuntary leakage, intermittent or continuous dribbling of urine) or retention (inability to empty the bladder completely).

2. Physical examination should include the observation of voiding with particular attention to stream size, duration of voiding, urine color, and the presence of accessory symptoms (e.g., dysuria, stranguria). Palpation of the bladder is fundamental for evaluating bladder tone, repletion status, and the possibility of achieving manual voiding.

3. A complete blood cell count, biochemistry profile, urinalysis, and urine culture should be carried out to evaluate signs of inflammation or urinary tract infection.

4. A complete neurologic examination is important to establish if there are neurological signs of lumbosacral spinal cord and/or cauda equina dysfunction (e.g., flaccid paraparesis, low-carried tail, reduced withdrawal reflex of the pelvic limbs, and a decreased perineal reflex) or signs of thoracolumbar spinal cord dysfunction (spastic paraparesis, proprioceptive ataxia, proprioceptive deficits).

5. Signs of lumbosacral spinal cord or cauda equina dysfunction, together with a flaccid bladder and easy manual voiding, with the dripping of urine or a normal stream size, indicate that the problem is a "lower motor neuron" bladder.

6. Signs of thoracolumbar spinal cord dysfunction, together with a bladder having normal to increased tone, turgid at manual palpation, and difficulty to the impossibility of voiding manually, indicate that the problem is an "upper motor neuron" bladder.

7. Based on the clinical signs, the clinicopathological and the neurological findings, the most appropriate diagnostic protocol should be carried out.
   7.1 Spine radiographs (signs of degenerative lumbosacral stenosis, spinal fractures, spinal luxation, vertebral malformations, discospondylitis).
   7.2. Abdominal ultrasound (cystitis, uroliths, prostatitis, ectopic ureter).
   7.3. CT and/or MRI (intervertebral disc herniation, spinal cord neoplasia, ischemic myelopathy, hemorrhage, meningitis/meningomyelitis, spinal cord malformation, ectopic ureter).

DIAGNOSIS

8. A "lower motor neuron" bladder is caused by traumatic (e.g., lumbosacral fractures and pull-tail injury), degenerative (e.g., degenerative lumbosacral stenosis, intervertebral disc disease, dysautonomia), neoplastic or anomalous-congenital diseases (e.g., caudal lumbar and/or sacral malformations).

9. The causes of non-neurogenic incontinence are associated with anatomical or functional disorders of the urinary tract, such as lower urinary tract inflammation-infection, ectopic ureter, urethral sphincter incompetence, urethral hypoplasia, and partial outflow obstruction.

10. An "upper motor neuron" bladder is most commonly a consequence of degenerative diseases (e.g., intervertebral disc disease) but can also be traumatic (primary, such as spinal fractures, luxation, or subluxation; or secondary, such as spinal cord contusion), vascular (ischemic myelopathy, hemorrhage), idiopathic (e.g., the detrusor-urethral dyssynergia), or inflammatory in origin (meningomyelitis, discospondylitis, empyema).

11. The non-neurogenic causes of retention are mainly associated with anatomical or functional obstruction (polyps, uroliths, neoplasia).

TREATMENT

12. Increased detrusor muscle contraction: bethanechol chloride: parasympathomimetic (cholinergic), directly stimulates cholinergic receptors. Dosage is empiric, 2.5-25 mg PO q8h for dogs and 1.5-5 mg PO q8h for cats.

13. Decreased external urethral sphincter contraction: diazepam relaxes the striated muscles, stimulating GABA-ergic inhibitory interneurons in the sacral spinal cord, relaxing the external urethral sphincter at 0.2 mg/kg PO q8h in dogs. Avoid using it in cats due to possible hepatic necrosis; in cats with an "upper motor neuron" bladder, use other benzodiazepines (such as alprazolam).

    Decreased internal urethral sphincter: phenoxybenzamine hydrochloride: α-adrenergic antagonist at 0.25-0.5 mg/kg PO q12h in dogs and cats. Tamsulosin: $\alpha1_A$-adrenergic antagonist, highly uroselective, at 10-13 μg/kg PO q12-24h in dogs and cats.

14. Phenylpropanolamine: mixed adrenergic agonist, increased internal urethral sphincter tone at 1.5 mg/kg PO q8-12h in dogs and cats.

SUGGESTED READINGS

- Dewey C, da Costa R (editors). Practical Guide to Canine and Feline Neurology 3rd edition. Ames, Wiley Blackwell, 2015.
- Elliot J, Grauer GF. BSAVA Manual of Canine and Feline Nephrology and Urology 2nd edition. British Small Animal Veterinary Association, 2007.
- Lorenz MD, Coates JR, Kent M. Handbook of Veterinary Neurology 5th edition. St. Louis, Elsevier, 2011.

VOMITING

Paolo Silvestrini

Vomiting is one of the most common reasons for a veterinary consultation in dogs and cats. Since owners often misinterpret regurgitation as vomiting, clinicians should obtain an accurate history and description of the episodes and carry out a complete physical examination to differentiate vomiting from regurgitation.

Vomiting is the active expulsion of ingesta from the stomach and sometimes from the proximal duodenum. It involves contractions of the stomach, diaphragm, and abdominal wall muscles while relaxing upper and lower esophageal sphincters and positional changes of the larynx and epiglottis to protect the airways. The vomiting reflex involves a complex circuit in which the vomiting center can be stimulated by pathways from the abdominal viscera, chemoreceptor trigger zone, vestibular apparatus, and central nervous system.

Vomited material generally has an acidic pH; however, it can be neutral or high when it contains bicarbonate-rich fluid refluxed from the duodenum. It is generally associated with signs of nausea, such as hypersalivation, burping, and lip-smacking. When asked, owners generally describe abdominal contraction and sometimes extension of the neck just before expulsion of the ingesta. Patients with vomiting, especially if chronic, are more commonly hypo- or anorexic. Since it is an active and coordinated reflex, vomiting is associated with the concurrent closure of the nasopharynx and glottis, which reduces the risk of aspiration pneumonia. Frequent vomiting can cause dehydration and hypovolemia, acid-base and electrolyte derangements, and esophagitis.

VOMITING

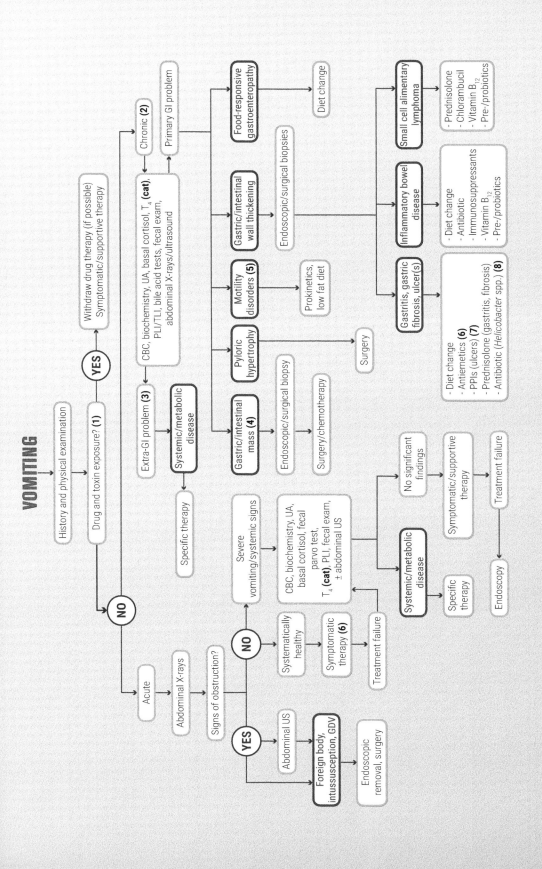

History and physical examination

Drug and toxin exposure? **(1)**

YES → Withdraw drug therapy (if possible)
Symptomatic/supportive therapy

NO

Acute

Abdominal X-rays

Signs of obstruction?

YES → Abdominal US → **Foreign body, intussusception, GDV** → Endoscopic removal, surgery

NO → Severe vomiting/systemic signs

Systematically healthy → Symptomatic therapy **(6)** → Treatment failure

CBC, biochemistry, UA, basal cortisol, fecal parvo test, T₄ **(cat)**, PLI, fecal exam, ± abdominal US

- No significant findings → Symptomatic/supportive therapy → Treatment failure → Endoscopy
- **Systemic/metabolic disease** → Specific therapy

Chronic **(2)**

- Extra-GI problem **(3)** → **Systemic/metabolic disease** → Specific therapy
- Primary GI problem

CBC, biochemistry, UA, basal cortisol, T₄ **(cat)**, PLI/TLI, bile acid tests, fecal exam, abdominal X-rays/ultrasound

Gastric/intestinal mass **(4)**
Endoscopic/surgical biopsy → Surgery/chemotherapy

Pyloric hypertrophy
→ Surgery

Motility disorders **(5)**
Prokinetics, low fat diet

Gastric/intestinal wall thickening
Endoscopic/surgical biopsies

Food-responsive gastroenteropathy
Diet change

Small cell alimentary lymphoma
- Prednisolone
- Chlorambucil
- Vitamin B₁₂
- Pre-/probiotics

Inflammatory bowel disease
- Diet change
- Antibiotic
- Immunosuppressants
- Vitamin B₁₂
- Pre-/probiotics

Gastritis, gastric fibrosis, ulcer(s)
- Diet change
- Antiemetics **(6)**
- PPIs (ulcers) **(7)**
- Prednisolone (gastritis, fibrosis)
- Antibiotic (*Helicobacter* spp.) **(8)**

1. The history should be evaluated for drugs, gastrointestinal irritants, and toxins. Some drugs can cause vomiting in some patients; these include non-steroidal anti-inflammatory drugs (NSAIDs), antimicrobials (e.g., erythromycin, tetracyclines), cardiac glycosides, and chemotherapeutics. Many toxins can cause vomiting (e.g., plant alkaloids, mushrooms, insecticides, and heavy metals [lead, zinc, iron]). Potential toxins in garbage (garbage intoxication) include preformed bacterial enterotoxins, mycotoxins, and fermentation products and can induce vomiting.

2. Vomiting is classified as chronic when it is >1-2 weeks duration.

3. Extragastrointestinal (GI) diseases that can cause vomiting include renal and hepatic diseases, hypoadrenocorticism, pancreatitis and exocrine pancreatic insufficiency in dogs and cats, and hyperthyroidism in cats.

DIAGNOSIS

4. Gastric tumors in dogs and cats represent <1% of the overall neoplasia. Adenocarcinoma affecting the lesser curvature and, less frequently, the pyloric region is the most common gastric neoplasia in dogs. Leiomyomas/sarcomas are often found around the cardias. In cats, lymphoma is the most common GI neoplasm, followed by adenocarcinoma and mast cell tumors.

5. Disorders of gastric emptying arise from mechanical obstruction or from defective propulsion. Malignancy, pyloric hyperplasia, and foreign bodies can cause mechanical obstruction. Gastroenteritis, pancreatitis, peritonitis, gastric ulceration, post-surgical gastroparesis, electrolyte disturbances (hypokalemia, hypocalcemia), endocrinopathies (hypothyroidism, hypoadrenocorticism, diabetes mellitus), uremia, dysautonomia, use of cholinergic antagonists, and adrenergic and opioid agonists can all cause defective gastric propulsion.

6. The most commonly used antiemetics in dogs and cats are
    1) Metoclopramide: D2 antagonist; site of action: chemoreceptor trigger zone (CRTZ), GI smooth muscle; dose: 0.2-0.4 mg/kg PO, SC, IM q8h or CRI 1-2 mg/kg/day IV. Metoclopramide is not a very effective antiemetic in cats as D2 receptors are scarce to absent in this species.
    2) Ondansetron: 5HT3 antagonist; site of action: CRTZ, vagal afferents; dose: 0.5-1 mg/kg PO, IV q12h.
    3) Maropitant: NK1 antagonist; site of action: CRTZ, emetic center; dose: 1 mg/kg SC, IV q24h, 2 mg/kg PO q24 h.

7. Proton pump inhibitors (PPIs) administered twice daily are superior to other gastroprotectants for treating acid-related gastroduodenal ulceration and erosion (GUE). There is no evidence to support the prophylactic use of PPIs in dogs and cats with non-erosive gastritis; this should be reserved only for those cases at high risk of GUE (concurrent use of NSAIDs

and steroids, hypovolemia, and use of NSAIDs, gastrinoma, intrahepatic porto-systemic shunt). When given for more than 3-4 weeks, a slow reduction in the dose is recommended. Intestinal dysbiosis and diarrhea are possible secondary effects.

8. A direct causal relationship between *Helicobacter* spp. and chronic gastritis and vomiting has not been established in dogs and cats. However, when vomiting persists despite symptomatic therapy and is associated with gastritis and the presence of numerous spiral bacteria (especially if in notable quantities and localized in the deep gastric wall layers), therapy for *Helicobacter* spp. should be considered. In humans, therapy against *H. pylori* includes two or three antimicrobials combined with a PPI, given for 1 to 2 weeks. The combination of clarithromycin (7.5 mg/kg PO q12h), amoxicillin (22 mg/kg PO q12h), and omeprazole (1 mg/kg PO q12h) for 2-3 weeks seems to be a good option in dogs. However, according to the recent American College of Veterinary Internal Medicine (ACVIM) Consensus Statement, there is no evidence that acid suppression treatment is beneficial or indicated in dogs or cats undergoing treatment for non-*H. pylori*.

SUGGESTED READINGS

- Gallagher A. Vomiting and regurgitation. In Ettinger SJ, Feldman EC, Côté E (editors). Textbook of Veterinary Internal Medicine 8th edition. St. Louis, Elsevier, 2017, pp 158-164.
- Leib MS. Gastric *Helicobacter* spp. and chronic vomiting in dogs. In Bonagura JD, Twedt DC (editors). Kirk's Current Veterinary Therapy XV 15th edition. St. Louis, Elsevier, 2014, pp 508-513.
- Marks SL, Kook PH, Papich MG, et al. ACVIM consensus statement: support for rational administration of gastrointestinal protectants to dogs and cats. *J Vet Intern Med* 32:1823-1840, 2018.

VULVAR DISCHARGE

Marco Cunto and Daniele Zambelli

Vulvar discharge in bitches and queens may be due to normal physiologic conditions, such as estrus (bitches) or parturition, or consequent to ovary, uterus, cervix, vagina, vestibule, or urinary tract disorders as well as to coagulation problems. The identification of its origin and etiology requires evaluation of the animal's history, physical examination, and reproductive tract diagnostic imaging findings, assessment of discharge features and duration, vaginal cytology, and evaluation of the reproductive hormone concentration. As an example, the increase in the cornification of the vaginal epithelial cells is correlated with high serum estrogen concentrations; this condition is observed during proestrus/estrus or in the case of ovarian remnant syndrome, cystic ovarian disease, or functional ovarian tumors. Differentiation of these conditions is based on the duration of the vulvar discharge and/or colpocytology consistent with proestrus/estrus; animals with cystic ovarian disease or functional ovarian tumors usually show increased estrogen concentrations for longer periods as compared to what is observed during a physiologic estrus cycle. If colpocytology is not indicative of high serum estrogens, signalment and history frequently provide data useful for the differentiation of non-estrogen dependent conditions. Uterine disorders are predominantly diagnosed in intact females or spayed females with ovarian remnant syndrome and/or uterine stump pyometra, while prepubertal bitches may show vaginal discharge due to juvenile vaginitis. Older animals are instead more predisposed to neoplasia. Postpartum conditions, such as subinvolution of placental sites (bitches) and metritis, also cause vaginal discharges. Cystic endometrial hyperplasia/pyometra is a diestrual disorder diagnosed by detection of uterine enlargement, purulent vulvar discharge (open cervix), and elevated white blood cell count with left shift. Even if some conditions determining vaginal discharge are more observed in bitches (e.g., vaginitis, vaginal neoplasia), it is also important to consider them in queens. All this information is crucial to reaching the diagnosis and choosing the most appropriate treatment. In some cases, the owner may request not to compromise the reproductive career of the animal; in these cases, when possible, the owner's will must also be considered.

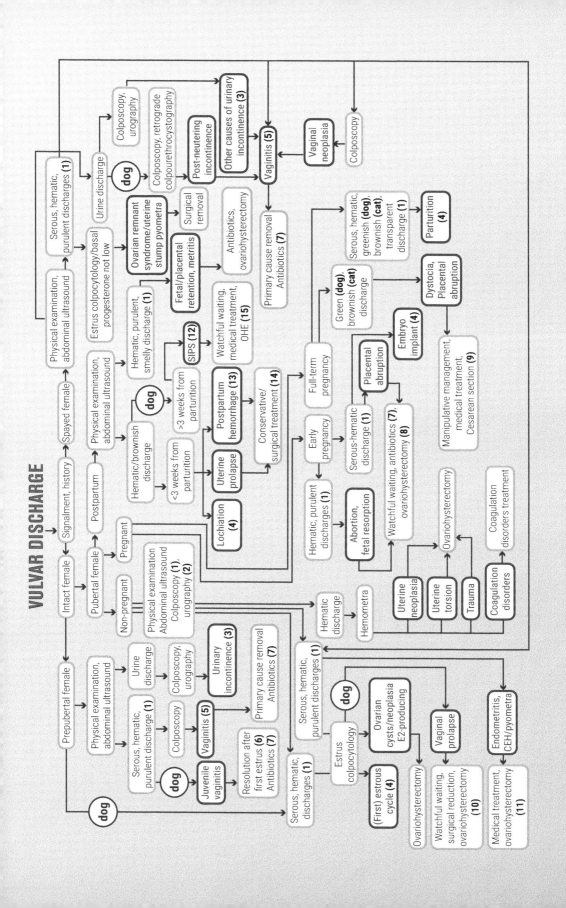

1. Colposcopy is not routinely performed in all cases in which vaginal discharge is observed; however, it could be necessary for the diagnosis of disorders indicated in the algorithm.

2. Urography is not routinely performed in all cases in which vaginal discharge is observed; however, it could be necessary for the diagnosis of disorders indicated in the algorithm.

DIAGNOSIS

3. There are several causes of urinary incontinence. In some cases (e.g., ectopic ureters), diagnosis is confirmed or made by colposcopy and/or urography with contrast.

4. Physiological condition, no treatment needed.

5. Vaginitis may be primary, caused by bacterial or viral infections, or secondary, subsequent to vaginal atrophy following ovariohysterectomy (OHE), urine or mucus pooling due to a congenital vaginal anomaly, the presence of vaginal neoplasia or foreign bodies, urinary tract disease, or systemic disease, such as diabetes mellitus.

12. Fetal trophoblasts or maternal decidual cells can be observed in the upper loose connective tissue of the lamina propria for the first two weeks after whelping; in normal bitches uterine involution is complete by 12 weeks postpartum. Subinvolution of the placental sites (SIPS) occurs when these processes are delayed.

13. Postpartum hemorrhage may occur for uterine/vaginal trauma during whelping or primarily, from placental sites, after puppies/kittens delivery.

6. Bitches affected by juvenile vaginitis are usually not systemically ill, and resolution is observed after the first estrus. In other cases, antibiotic administration could be considered.

7. Antibiotics should be administered only in case of bacterial causes and based on culture and sensitivity tests.

8. In the early stage of pregnancy, in the case of abortion, fetal resorption and placental abruption, systemic illness is not usually observed, and spontaneous resolution is obtained. When a purulent discharge is present and/or the animal is systemically ill, antibiotics are recommended, and, if not resolutive, ovariohysterectomy should be performed.

9. The aim of medical treatment is to induce fetal expulsion and is generally based on oxytocin (5-20 IU IM repeated at 30-40 minute intervals in bitches; 3-5 IU IM repeated at 20-30 minute intervals in queens) and/or 10% calcium gluconate (0.2 mL/kg IV or 1-5 mL/bitch SC;

controversial use in queens). It should be avoided if the birth canal is not patent or if its patency conditions are unknown. Cesarean section should be performed if manipulative management and/or medical treatment are not resolutive or if fetal/mother conditions require it.

10. Vaginal prolapse treatment involves either decreasing the estrogen stimulus, removing the prolapsed tissue, or both. Waiting for decreased estrogen influence on vaginal tissue prolapse could lead to spontaneous regression. In this case, exposed tissue should be kept clean and protected. If a vaginal prolapse is allowed to regress spontaneously, recurrence at the subsequent estrus cycle is common.

11. Ovariohysterectomy (OHE) is the elective therapy. Cystic endometrial hyperplasia (CEH)/ pyometra medical treatment is generally suggested in young breeding bitches, which are of breeding age and inserted in a breeding program, not systemically ill, and with an open cervix. In other cases, medical therapy is discouraged. Different protocols have been proposed. Antibiotic administration is an integral part of CEH/pyometra medical treatment but usually is not resolutive if uterine fluid content is present and the uterine diameter is increased. In these cases, association with antiprogestins (e.g., aglepristone 10 mg/kg SC at days 1, 2, 8, 15, 22, 29; success rate 63%) or antiprogestins and prostaglandins (e.g., aglepristone 10 mg/kg SC at days 1, 2, 8, 15, 22 and cloprostenol 1µg/kg/day SC from third to seventh day; success rate: 84.4%) is suggested.

14. Conservative management after uterine prolapse (uterine replacement) should be attempted only if the status of the uterus is not compromised. With postpartum hemorrhage, conservative treatment may be resolutive if not caused by uterine rupture and if the hemorrhage is not severe. Ecbolic agents (e.g., oxytocin, ergonovine) are usually used to cause uterine contraction and vasoconstriction.

15. Since spontaneous remission is usually observed, medical or surgical therapy is generally not required. Antibiotics should not be used unless secondary metritis occurs. Ovariohysterectomy (OHE) should be taken into consideration only if severe hemorrhage or ulceration of the endometrium/myometrium occurs.

SUGGESTED READINGS

- De Gier J, Schaefers-Okkens AC. Vulvar and preputial discharge. In Ettinger SJ, Feldman EC, Côté E (editors). Textbook of Veterinary Internal Medicine 8th edition. St. Louis, Elsevier, 2017, pp 178-184.
- England G, Von Heimendahl A. BSAVA Manual of Canine and Feline Reproduction and Neonatology. British Small Animal Veterinary Association, 2010.
- Johnston SD, Root Kustritz MV, Olson PN. Canine and Feline Theriogenology. WB Saunders, 2001.

WEIGHT GAIN

Alexander German

Weight gain is usually the result of fluid accumulation or increased tissue mass. Fluid usually accumulates rapidly, either within body cavities or subcutaneously. Weight gain that arises from increased tissue mass typically comprises both adipose, lean tissue (e.g., skeletal structures and soft tissues such as internal organs and muscle), or both. The process is more gradual, typically taking weeks to months. By far, the most common cause of weight gain is obesity, which is associated with multiple comorbidities, decreased longevity, and a poorer quality of life; therefore, it is now formally recognized as a disease by the veterinary profession. The weight gain seen in obesity mainly arises from increased adipose tissue mass, although some lean tissue accumulation also occurs (e.g., abdominal organomegaly size, increased muscle mass). Obesity results from disordered energy homeostasis, resulting from an imbalance between energy intake and energy use. Multiple risk factors influence this process, including genetics, dietary factors, owner factors, comorbidities, environmental factors, and neutering. Drugs can also predispose to weight gain through appetite stimulation, with examples including corticosteroids, anticonvulsants (phenobarbital and potassium bromide), and progestins. Energy homeostasis can also be disrupted by some comorbidities of obesity, for example, musculoskeletal diseases, where immobility results in decreased energy expenditure. Endocrinopathies can also predispose to weight gain, with examples including hyperadrenocorticism (both dogs and cats), hypothyroidism (dogs only), acromegaly (cats only), and insulinoma (dogs only). Hypothyroidism disrupts energy homeostasis as a result of decreased metabolism, whilst both acromegaly and hyperadrenocorticism cause weight gain both from increased food intake (due to polyphagia), fat redistribution (increased visceral fat), and organomegaly. Finally, weight gain can also arise from large tumors, most likely arising within the abdominal cavity.

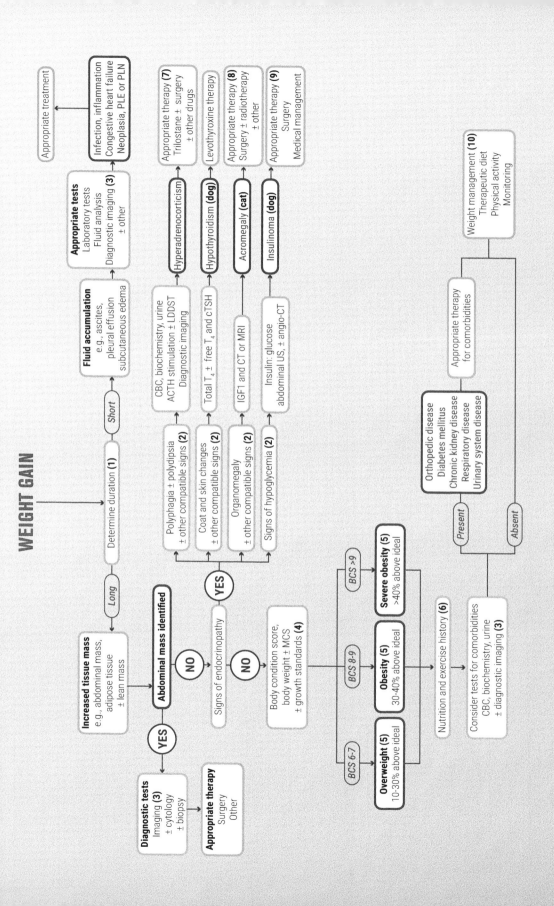

WEIGHT GAIN

Determine duration (1)

Long

Increased tissue mass
e.g., abdominal mass,
adipose tissue
± lean mass

Abdominal mass identified

YES → **Diagnostic tests (3)**
Imaging (3)
± cytology
± biopsy

→ **Appropriate therapy**
Surgery
Other

NO → Signs of endocrinopathy

YES →

Polyphagia ± polydipsia
± other compatible signs (2) → CBC, biochemistry, urine
ACTH stimulation ± LDDST
Diagnostic imaging → **Hyperadrenocorticism** → Appropriate therapy (7)
Trilostane ± surgery
± other drugs

Coat and skin changes
± other compatible signs (2) → Total T$_4$ ± free T$_4$ and cTSH → **Hypothyroidism (dog)** → Levothyroxine therapy

Organomegaly
± other compatible signs (2) → IGF1 and CT or MRI → **Acromegaly (cat)** → Appropriate therapy (8)
Surgery ± radiotherapy
± other

Signs of hypoglycemia (2) → Insulin: glucose
abdominal US, ± angio-CT → **Insulinoma (dog)** → Appropriate therapy (9)
Surgery
Medical management

NO →

Body condition score,
body weight ± MCS
± growth standards (4)

BCS 6-7 → **Overweight (5)**
10-30% above ideal

BCS 8-9 → **Obesity (5)**
30-40% above ideal

BCS >9 → **Severe obesity (5)**
>40% above ideal

→ Nutrition and exercise history (6)

→ Consider tests for comorbidities
CBC, biochemistry, urine
± diagnostic imaging (3)

→ Orthopedic disease
Diabetes mellitus
Chronic kidney disease
Respiratory disease
Urinary system disease

Present → Appropriate therapy
for comorbidities

Absent →

Weight management (10)
Therapeutic diet
Physical activity
Monitoring

Short

Fluid accumulation
e.g., ascites,
pleural effusion
subcutaneous edema

→ **Appropriate tests**
Laboratory tests
Fluid analysis
Diagnostic imaging (3)
± other

→ Infection, inflammation
Congestive heart failure
Neoplasia, PLE or PLN

→ Appropriate treatment

DIAGNOSTIC PROTOCOL

1. Both the duration of weight gain and its magnitude (percentage change in body weight) can be accurately determined by reviewing weight measurements recorded in the electronic patient records. Rapid body weight increases suggest fluid accumulation and prompt the veterinarian to look for possible cardiac, hepatic, infectious, inflammatory, or protein-losing conditions. In contrast, weight gain arising more gradually suggests increased tissue mass, with the most likely causes being either endocrinopathy or abdominal mass.

2. Signs of a possible endocrinopathy include polyphagia (e.g., hyperadrenocorticism, insulinoma, or acromegaly), polyuria, and polydipsia (hyperadrenocorticism or acromegaly, if concurrent diabetes mellitus); coat and skin changes such as alopecia, scale, myxedema, thin skin, hyperpigmentation and comedones (hyperadrenocorticism, hypothyroidism); and seizures or other neurological signs (insulinoma). Other possible signs of hyperadrenocorticism include lethargy, exercise intolerance, excess panting, and pot-belly appearance, whilst other signs seen with acromegaly include coarsened facial features.

3. The diagnostic imaging modality used depends upon the reason that it is deployed. For example, cardiac disorders and pleural effusion can be identified with thoracic radiography and ultrasonography (including echocardiography); abdominal neoplasia, organomegaly, adrenal gland changes, and ascites can be identified with abdominal radiography and ultrasonography. However, the body cavities of large dogs are arguably better assessed with whole-body computed tomography (CT), and either MRI or CT are indicated for possible pituitary masses.

4. The WSAVA recommends the 9-point body condition score (BCS) system. However, since BCS systems are not fully validated for puppies and kittens, weight gain from growth is best monitored by regular weight measurements with reference to evidence-based growth standards. Such measures confirm whether the rate of weight gain is appropriate or excessive.

6. Where obesity is suspected, detailed information should be gathered about food intake, details of the family unit, and physical activity (intensity and amount). Details of drug therapy and known comorbidities are also important.

DIAGNOSIS

5. Although obesity is assumed when a dog or cat is >30% above its ideal weight (BCS 8-9) a continuum exists, with dogs and cats defined as overweight when a lesser accumulation of adipose tissue has occurred (10-30% above ideal weight, corresponding to BCS 6-7). Some dogs and cats have "severe obesity" (>40% above ideal weight), where the degree of adiposity exceeds that depicted by the BCS 9 category.

TREATMENT

7. If hyperadrenocorticism is pituitary-dependent, medical management is indicated, usually with trilostane, and therapeutic efficacy is monitored by either pre-pill cortisol or ACTH stimulation test. If hyperadrenocorticism is due to an adrenal gland tumor, adrenalectomy should be

performed. However, if surgery is not feasible (e.g., tumor invading major abdominal blood vessels), medical management is an alternative, typically with trilostane.

8. The most effective treatment modality for acromegaly is hypophysectomy, although radiotherapy could be considered if there are cost or availability issues. If these treatments are not feasible, treating at least concurrent diabetes mellitus with subcutaneous insulin therapy is recommended (albeit requiring high insulin doses).

9. Surgical removal provides the best guarantee of a positive long-term outcome. However, if this is not possible (due to cost or other limitations), medical management is advised. This includes feeding food over multiple small meals, controlling exercise, and giving prednisolone at 0.5 mg/kg PO q24h.

10. The key components of successful weight management include decreasing energy intake whilst ensuring all essential nutrient requirements and increasing physical activity. Regular monitoring of the program is vital. Evidence suggests that purpose-formulated therapeutic diets improve owner compliance and outcomes whilst decreasing the risk of nutrient deficiencies and weight regain after reaching the target. Increasing physical activity alone does not lead to meaningful weight loss but provides other improvements, including minimizing lean tissue loss.

SUGGESTED READINGS

- German AJ. 11.5 Adipositas/obesity. In Heilmann RM, Lidbury JA, Steiner J (editors). Small Animal Gastroenterology 2nd edition. Hanover, Schlütersche, In press.
- Murphy M, Cline M (editors). Obesity in Small Animal Practice. Boca Raton, CRC Press, 2019.

WEIGHT LOSS

Francesca Del Baldo

Maintaining body weight is a reflection of nutrient intake, absorption, and utilization. Weight loss occurs when energy expenditure exceeds dietary energy intake. The predominant body tissue lost is adipose tissue. Initially, lean tissue loss is limited. However, lean tissue loss becomes inevitable when the energy deficit is severe. Cachexia is the term used to describe weight loss, loss of muscle, and anorexia associated with many chronic diseases. Cachexia is not simply caused by inadequate nutrient intake; it can be differentiated from starvation by two biochemical features. First, unlike starvation, inflammation is a consistent feature of cachexia. Cachexia causes marked activation of the inflammatory cascade, characterized by a pronounced acute-phase inflammatory response and excessive production of proinflammatory cytokines (interleukins and tumor necrosis factor-alpha). These cytokines stimulate the ubiquitin pathway, a central pathway in protein turnover. Ubiquitin complexes target cellular proteins and stimulate their metabolism via the proteasome system. Second, cachexia is also associated with a rise in resting energy expenditure which increases as a consequence of alteration in the protein, fat, and carbohydrate metabolism. There is marked loss of body muscle and adipose tissue, and an insulin-resistant condition may develop. A diagnosis of cachexia should be considered in any dog or cat with marked weight loss, severe muscle loss, and decreased appetite in the setting of a chronic inflammatory response or cancer.

Clinically relevant weight loss has not been defined for dogs and cats; however, unintentional weight loss >5% is a reasonable benchmark. Weight loss is a well-recognized clinical sign in numerous disorders. It can be the primary or sole complaint, or, more commonly, it accompanies other signs associated with an underlying condition.

Common mechanisms leading to weight loss include decreased caloric intake, increased metabolic demand, accelerated energy loss, inability to utilize ingested calories, and inappetence. Etiologies determining weight loss typically act by means of several mechanisms, each of which should be evaluated for weight loss.

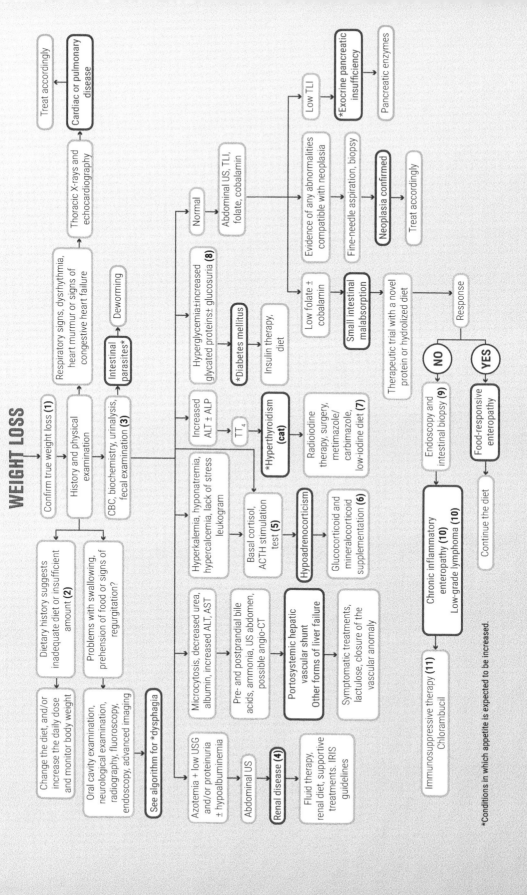

WEIGHT LOSS

Confirm true weight loss (1)

History and physical examination

Dietary history suggests inadequate diet or insufficient amount (2)
- Change the diet, and/or increase the daily dose and monitor body weight

Problems with swallowing, prehension of food or signs of regurgitation?
- Oral cavity examination, neurological examination, radiography, fluoroscopy, endoscopy, advanced imaging
- See algorithm for *dysphagia

Respiratory signs, dysrhythmia, heart murmur or signs of congestive heart failure
- Thoracic X-rays and echocardiography
  - Treat accordingly
  - **Cardiac or pulmonary disease**

CBC, biochemistry, urinalysis, fecal examination (3)

Intestinal parasites*
- Deworming

Azotemia + low USG and/or proteinuria ± hypoalbuminemia
- Abdominal US
  - **Renal disease (4)**
    - Fluid therapy, renal diet, supportive treatments. IRIS guidelines

Microcytosis, decreased urea, albumin, increased ALT, AST
- Pre- and postprandial bile acids, ammonia, US abdomen, possible angio-CT
  - **Portosystemic hepatic vascular shunt / Other forms of liver failure**
    - Symptomatic treatments, lactulose, closure of the vascular anomaly

Hyperkalemia, hyponatremia, hypercalcemia, lack of stress leukogram
- Basal cortisol, ACTH stimulation test (5)
  - **Hypoadrenocorticism**
    - Glucocorticoid and mineralocorticoid supplementation (6)

Increased ALT ± ALP
- TT₄
  - ***Hyperthyroidism (cat)**
    - Radioiodine therapy, surgery, metimazole/carbimazole, low-iodine diet (7)

Hyperglycemia±increased glycated proteins± glucosuria (8)
- ***Diabetes mellitus**
  - Insulin therapy, diet

Normal
- Abdominal US, TLI, folate, cobalamin
  - Low TLI
    - ***Exocrine pancreatic insufficiency**
      - Pancreatic enzymes
  - Evidence of any abnormalities compatible with neoplasia
    - Fine-needle aspiration, biopsy
      - **Neoplasia confirmed**
        - Treat accordingly
  - Low folate ± cobalamin
    - **Small intestinal malabsorption**
      - Therapeutic trial with a novel protein or hydrolized diet
        - **NO**
          - Endoscopy and intestinal biopsy (9)
            - **Chronic inflammatory enteropathy (10) / Low-grade lymphoma (10)**
              - Immunosuppressive therapy (11) / Chlorambucil
        - **YES**
          - **Food-responsive enteropathy**
            - Continue the diet
          - Response

*Conditions in which appetite is expected to be increased.

1. Weight loss can also result from dehydration. Before considering the weight loss relevant, evaluate the animal's hydration status. If the dog or cat is dehydrated, investigate possible causes and correct the hydration state by administering fluid therapy or by augmenting water consumption.

2. Dietary history should include all food currently fed and consumed, how the proportions are measured, how the food is fed, and any recent dietary changes. If necessary, the owners should be asked to provide label information. For home-prepared food, it might be necessary to contact a veterinary nutritionist. It is also important to consider whether the animal's energy demand has been increased (e.g., due to extreme exercise or lactation). In this case, a specific diet should be administered or, alternatively, the quantity of food should be increased to satisfy the increased energy demand. Determining whether appetite is increased, decreased, or unchanged can help in narrowing down the list of differential diagnoses.

3. In cats, additional tests required are serology for feline leukemia virus and feline immunodeficiency virus.

5. If no causes of weight loss are found, it may also be useful to carry out an ACTH stimulation test in normokalemic and normonatremic dogs. Serum basal cortisol assessment can also be useful. A basal serum cortisol >2 µg/dL excludes hypoadrenocorticism. If basal cortisol is <2 µg/dL, the ACTH stimulation test should be carried out to confirm or exclude the disease.

8. In cats, the potential for stress hyperglycemia warrants caution in the interpretation of hyperglycemia of any magnitude. Diabetes mellitus in cats is diagnosed when hyperglycemia is associated with the classical clinical signs of hyperglycemia (with no other possible cause), increased glycated proteins, and glucosuria on more than one occasion on a naturally voided sample acquired in a home environment at least 2 days after any stressful events.

9. By definition, idiopathic chronic inflammatory enteropathy is a diagnosis of exclusion. If no causes of weight loss are found, it may be recommended to perform endoscopy even if folate and cobalamin are normal, in particular in dogs that present diarrhea and vomiting.

DIAGNOSIS

4. In protein-losing nephropathy, creatinine and urea can be within the reference range, and biochemistry usually shows low albumin and high cholesterol due to the excessive loss of albumin through the glomerulus and increased synthesis of lipoproteins.

10. Chronic inflammatory enteropathies can be classified according to the predominant inflammatory cell type and anatomical location. Lymphoplasmacytic enteritis is seen most frequently, followed by eosinophilic enteritis; the granulomatous and neutrophilic forms occur less commonly. Both chronic inflammatory enteropathies and low-grade lymphoma

can be associated with panhypoproteinemia (protein-losing enteropathies) due to excessive loss of proteins through the gastrointestinal tract. In this case, biochemistry usually also shows low cholesterol, and on CBC, lymphopenia can be detected.

TREATMENT

6. In the case of normokalemic and normonatremic hypoadrenocorticism, it is possible to administer only glucocorticoids without the addition of mineralocorticoids.

7. Radioiodine therapy is the mainstay of treatment. If this therapy is declined or is not available, surgical removal of the thyroid lobe/lobes affected by the adenoma can be considered a definitive treatment. In this case, it is important to carry out scintigraphy in order to plan the correct surgical approach. If surgery is declined, medical treatment with antithyroid drugs or a specific diet can be chosen.

11. Glucocorticoids, typically prednisolone, are generally used as the first-line treatment. The recommended dose is 1-2 mg/kg orally q24h in dogs and 2-4 mg/kg orally q24h in cats. In cases that appear refractory to glucocorticoids, adjunctive immunosuppressive therapy should be considered. Options include cyclosporine, azathioprine, and chlorambucil.

SUGGESTED READINGS
- Ettinger SJ, Feldman EC, Côté E (editors). Textbook of Veterinary Internal Medicine 8th edition. St. Louis, Elsevier, 2017.
- Hall EJ, Williams DA, Kathrani A (editors). BSAVA Manual of Canine and Feline Gastroenterology 3rd edition. British Small Animal Veterinary Association, 2020.